KU-124-499

CLINICAL ATLAS OF
Cerebrovascular
Disorders

DISCARDED

CLINICAL ATLAS OF
Cerebrovascular Disorders

EDITED BY
Marc Fisher, MD
Chief of Neurology
The Medical Center
    of Central Massachusetts
Professor of Neurology and Radiology
University of Massachusetts Medical School
Worcester, Massachusetts

FOREWORD BY
James F. Toole, MD
Wake Forest University Medical Center
Winston-Salem, North Carolina

Original Illustrations by Laura Pardi Duprey

NM WOLFE
London • St. Louis • Boston • Chicago • Philadelphia • Sydney • Toronto

For full details of all Mosby-Year Book Europe, Ltd. titles please write to:
Mosby-Year Book Europe, Ltd., Lynton House, 7-12 Tavistock Square, London
WC1H 9LB, England.

LIBRARY OF CONGRESS CATALOGING-IN-PUBLICATION DATA
Clinical Atlas of Cerebrovascular Disorders / edited by Marc Fisher.
    p. cm.
    Includes bibliographical references and index.
       ISBN 1-56375-091-0
       1. Cerebrovascular disease. I. Fisher, Marc, 1948-
       [DNLM: 1. Cerebrovascular Disorders—diagnosis.
    2. Cerebrovascular Disorders—therapy. WL 355 S92128]
    RC388.5.S85235 1993
    616.8'1—dc20 92-49808

BRITISH LIBRARY CATALOGUING IN PUBLICATION DATA
A catalogue record for this book is available from the British Library

9/1/95
WL 355
THE LIBRARY
POSTGRADUATE CENTRE
MAIDSTONE HOSPITAL
37,973
DO 17198
95 01067

Project Manager: Alison Marek
Illustrator: Laura Pardi Duprey
Art Director/Designer: Kathryn Greenslade
Editorial Assistants: Jean Unger, Demetrius McDowell
Typesetters: Madeline Carroll, Erick Rizzotto

The right of Marc Fisher to be identified as author of this work has been asserted
by him in accordance with the Copyright, Design and Patents Act 1988.

COPYRIGHT © 1994 MOSBY-YEAR BOOK EUROPE, LTD. All rights reserved.
No part of this publication may be reproduced, stored in a retrieval system, copied
or transmitted, in any form or by any means, electronic, mechanical, photocopying,
recording or otherwise without written permission from the Publisher or in
accordance with the provisions of the Copyright Act 1988, or under the terms of
any license permitting limited copying issued by the Copyright Licensing Agency,
33-34 Alfred Place, London, WC1E 7DP.

Any person who does any unauthorized act in relation to this publication may be
liable to criminal prosecution and civil claims for damages.

Permission to photocopy or reproduce solely for internal or personal use is
permitted for libraries or other users registered with the Copyright Clearance
Center, provided that the basc fee of $4.00 per chapter plus $ .10 per page is paid
directly to the Copyright Clearance Center, 21 Congress Street, Salem, MA 01970.
This consent does not extend to other kinds of copying, such as for general
distribution, for advertising or promotional purposes, for creating new collected
works, or for resales.

Originated in Singapore by Colourscan Overseas Co.
Printed and bound in Spain
Produced by Grafos

Acknowledgments

I would like to thank my wife Deborah, and sons David and Matthew for their support. I would also like to thank my teachers and, most important, my stroke patients for giving me insight into cerebrovascular problems. I share the widespread hope and enthusiasm that effective treatment to improve outcome after ischemic stroke will be available in the near future.

Table of Contents

8. LACUNAR STROKE

9. UNUSUAL CAUSES OF STROKE

10. STROKE IN YOUNGER PATIENTS

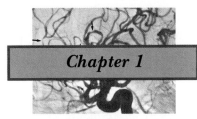

Chapter 1

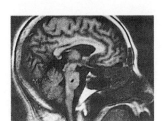

RALPH L. SACCO

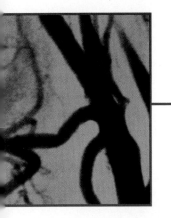

Frequency and Determinants of Stroke

STROKE IS A MAJOR PUBLIC HEALTH problem in the United

States, ranking among the top three causes of death. More

often disabling than fatal, stroke resulted in expenditures of

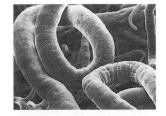

approximately $16.8 billion for health care and lost productiv-

ity in 1992 (Fig. 1.1). A major goal of the Public Health

Service, and one of its National Health Promotion and Disease

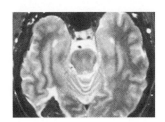

Prevention Objectives, is "to reduce stroke deaths to no more

than 20 per 100,000" by the year 2000.

MORTALITY, PREVALENCE, AND INCIDENCE OF STROKE

MORTALITY

Measures of stroke magnitude include mortality, prevalence, and incidence. Mortality data is available from many countries, but may provide an inaccurate description because fatal cases may be disproportionately represented, death certificates may not accurately depict the underlying cause of death, and the international coding of diseases has been modified over the years. The average age-adjusted stroke mortality in the United States is 50 to 100 out of 100,000 per year. Stroke mortality is lower in the United States than it is in Japan and China, but greater than in the Philippines.

Stroke mortality rises exponentially with age, virtually doubling every 5 years (Fig. 1.2). An excess stroke mortality rate has been reported in men and among blacks of the same age and sex. The rates for Hispanics are not known. Most countries exhibit regional variations in mortality rates. In the United States, the southeast and west are the hardest hit (Fig. 1.3). Much of the regional and racial variations are probably due to differences in stroke incidence.

INCIDENCE AND PREVALENCE

Stroke incidence, the number of new cases over a defined time interval in a specific population, and stroke prevalence, the total number of cases measured at one time in a defined population, are often difficult to determine because of incomplete case ascertainment or inadequate knowledge of the underlying numbers for the population at risk. The annual incidence of new strokes in the United States is estimated at 500,000 and the prevalence of stroke survivors is nearly 3 million (see Fig. 1.1). Stroke preva-

---

FIGURE 1.1 → ESTIMATED PUBLIC HEALTH IMPACT OF STROKE IN THE UNITED STATES, 1992

INCIDENCE	PREVALENCE	MORTALITY	COST
500,000 new strokes each year	2,980,000 survivors of stroke	150,000 stroke deaths each year (third leading cause of mortality)	$16.8 billion for stroke-related care • hospital/nursing home 12.3 • lost productivity 2.6 • physician services 1.6 • medication 0.3

FIGURE 1.2 → INCIDENCE, PREVALENCE AND MORTALITY OF STROKE BY AGE

	AGE< 45	45–54	55–64	65–74	75–84	≥ 85
AGE-SPECIFIC RATE PER 100,000						
INCIDENCE[1]	10	104	209	681	1113	1837
PREVALENCE[2]	66	——— 998 ———		——— 5063 ———		
MORTALITY[3]			75	250	800	

[1]Average annual stroke incidence per 100,000, Rochester, 1980–84 Adapted from Broderick JP, et al. 1989.
[2]National Survey of Stroke, 1976
[3]US vital statistics, 1980

lence ranges between 500 to 600 per 100,000. Age-adjusted incidence rates, which range between 100 to 300 per 100,000 each year, depend on the study methodology and population demographics. Captive populations such as that in Rochester, Minnesota, have led to estimates of the overall age- and sex-adjusted average annual incidence of stroke as being 105/100,000. Using community-wide, hospital-based stroke registries in Pennsylvania's Lehigh Valley, as well as in northern Manhattan, overall age-adjusted stroke incidence estimates were 167 and 372 per 100,000, respectively.

Variation by Age and Sex
Stroke incidence and prevalence rise dramatically with age (see Fig. 1.2). The majority of strokes occur in persons over 65 years of age, with a slight preponderance toward men. Prospective studies, such as the one in Framingham, Massachusetts, have indicated that the age-adjusted, average annual incidence of atherothrombotic brain infarction over age 30 was 270 per 100,000 for men and 210 per 100,000 for women. The male to female ratio has been estimated at 1.3:1 and may differ by stroke subtype. Men are more prone to cerebral infarction; subarachnoid hemorrhage (SAH) seems to have a female predilection, and both sexes are equally susceptible to intracerebral hemorrhage (IH).

Variation by Race
Studies have found that blacks are more vulnerable to stroke than are whites of comparable age, sex, and residence. In a population-based Alabama stroke study, the age-adjusted incidence of hospitalized stroke was twice as high among blacks. Recent evidence from the Lehigh Valley reported a standardized morbidity rate of 2.43 in blacks as compared to whites. In northern

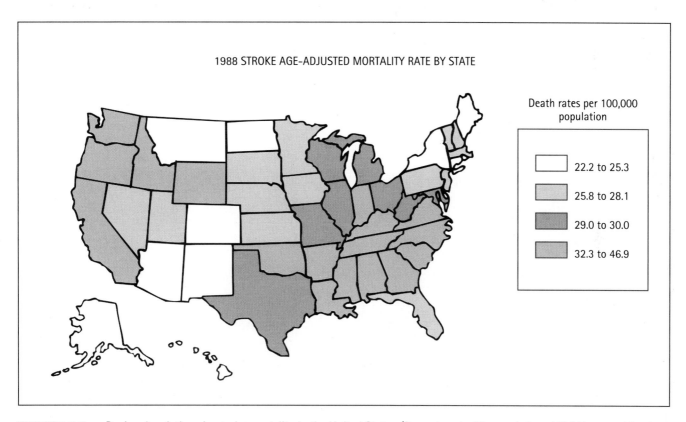

FIGURE 1.3 → Regional variations in stroke mortality in the United States. (Reproduced with permission. *1992 Heart and Stroke Facts,* 1991. Copyright American Heart Association)

Manhattan, stroke in both men and women was twice as frequent in blacks as compared to whites (Fig. 1.4).

Some of the increased incidence in blacks may be due to a higher prevalence of hypertension in that population. Mean blood pressures and the frequency of hypertension have been reported to be higher in black cohorts. However, in the National Health and Nutrition Survey, the relative risk of stroke among blacks was higher despite adjustment for age, hypertension, and diabetes.

By contrast, Hispanics are rarely categorized in epidemiologic stroke studies. In the Lehigh Valley, where Hispanics reportedly account for 3.3% of the population, the standardized morbidity ratio of 0.73 suggested that stroke occurrence was less in Hispanics than in whites. In northern Manhattan, however stroke incidence was similar in Hispanics and whites.

TEMPORAL TRENDS IN MORTALITY AND INCIDENCE

Stroke mortality has decreased overall since the early 1900s. The rate of decline was a constant 1% per year until 1969, when it accelerated to nearly 5% per year (Fig. 1.5). The greatest decline was in the older age groups. Reduction in stroke mortality occurred in each race-sex group, but the relative difference between the races has remained fairly uniform, with a nearly twofold increase in stroke mortality among blacks.

The reasons for this trend remain a subject of speculation. Epidemiologic data supports various possibilities, including declining stroke incidence, improved survival and case-fatality, reduction in the severity of stroke, changing diagnostic criteria, and better stroke risk-factor control. In Rochester, declining stroke mortality was attributed more to declining incidence than to improved survival. Age- and sex-adjusted stroke incidence had declined in each of the 5-year periods since 1945–49 (Fig. 1.6). Incidence began dropping in 1955 and in 1969 for men. SAH incidence in women has remained stable, while the rates for IH and cerebral infarction have dropped. More recently, however, the decline of stroke incidence in Rochester has ended, with rates in both men and women increasing between 1975–79 and 1980–84.

Case-fatality rates have fallen, and long-term survival rates after stroke have improved in various studies. In Rochester, 30-day case-fatality decreased by

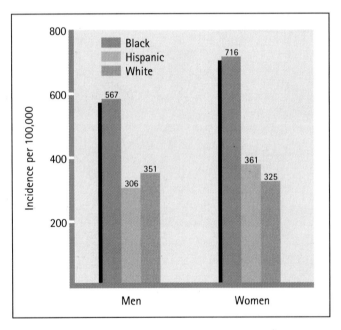

FIGURE 1.4 → Age-adjusted, hospitalized stroke incidence in northern Manhattan whites, blacks, and Hispanics who were over age 40, 1983–1986.

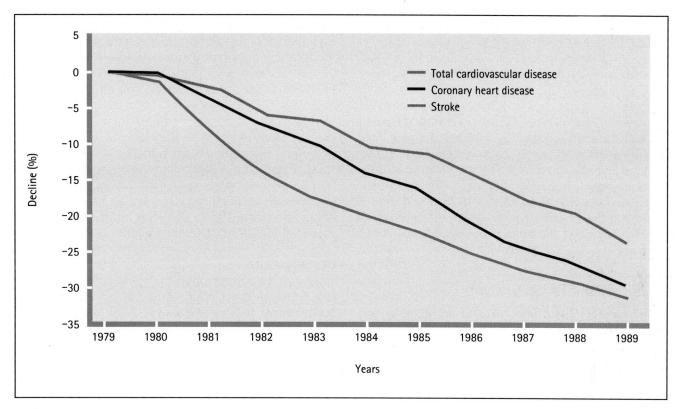

FIGURE 1.5 → Declining mortality from stroke and cardiovascular diseases in the United States. (Reproduced with permission. *1992 Heart and Stroke Facts*, 1991. ©Copyright American Heart Association)

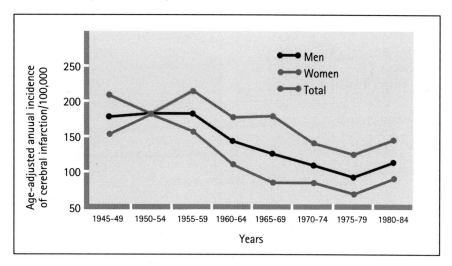

FIGURE 1.6 → Temporal trends in 5-year stroke incidence in men and women over a forty year period. (Adapted from Broderick JP, et al. 1989)

50% from 1945–49 to 1980–84. Survival after cerebral infarction improved from 42% survival for only 3 years in 1945–49 to 45% at 6 years in 1975–79. In Framingham, 1-year case-fatality in men decreased from 35% to 14%. Hospital case-fatality rates in the Hospital Discharge Survey have declined nearly 50% between 1971 and 1982. Stroke severity decreased in some surveys, as indicated by a drop in the percentage of patients presenting with coma; this helps to explain some of the reduction in stroke mortality rates. Some have attributed the reduced stroke mortality to better control of hypertension. Others have noted that the decline began before the widespread use of anti-hypertensives and that indexes of hypertension control have not correlated with stroke mortality.

DETERMINANTS OF STROKE

Besides the reported differences in stroke occurrence by age, sex, and race, numerous stroke risk factors that are potentially modifiable have been identified in asymptomatic populations. Major reductions in stroke morbidity and mortality are more likely to arise from the identification and control of environmental factors in the stroke-prone individual. Stroke risk factors, as determined by prospective cohort and case-control studies, include: hypertension, diabetes, cardiac disease (particularly atrial fibrillation), hypercholes-terolemia, cigarette use, and alcohol abuse (Fig. 1.7). Specific high stroke risk subgroups have been identified as persons with atrial fibrillation (AF), recent myocardial infarction, transient ischemic attacks (TIAs) or carotid stenosis. The latter two are discussed at length in Chapters 4 and 5.

HYPERTENSION

After age, hypertension is the most powerful stroke risk factor in the United States, affecting both men and women. It is especially prevalent among blacks (Fig. 1.8). The risk of stroke rises with higher blood

---

FIGURE 1.7 → MODIFIABLE STROKE RISK FACTORS

STROKE RISK FACTOR	ESTIMATED RELATIVE RISK	ESTIMATED PREVALENCE (%)*
Hypertension	4.0–5.0	25–40
Cardiac disease	2.0–4.0	10–20
Atrial fibrillation	5.6–17.6	1
Diabetes mellitus	1.5–3.0	4–8
Cigarette smoking	1.5–2.9	20–40
Alcohol abuse	1.0–4.0	5–30
Hyperlipidemia	1.0–2.0	6–50
Asymptomatic carotid stenosis	2.0–3.0	5

*Prevalence varies by age, sex, race/ethnicity, and definition of the stroke risk factor.

FIGURE 1.8 → HYPERTENSION IN UNITED STATES ADULTS, AGES 18–74

	% HYPERTENSIVE*	
	MEN	WOMEN
WHITE	33%	25%
AFRICAN-AMERICAN	38%	39%

*Persons with a systolic level ≥ 140 and/or a diastolic level ≥90 or who report using antihypertensive medication.

©Reproduced with permission. 1992 Heart and Stroke Facts, 1991. Copyright American Heart Association.

pressure. In Framingham, the age-adjusted relative risk of stroke among those with definite hypertension (BP > 160/95) was 4.0 for men and 4.4 for women. Even among borderline hypertensives, the relative risk is 2.0 compared to normotensives (Fig. 1.9). Both elevated diastolic and systolic blood pressures are associated with increased stroke risk. Isolated systolic hypertension becomes more common with age, increasing the risk of stroke by 2 to 4 times, independent of other risk factors.

CARDIAC DISEASE

Cardiac disease ranks third as a stroke risk factor. Various types of cardiac disease that have been clearly associated with increasing the risk of ischemic stroke include: AF, valvular heart disease, myocardial infarction, coronary artery disease, congestive heart failure, left ventricular thrombus, electrocardiographic evidence of left ventricular hypertrophy, and perhaps mitral valve prolapse.

Atrial Fibrillation

Chronic AF affects more than 1 million Americans and 1% of those over 60 years old. AF is easily detected by electrocardiography or Holter monitor. It is usually associated with subjective complaints of palpitations. AF increases the relative risk of stroke to 5.6 in nonvalvular AF and to 17.6 in patients with rheumatic heart disease. The effect persists even after accounting for coexisting factors such as age, hypertension, and other cardiac impairments. AF appears to account for 7% to 30% of all strokes in patients over the age of 60 years as well as for more than 75,000 cases of stroke per year. The duration of AF may be an important determinant of stroke risk; stroke occurrence is clustered in the initial year after AF onset.

Coronary Artery Disease and Congestive Heart Failure

Stroke risk nearly doubles in those with antecedent coronary artery disease or congestive heart failure

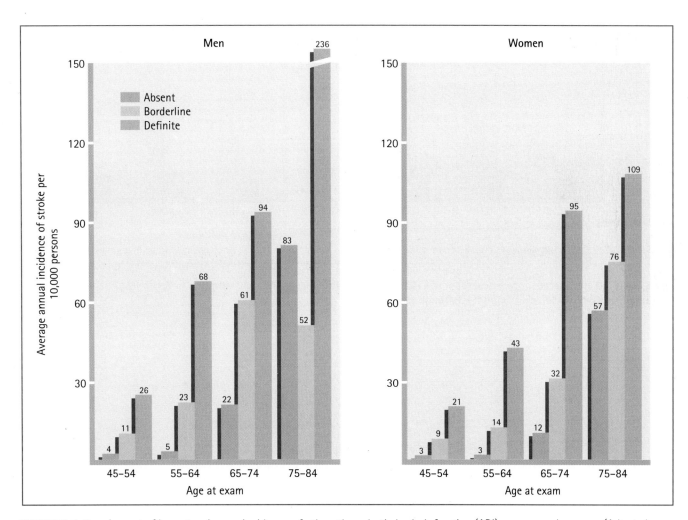

FIGURE 1.9 → Impact of hypertension on incidence of atherothrombotic brain infarction (ABI) on men and women. (Adapted from Wolf PA, et al. In: Barnett HJM, et al. 1992)

(Fig. 1.10). Acute myocardial infarction has also been associated with stroke, particularly when the anterior wall is involved. There is good evidence that patients with acute myocardial infarction and mural thrombus may have a greater risk of cerebral emboli. Electrocardiographic evidence of left ventricular hypertrophy is more prevalent with advancing age and high blood pressure. It increases the risk of stroke nearly fourfold.

DIABETES MELLITUS
Diabetes has also been associated with increased stroke risk, ranging from relative risks of 1.5 to 3.0, depending on the type and severity. This relative risk is found in both men and women and does not diminish with age (Fig. 1.11). The effect of diabetes is independent of hypertension and has been attributed to microvascular angiopathy as well as to the progression of cerebral atherosclerosis. Serum hyperglycemia has been found to be related to stroke severity and early stroke recurrence.

LIPIDS
Elevated serum lipids (triglyceride, cholesterol, LDL) are more notable for their effect on coronary disease than on cerebrovascular disease. In prior studies from Framingham, a quadratic or U-shaped relationship

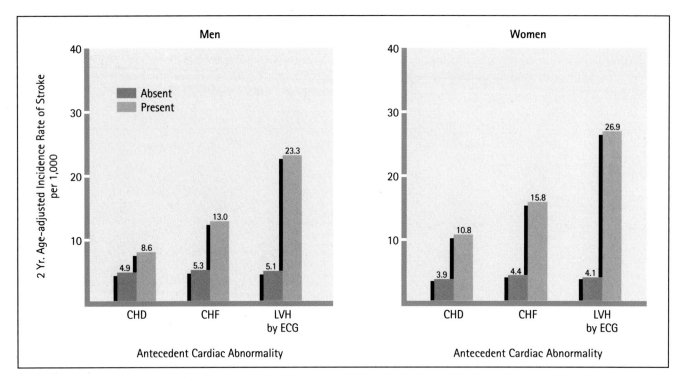

FIGURE 1.10 → Antecedent cardiac disease and ischemic stroke incidence in men and women. Thirty-six year follow-up. (Adapted from Wolf PA, et al. In: Barnett HJM, et al. 1992)

was found between serum total cholesterol and stroke incidence. Degree and progression of carotid atherosclerosis were directly related to cholesterol and LDL and inversely related to HDL. In some autopsy studies, small-vessel cerebrovascular disease was associated with triglycerides. The true relationship between blood lipids and ischemic stroke needs further clarification, which may require examining the effect of lipids upon certain atherosclerotic stroke subtypes.

CIGARETTE SMOKING
Once classified as a "treatable, but value not established" stroke risk factor, smoking has recently been established as an independent determinant of stroke. In Framingham, cigarette smoking accounted for adjusted relative risks of brain infarction of 1.56 in men and 1.86 in women after controlling for other cardiovascular risk factors. Ex-smokers developed stroke at the level of nonsmokers within 5 years after quitting. The dose-response relationship indicated that persons smoking more than 40 cigarettes per day had nearly twice the stroke risk of those smoking fewer than 10 cigarettes per day. Hemorrhagic stroke, particularly SAH, has also been associated with smoking. A meta-analysis of 32 separate studies demonstrated an overall relative stroke risk of 1.5 (95% CI

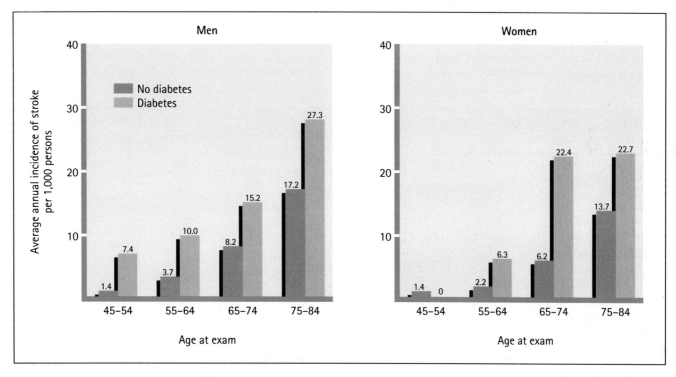

FIGURE 1.11 → The connection between diabetes and incidence of ischemic stroke in men and women. Thirty-six year follow-up. (Adapted from Wolf PA, et al. In: Barnett HJM, et al. 1992)

1.4–1.6) in cigarette smokers. The risk was greatest for SAH, intermediate for cerebral infarction, and lowest for cerebral hemorrhage (Fig. 1.12). A dose-response relationship was noted. The risk decreased with age; a small increased risk was noted in women compared to men.

ALCOHOL

Alcohol's role as a stroke risk factor is controversial. Results range from a definite independent effect in both men and women, an effect only in men, and no effect after controlling for other confounding risk factors such as cigarette smoking. Early Framingham data found an association between alcohol intake and the incidence of stroke, but only in men. More recently, Framingham and other studies have noted a J-shaped relationship between alcohol and stroke. Moderate to heavy alcohol consumption was associated with an increased relative risk of stroke, while light drinking was associated with reduced relative risk when compared to nondrinkers. In one study of men, the relative risk of stroke adjusted for hypertension, cigarette smoking, and medication was lower in light drinkers than in nondrinkers, but was 4 times greater in heavy drinkers (Fig. 1.13). In a large prospective study of middle-aged women, moderate alcohol consumption decreased the risk of ischemic stroke, but increased the risk of SAH. One case-control study found that the joint effects of cigarette smoking and alcohol consumption led to an odds ratio of 6.7 for the risk of stroke. More data is needed to clarify the relationship between alcohol and hemorrhagic or ischemic stroke types.

ASYMPTOMATIC CAROTID DISEASE

Asymptomatic carotid artery disease, which includes a bruit, ulcerative plaque, and hemodynamic stenosis, is associated with a 1% to 2% annual stroke risk.

FIGURE 1.12 → CIGARETTE SMOKING AND STROKE RISK

VARIABLE	POOLED RELATIVE RISK (95% CONFIDENCE INTERVAL)
STROKE SUBTYPE	
Cerebral infarction	1.92 (1.71–2.16)
Subarachnoid hemorrhage	2.93 (2.48–3.46)
Intracerebral hemorrhage	0.74 (0.56–0.98)
SEX	
Men	1.43 (1.35–1.52)
Women	1.72 (1.59–1.86)
AGE	
< 55	2.94 (2.40–3.59)
55–74	1.75 (1.56–1.97)
≥ 75	1.11 (0.96–1.28)
CIGARETTES PER DAY	
Low (< 10)	1.37 (1.24–1.52)
Intermediate (10–20)	1.45 (1.33–1.57)
High (> 20)	1.82 (1.70–1.96)

Adapted from Shinton R, Beevers G, 1989.

FIGURE 1.13 → ALCOHOL USE AND STROKE RISK*

ALCOHOL INTAKE (DRINKS PER WEEK) MEN	RELATIVE RISK	95% CONFIDENCE INTERVAL
None	1.0	0.2–1.0
1–9	0.5	0.6–2.1
10–29	1.1	1.7–10.0
≥ 30	4.2	

*Relative risk of stroke among men with increasing alcohol intake, adjusted for treatment of hypertension, cigarette smoking and medication.

Reprinted by permission of The New England Journal of Medicine, In: Gill JS, et al. Stroke and alcohol consumption. 1986; 315:1041–1046.

Asymptomatic carotid bruit occurs in about 5% of patients over age 50 and has a stroke risk twice that of the general population, but more often the stroke is not ipsilateral to the carotid bruit. The development of symptoms may depend on the adequacy of collateral circulation, the character of the atherosclerotic plaque, and the plaque's propensity to form thrombus at the site of stenosis. The severity, type, distribution, and progression of carotid artery disease in the asymptomatic patient help define the subsequent stroke risk.

TRANSIENT ISCHEMIC ATTACKS

Transient ischemic attacks (TIAs) are a strong indicator of subsequent stroke, with annual stroke risks of 1% to 15%. They occur prior to stroke in about 10% to 20% of patients. The first year after a TIA appears to have the greatest stroke risk (5%). In Rochester, after accounting for other factors, the relative risk of stroke following TIA has been estimated as 3.9%. Approximately half of TIA patients have ipsilateral carotid disease, which can be detected by carotid bruits or noninvasive vascular imaging. Age, cigarette smoking, and history of ischemic heart disease clearly influenced the outcome following a TIA, while distribution of the TIA, history of prior stroke, and history of diabetes did not. The number, duration, tempo of TIAs, the degree of underlying carotid stenosis, presence of ulceration, and severity of cerebral perfusion deficit help predict the subsequent stroke risk.

OTHER POTENTIAL STROKE RISK FACTORS

Other potential stroke risk factors have been identified by some studies, but they need confirmation and clarification in further epidemiologic investigations (Fig. 1.14). A family history of stroke (first-degree or maternal relative) has been found to be a predictor in a few studies, as have obesity and physical inactivity.

FIGURE 1.14 → OTHER POTENTIAL STROKE RISK FACTORS

Family history	HEMATOLOGIC	CARDIAC
Obesity	Hematocrit	Mitral valve prolapse
Physical Inactivity	Polycythemia	Patent foramen ovale
Oral Contraceptive Use	Sickle cell disease	Aortic arch disease
Migraine	White blood cell count	Atrial septal aneurysm
	Fibrinogen	Spontaneous echo
	Hyperuricemia	contrast
	Hyperhomocysteinemia	
	Protein C	
	Free protein S	
	Lupus anticoagulant	
	Antiphospholipid antibodies	

Migraine and oral contraceptive use have been associated with a higher stroke risk, although recent epidemiologic studies have questioned the relation between stroke and newer oral contraceptives. Laboratory abnormalities that have been identified as stroke precursors include: hematocrit, polycythemia, sickle cell anemia, white blood count, fibrinogen, hyperuricemia, Protein C and Free Protein S deficiencies, Lupus anticoagulant, and anticardiolipin antibodies. Improved cardiac imaging has led to the detection of potential stroke risk factors such as mitral valve prolapse, patent foramen ovale, aortic arch disease, atrial septal aneurysms, and spontaneous echo contrast.

Many people exhibit multiple stroke risk factors, which may lead to synergistically increased subsequent stroke risk. Stroke-prone profiles developed from the Framingham Study help estimate the risk of stroke for a person with a combination of factors. Identifying the independence or codependence of factors is important in estimating the probability of stroke. The underlying frequency of the condition is another integral component. A risk factor may greatly increase an individual's risk of stroke, but if it is exceedingly rare in the general population it may only be responsible for a small proportion of strokes. Examining the attributable risk of a given factor is one way of accounting for this. Despite the multitude of identified stroke risk factors, however, a large proportion of strokes still defy adequate explanation and mandate future epidemiologic investigations.

NATURAL HISTORY OF ISCHEMIC STROKE

Outcomes among patients who have an acute stroke include: worsening, survival with minimal deficit, death, stroke recurrence, myocardial infarction, functional disability, and dementia. Since the majority of strokes are cerebral infarcts, most of the discussion of prognosis pertains to this group.

SURVIVAL

The period immediately following an ischemic stroke carries the greatest risk of death from the initial infarc-

FIGURE 1.15 → EARLY HOSPITAL COURSE AFTER ACUTE CEREBRAL INFARCTION BY STROKE DIAGNOSTIC SUBTYPE: STROKE DATA BANK

| | STROKE SUBTYPE | | | | | |
CHARACTERISTIC	ATH	EMB	LAC	TAP	IUC	TOTAL
Number of patients	113	246	337	68	507	1271
30-day mortality	13.3%	11.4%	0.6%	1.5%	11.4%	8.2%
Unstable hospital course	44.3%	22.0%	13.4%	25.0%	27.4%	24.0%
Medical complication	11.6%	5.7%	1.2%	4.4%	9.3%	6.4%
Stroke evolution	33.6%	16.3%	12.5%	11.8%	17.8%	17.2%
Proportion of worsening from stroke evolution	76.0%	74.1%	93.3%	47.1%	64.7%	71.5%

(ATH = atherosclerosis; EMB = cardioembolism, IUC = infarction of undetermined cause; LAC = lacune; TAP = tandem arterial pathology)

tion. Fatality rates, which range from 8% to 20% in the first 30 days, are more likely due to cardiopulmonary complications, rather than brain death from transtentorial herniation. In Framingham, the 30-day case-fatality for men and women with atherothrombotic infarction was 15%, increasing directly with age. Survival is worse for the hemorrhagic strokes, with mortality ranging from 30% to 80% for intracerebral, and 20% to 50% for subarachnoid hemorrhage. Thirty-day mortality differs by infarct subtype (Fig. 1.15). Cardioembolism and infarcts of undetermined cause have a similar early mortality, while lacunar stroke and artery-to-artery embolism are less often fatal.

Survivors of the initial ictus continue to have a 3 to 5 times greater risk of death compared to the age-matched general population. In the National Survey, 53% of stroke patients who survived the initial 6 months lived for 5 years. Five year survival was 75% in those under 65, and fell to 23% in those 85 or older. In Framingham, five year survival rates after atherothrombotic brain infarction were 56% and 64% for men and women (Fig. 1.16).

WORSENING

Overall, ischemic stroke is more likely to worsen and incapacitate than it is to be fatal. Worsening after acute stroke is common, and is usually caused by stroke evolution rather than medical complications. Worsening also varies by infarct subtype (see Fig. 1.15). Atherosclerotic stroke has the greatest propensity to evolve. Cardioembolism and infarcts of undetermined cause have a similar frequency of in-hospital worsening.

STROKE RECURRENCE

Recurrent stroke, which is frequent, is responsible for most stroke morbidity and mortality. Despite the reported decline in stroke incidence, no decline is consistently reported for stroke recurrence. With the declining mortality from stroke and the increased longevity of the United States population, stroke recurrence may account for a greater share of the annual cost of stroke-related health care.

The period immediately following a stroke carries the highest risk for early recurrence. According to the Stroke Data Bank, 40 out of 1273 patients with

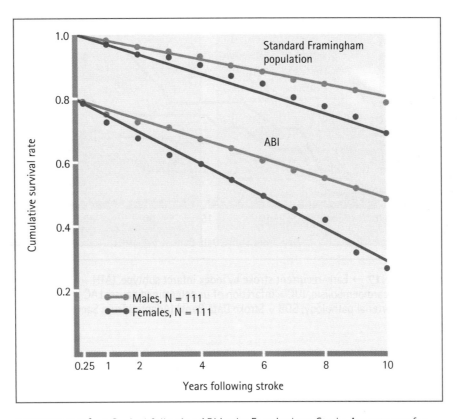

FIGURE 1.16 → Suvival following ABI in the Framingham Study. Average age for males in study was 66.6 years. Females averaged at 66.8 years. (Adapted from Sacco RL, et al. 1982)

REFERENCES

American Heart Association. The National Health and Nutrition Examination Survey II, 1976-80. In: *1992 Heart and Stroke Facts*. Dallas, 1991.

Bogousslavsky J, Van Melle G, Regli F. The Lausanne Stroke Registry: analysis of 1000 consecutive patients with first stroke. *Stroke* 1988; 19:1083–1092.

Broderick JP, Phillips SJ, Whisnant JP, et al. Incidence rates of stroke in the eighties: the end of the decline in stroke? *Stroke*. 1989; 20:577–582.

Camargo CA. Moderate alcohol consumption and stroke: the epidemiologic evidence. *Stroke* 1989; 20:1611–1626.

Cooper R, Sempos C, Hsieh SC, Kovar MG. Slowdown in the decline of stroke mortality in the United States, 1978–1986. *Stroke*. 1990; 21:1274–1279.

Davis PH, Hachinski V. Epidemiology of Cerebrovascular Disease. In: Anderson DW (ed). *Neuroepidemiology: A Tribute to Bruce Schoenberg*. Boca Raton: CRC Press. 1991; 27–53.

Foulkes MA, Wolf PA, Price TR, Mohr JP, Hier DB. The Stroke Data Bank: design, methods, and baseline characteristics. *Stroke*. 1988; 19:547–54.

Garraway WM, Whisnant JP. The changing pattern of hypertension and the declining incidence of stroke. *JAMA*. 1987; 258:214–17.

Gill JS, Zezulka AV, Shipley MJ, et al. Stroke and alcohol consumption. *N Engl J Med*. 1986; 315:1041–6.

Gillum RF. Stroke in blacks. *Stroke*. 1988; 19:1–9.

Gross CR, Kase CS, Mohr JP, et al. Stroke in south Alabama: incidence and diagnostic features—a population based study. *Stroke*. 1984; 15:249–255.

Hier DB, Foulkes MA, Swiontoniowski M, et al. Stroke recurrence within two years after ischemic infarction. *Stroke*. 1991; 22:155–161.

Matsumoto N, Whisnant JP, Kurland LT, Okazaki H. Natural history of stroke in Rochester, Minnesota, 1955 through 1969: an extension of a previous study. *Stroke*. 1973; 4:20–29.

Mohr JP, Caplan LR, Melski JW, et al. The Harvard cooperative stroke registry: a prospective registry. *Neurology*. 1978; 28:754–762.

Sacco RL, Foulkes MA, Mohr JP, et al. Determinants of early recurrence of cerebral infarction: Stroke Data Bank. *Stroke*. 1989; 20:983–89

Sacco RL, Hauser WA, Mohr JP. Hospitalized stroke in blacks and Hispanics in northern Manhattan. *Stroke*. 1991; 22:1491–96.

Sacco RL, Wolf PA, Kannel WB, McNamara PM. Survival and recurrence following stroke: the Framingham Study. *Stroke*.1982; 13:290–295.

Schoenberg BS, Schulte BPM. Cerebrovascular disease: epidemiology and geopathology. In: Toole JF (ed). *Vascular Diseases Part I*. In: Vinken PJ, Bruyn GW, Klawans HL (eds). *Handbook of Clinical Neurology*, New York: Elsevier Publishers. 1988; 53:1–26.

Shinton R, Beevers G. Meta-analysis of relation between cigarette smoking and stroke. *Br Med J*. 1989; 298:789–94.

Whisnant JP, Fitzgibbons JP, Kurland LT, Sayre GP. Natural history of stroke in Rochester, Minnesota, 1945 through 1954. *Stroke*. 1971; 2:11–22.

Wolf PA, Cobb JL, D'Agostino RB. Epidemiology of Stroke. In: Barnett HJM, Mohr JP, Stein BM, Yatsu FM (eds). *Stroke: Pathophysiology, Diagnosis, and Management*. New York: Churchill Livingstone. 1992.

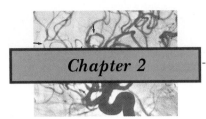

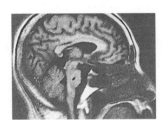

Chapter 2

RALPH L. SACCO

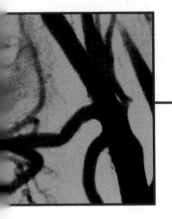

Classification of Stroke

STROKE IS BROADLY DEFINED as the abrupt onset of focal or global neurologic symptoms caused by ischemia or hemorrhage into or around the brain as a result of cerebral blood vessel diseases. The presenting neurologic syndrome reflects the location, size, and type of stroke. Part of the challenge of understanding stroke is localizing the lesion by its clinical symptoms and signs. The aim is to identify precisely the affected anatomic region of the brain, the corresponding vascular territory and, subsequently, the mechanism of the stroke or stroke subtype in an effort to plan specific therapies.

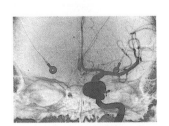

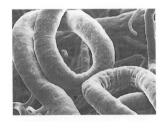

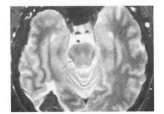

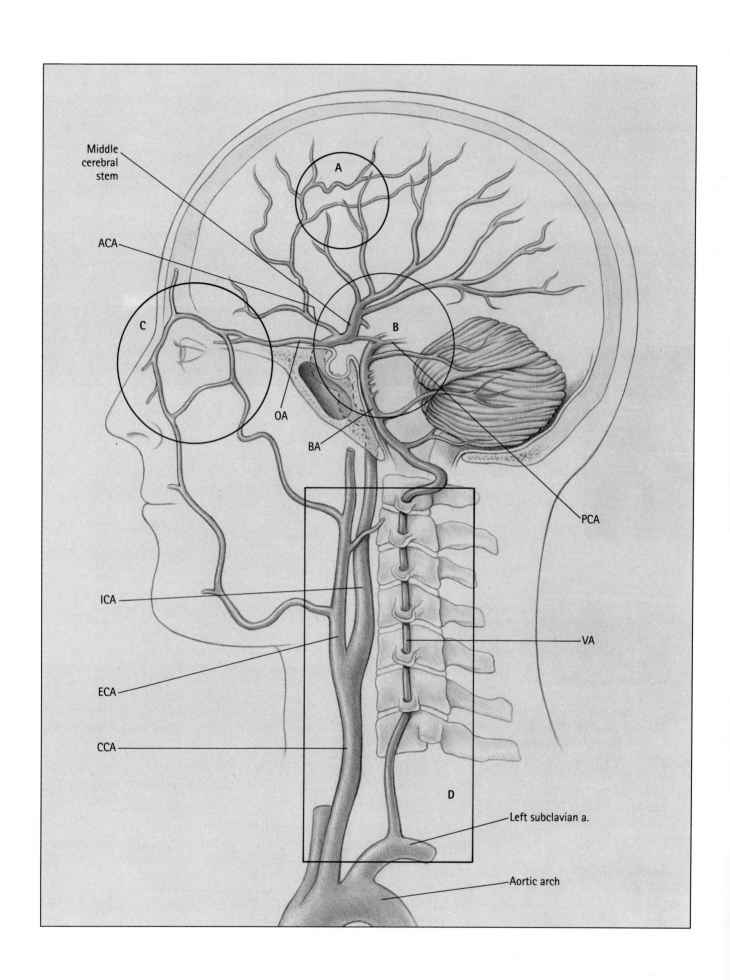

Middle cerebral stem

ACA

A

C

B

OA

BA

PCA

ICA

ECA

CCA

VA

D

Left subclavian a.

Aortic arch

Localizing a stroke can be difficult. Individual vascular variations exist, and symptoms are sometimes fleeting. Disturbances in consciousness, language, or behavior may camouflage important localizing signs; coexisting prior neurologic deficits can lead to confounding presenting syndromes. Even when modern imaging techniques locate the lesion, the neurologic syndrome may fail to conform to the functional anatomic and vascular correlations enumerated in classic neurologic teaching. As neuroimaging modalities become more sophisticated, new clinicoradiologic correlations may help to reshape our view of the functional anatomy and vascular supply of the brain.

VASCULAR ANATOMY

The brain is perfused by the carotid and vertebral arteries, which begin as extracranial arteries off the aorta or other great vessels and course through the neck and base of the skull to reach the intracranial cavity. A rich anastomotic network includes various extracranial intercommunicating systems, intracranial connections through the circle of Willis, and distal intracranial connections through meningeal anastomoses throughout the border zones over the cortical and cerebellar surfaces (Fig. 2.1).

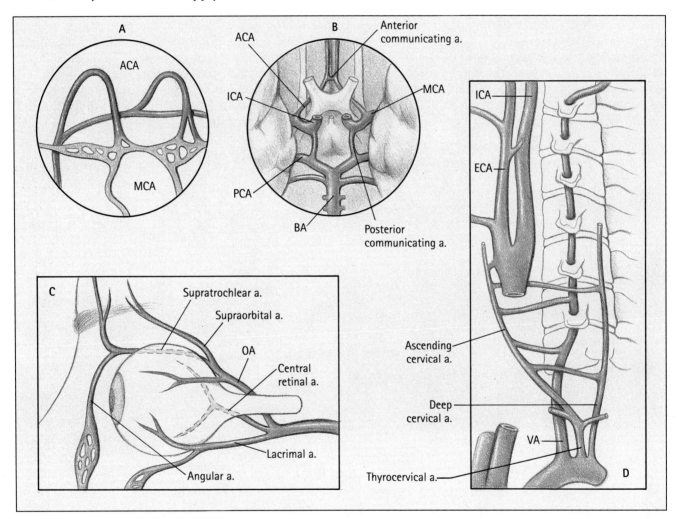

FIGURE 2.1 → Arterial supply to the brain with enlarged detail of the sites of anastomosis in the cerebral circulation. **A,** Over the convexity, subarachnoid interarterial anastomoses link the middle, anterior, and posterior cerebral arteries (MCA, ACA, PCA) through the border zone. **B,** The Circle of Willis provides communication between the anterior and posterior cerebral circulation via the anterior and posterior communicating arteries. **C,** Through the orbit, anastomoses occur between the external and internal carotid arteries (ECA, ICA). **D,** Extracranial anastomoses connect the muscular branches of the cervical arteries to the vertebral arteries (VAs) and the ECAs. (OA = ophthalmic artery; BA = basilar artery; CCA = common carotid artery)

CAROTID CIRCULATION

Internal Carotid Artery

The right common carotid originates from the bifurcation of the innominate artery, while the left originates directly from the aortic arch. The internal carotid arteries (ICAs) stem from the common carotid, usually at the level of the upper border of the thyroid cartilage at the fourth cervical vertebral body. They do not branch into the neck or face; they enter the cranium through the carotid canal. Figure 2.2 illustrates the four main segments: 1) the *cervical,* which runs from the bifurcation to the entrance of the carotid canal; 2) the *petrous,* which continues into the carotid canal of the petrous bone to pierce the dura at the foramen lacerum, giving off the caroticotympanic and pterygoid branches; 3) the *cavernous,* which runs from the foramen lacerum and cavernous sinus entrance to just medial of the anterior clinoid process, giving off three main branches (meningohypophyseal trunk, artery to the inferior

portion of the cavernous sinus, capsular artery of McConnell); and 4) the *supraclinoid,* which enters the intracranial space at the anterior clinoid after passing between the 2nd and 3rd cranial nerves. The supraclinoid continues to the termination just below the anterior perforated substance into the middle and anterior cerebral arteries, after segmenting into the ophthalmic, superior hypophyseal, posterior communicating, and anterior choroidal arteries. The siphon is the term used to describe the series of turns made by the cavernous and supraclinoid segments of the ICA. The *anterior choroidal artery* supplies the optic tract, the inferior portion of the posterior limb of the internal capsule, the medial portion of the globus pallidus, the pyriform cortex and uncus of the temporal lobe, the hippocampal and dentate gyri, the tail of the caudate nucleus, the posteromedial half of the amygdala, the middle third of the cerebral peduncle, the substantia nigra, parts of the red nucleus, a portion of the subthalamus, and the lateral geniculate.

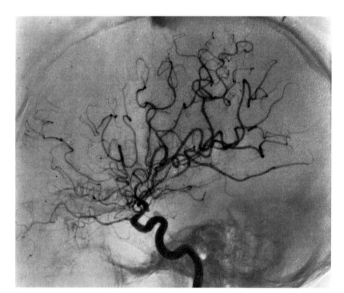

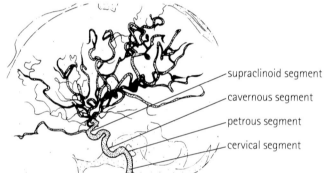

FIGURE 2.2 → Segments of the ICA are shown on this x-ray.

Middle Cerebral Artery

The ICA's largest branch, the middle cerebral artery (MCA), appears almost as its direct continuation. The MCA begins as a single trunk (stem or M1 segment), passing laterally to the sylvian fissure where it becomes the M2 (insular) segment, which gives rise to the 12 cerebral surface branches that continue as the M3 (opercular) and M4 (cortical) segments (Fig. 2.3). The stem branches into the medial and lateral lenticulostriates, which supply the extreme capsule, claustrum, putamen, most of the globus pallidus, part of the head and the entire body of the caudate, as well as the superior portions of the internal capsule's ante-

rior and posterior limbs. The stem usually ends in either a bifurcation into the upper and lower divisions, or a trifurcation into three major trunks (upper, middle, and lower divisions). The upper division most often gives rise to the lateral orbitofrontal, ascending frontal, precentral (prerolandic), central (rolandic), and anterior parietal, while the lower division usually contains the temporal polar, temporo-occipital, anterior, middle, and posterior temporal branches (Fig. 2.4A,B). The posterior parietal and angular branches are more variable. The cortical divisions supply almost the entire cortical surface of the brain, including the insula, operculum, frontal, parietal, temporal, and part

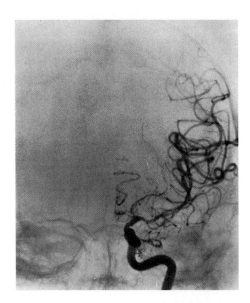

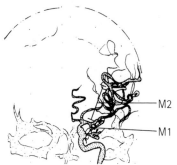

FIGURE 2.3 → This x-ray delineates the segments of the MCA.

of the occipital cortex, but spare the frontal pole, the superior and extreme posterior rim of the convex surface, and medial cortical surfaces.

Anterior Cerebral Artery

The anterior cerebral (ACA) artery begins as a medial branch of the ICA, forming the A1 (proximal) segment to the junction of the anterior communicating artery, where it continues as the A2 (distal) segment. It is referred to as the A3 segment when it runs over the genu of the corpus callosum, becoming the A4 segment just distal to the coronal suture, and terminating as the A5 segment (Fig. 2.4C,D). Perforating arteries arise from the A1 and A2 segments to supply the paraolfactory structures, medial anterior commissure, anteroinferior portions of the globus pallidus, caudate, putamen, anterior hypothalamus, the anterior limb of the internal capsule, and sometimes part of the thalamus's anterior nucleus and genu of the internal capsule's posterior limb. The largest branch is the recurrent artery of Heubner. The other branches are 1) the *medial orbitofrontal,* which supplies the frontal lobe's medial and orbital surfaces; 2) the *frontopolar,* supplying the medial parts of the frontal lobe, extending to the convexity of the anterior portion of the superior frontal gyrus; 3) the *callosomarginal,* supplying the posterior part of the superior frontal gyrus, the medial surface of the frontal lobe, parts of the cingulate gyrus, and paracentral lobule; and 4) the *pericallosal,* which supplies the medial surface of the parietal lobe, including the anterior portion of the precuneus.

VERTEBROBASILAR CIRCULATION

Vertebral Artery

The vertebral artery (VA) usually arises from the subclavian artery and is commonly divided into 4 segments: 1) the *prevertebral,* which runs from its origin to the transverse foraminal entrance at the level of the sixth cervical vertebral body; 2) the *cervical,* which courses through the transverse foramina; 3) the *atlantic,* which exits from the transverse foramen of C2; and 4) the *intradural or intracranial,* which pierces the dura, entering the cranial cavity to join the contralateral VA. At the upper end of the cervical and atlantic segments, the anterior and posterior meningeal branches originate (Fig. 2.4E). The intracra-

nial segment is the origin for the anterior and posterior spinal arteries as well as the posterior inferior cerebellar artery (PICA). The latter bifurcates into medial and lateral branches that supply the inferior surface of the cerebellum. The lateral medulla is supplied by the multiple perforating branches of the PICA or direct medullary branches of the VA.

Basilar Artery

The basilar artery (BA) is formed by the joining of the right and left VAs, usually at the level of the pontomedullary junction (Fig. 2.4E,F). It gives rise to medial penetrators, short and long lateral circumferential penetrators, the anterior inferior cerebellar (AICA) and superior cerebellar arteries, terminating into the two posterior cerebral arteries. The penetrators supply the pons, the inferior portion of the midbrain, and the ventrolateral aspect of the cerebellar cortex. The internal auditory (labyrinthine) artery either arises directly from the BA or from the AICA to supply the cochlea, labyrinth, and a portion of the facial nerve. The AICA supplies the middle cerebellar peduncle as well as the anteroinferior aspect of the cerebellum. Just proximal to the basilar termination, the superior cerebellar artery arises, sending perforating branches to the midbrain and adjacent pons, ending in medial and lateral branches that supply the superior half of the cerebellum.

Posterior Cerebral Artery

The BA usually terminates into the posterior cerebral arteries (PCAs) (Fig. 2.4G,H). They are joined to the ICA by the posterior communicating artery. In approximately 15% of patients, the PCA is a direct continuation of the posterior communicating artery. A series of penetrators (posteromedial, thalamoperforates, thalamogeniculate, tuberothalamic) arise from the posterior communicating artery and the PCA to supply the hypothalamus, dorsolateral midbrain, lateral geniculate, and thalamus. The PCA also gives rise to the medial and lateral posterior choroidal arteries, which supply the posterior portion of the thalamus and choroid plexus. The PCA splits into the anterior division, which gives rise to the anterior and posterior temporal arteries that supply the inferior surface of the temporal lobe, as well as the posterior division (internal occipital artery), which gives rise to the pos-

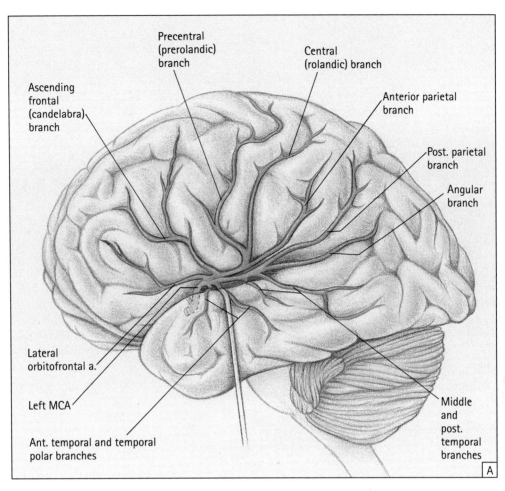

Precentral (prerolandic) branch

Central (rolandic) branch

Anterior parietal branch

Post. parietal branch

Angular branch

Ascending frontal (candelabra) branch

Lateral orbitofrontal a.

Left MCA

Ant. temporal and temporal polar branches

Middle and post. temporal branches

A

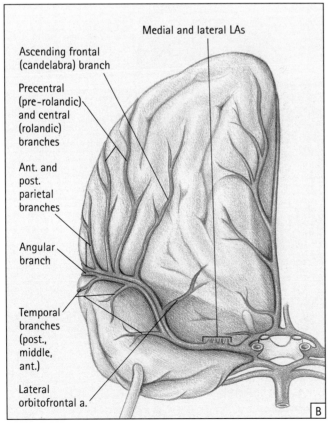

Medial and lateral LAs

Ascending frontal (candelabra) branch

Precentral (pre-rolandic) and central (rolandic) branches

Ant. and post. parietal branches

Angular branch

Temporal branches (post., middle, ant.)

Lateral orbitofrontal a.

B

FIGURE 2.4 → The cerebral circulation as viewed from different angles. **A,** MCA branches, lateral view. **B,** MCA branches, frontal view. (LA=lentriculostriate arteries)

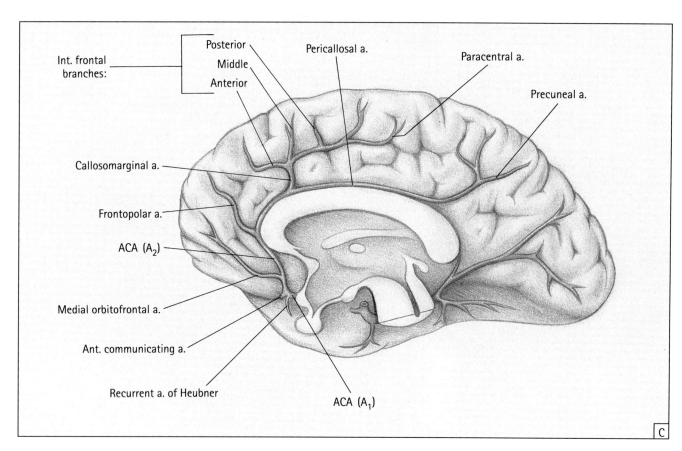

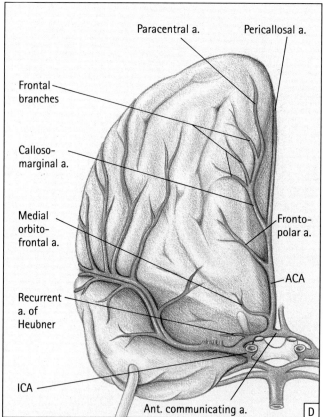

FIGURE 2.4 → **C**, ACA branches, medial view. **D**, ACA branches, frontal view.

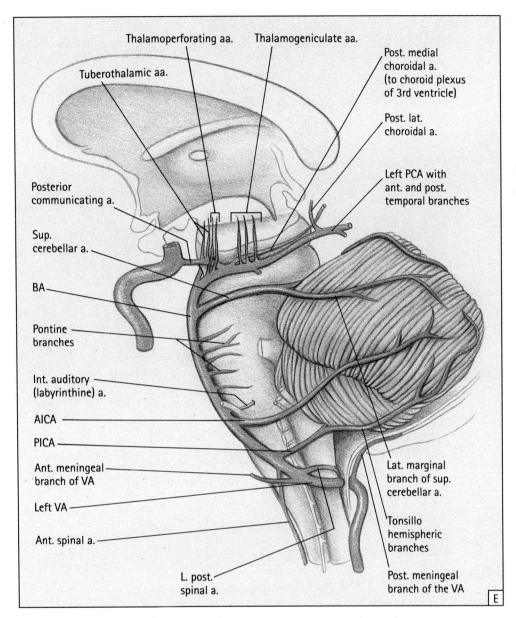

Thalamoperforating aa.

Thalamogeniculate aa.

Tuberothalamic aa.

Post. medial
choroidal a.
(to choroid plexus
of 3rd ventricle)

Post. lat.
choroidal a.

Posterior
communicating a.

Left PCA with
ant. and post.
temporal branches

Sup.
cerebellar a.

BA

Pontine
branches

Int. auditory
(labyrinthine) a.

AICA

PICA

Ant. meningeal
branch of VA

Lat. marginal
branch of sup.
cerebellar a.

Left VA

Tonsillo
hemispheric
branches

Ant. spinal a.

L. post.
spinal a.

Post. meningeal
branch of the VA

E

FIGURE 2.4 → **E,** VA and BA, lateral view. (AICA = anterior inferior cerebellar artery;
PICA = posterior inferior cerebellar artery)

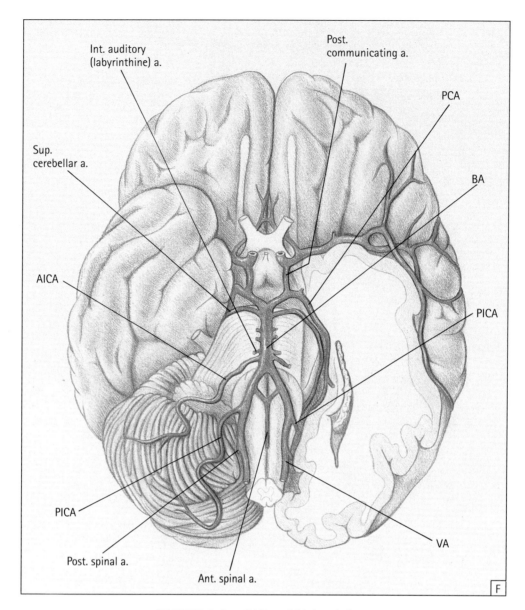

Int. auditory (labyrinthine) a.

Post. communicating a.

PCA

Sup. cerebellar a.

BA

AICA

PICA

PICA

Post. spinal a.

Ant. spinal a.

VA

FIGURE 2.4 → **F**, VA and BA, basal view.

Cerebrovascular Disorders

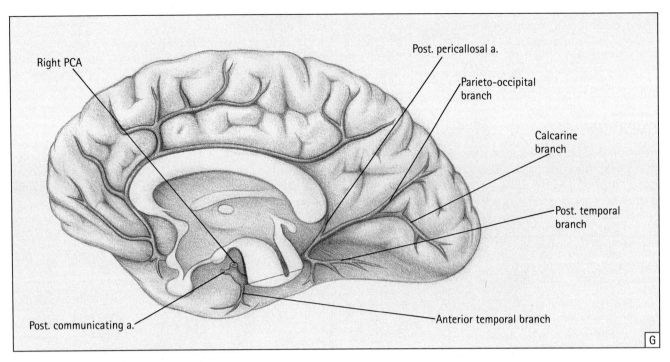

Right PCA

Post. pericallosal a.

Parieto-occipital branch

Calcarine branch

Post. temporal branch

Post. temporal branch

Post. communicating a.

Anterior temporal branch

G

FIGURE 2.4 → G, PCA branches, medial view. **H,** PCA branches, inferior view.

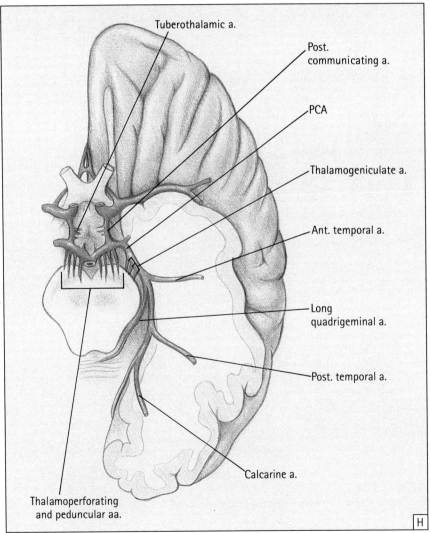

Tuberothalamic a.

Post. communicating a.

PCA

Thalamogeniculate a.

Ant. temporal a.

Long quadrigeminal a.

Post. temporal a.

Calcarine a.

Thalamoperforating and peduncular aa.

H

terior pericallosal, occipitoparietal, posterior parietal, and calcarine branches. These supply the undersurface of the occipital lobe, including the lingual and fusiform gyrus, the medial surface of the occipital cortex, and the precuneus.

OVERVIEW OF VASCULAR SUPPLY

Individual variations exist in the arterial supply of the brain, but there are generally agreed upon regions of perfusion (Fig. 2.5). Infarction may occur in more than one vascular territory if the occlusion is more proximal in the arterial tree and the ischemia is widespread. Given the vast array of collateral supply, however, border-zone ischemia may result with limited infarction in the distal fields of the vascular supply. Intracranial proximal occlusions may cause penetrant artery ischemia and coexisting surface branch territory infarction, while single branch occlusions are more likely to occur when an embolism reaches its most distal resting place. Knowledge of the vascular and functional anatomy is a prerequisite to unraveling the pathophysiology of stroke in an individual patient.

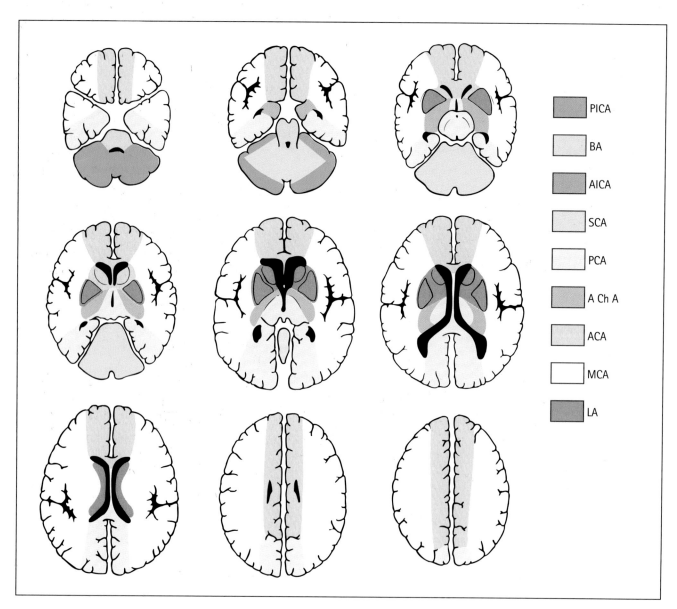

FIGURE 2.5 → The vascular territories of the PICA, the BA, the AICA, the superior cerebral artery (SCA), the PCA, and the anterior choroid artery (AChA) are shown in this diagram, as are the territories of the ACA, the MCA, and the LAs. (Adapted with permission from Savoiardo M. The vascular territories of the carotid and vertebrobasilar system. *Ital J Neurol Sci* 1986; 7:405)

FUNCTIONAL ANATOMY

FRONTAL LOBES

The frontal lobes are defined as the cerebral hemispheres anterior to the Rolandic fissure, superior to the Sylvian fissure, and connected by the corpus callosum (Fig. 2.6). Areas of clinical importance include the motor strip (precentral gyrus, Area 4), the supplemental motor areas (Area 6), frontal eye fields (Area 8), micturition center on the medial surface, and Broca's speech area (Area 44). The motor strip has a homuncular organization, with a large lateral representation of the face, hand, and arm; the trunk and leg are represented in the superolateral and sagittal surfaces (Fig. 2.7). Personality, drive, and social inhibition are some of the other functions attributed to the frontal lobes.

PARIETAL LOBES

From the Rolandic fissure, the parietal lobes extend posteriorly to the parieto-occipital fissure and superiorly to the temporal lobes, separated by the Sylvian fissure (see Fig. 2.6). Sensory function is localized to the postcentral gyrus and is organized similarly to the motor strip. Cortical sensory modalities include graphesthesia, two-point discrimination, and stereognosis. Speech and language function are often localized to the supramarginal and angular gyri (Areas 39 and 40), in conjunction with

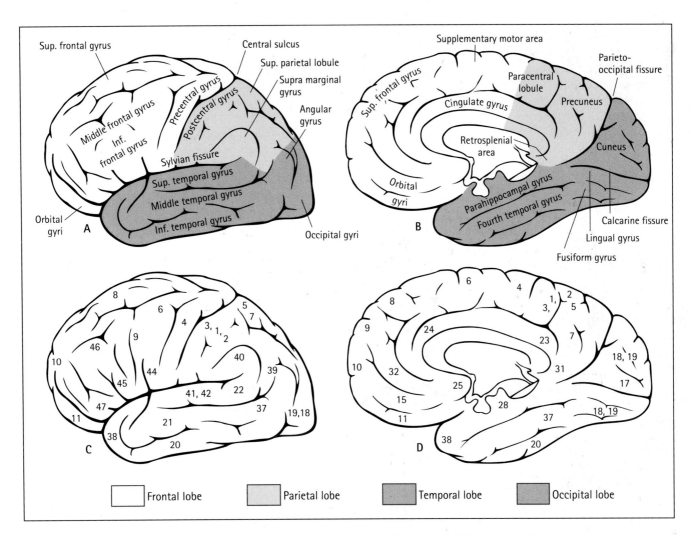

FIGURE 2.6 → The cerebral cortex. **A,** Lateral view. **B,** Medial view. **C,D:** Brodmann's areas are clearly labeled in these diagrams.

the superior temporal lobe. Praxis and spatial orientation are also attributed to parietal lobe function.

OCCIPITAL LOBES

The occipital cortex extends posteriorly from the parieto-occipital fissure, forming the posterior pole of the cerebral hemispheres (see Fig. 2.6). Vision is processed by the calcarine or striate cortex (Area 17) and the visual association cortex (Areas 18, 19). Reading, writing, naming—particularly for colors or faces—and topographic orientation are some of the functions attributed to the occipital lobes in association with the temporal lobes.

TEMPORAL LOBES

The temporal cortex is inferior to the parietal and frontal lobes and folds in on itself (see Fig. 2.6). The extensive connections between the cingulate gyrus and the hippocampal area form the basis of the "limbic" system. Functions attributed to the temporal lobe include central auditory processing, memory, visual association, speech, and language. The temporal lobes are also responsible for the upper visual pathways and supplemental motor areas concerning emotional facial expression, and behavior, as well as the central control of autonomic functions.

BASAL GANGLIA AND THALAMUS

The caudate, claustrum, amygdaloid body, putamen, and globus pallidus make up the basal ganglia. The latter two are often called the lentiform nucleus. The corpus striatum is formed by the caudate and lentiform nucleus (see Fig. 2.7). Control of movement is its prime function through the extrapyramidal motor system, which has rich connections with other areas, including the frontal lobes, thalamus, and cerebellum. The thalamus is a large, central, deep, nuclear area that makes up the diencephalon. Various nuclear groups (e.g., ventral posterior lateral nuclei, etc.) serve as relays to other areas and function with processing of sensation, vision, movement, language, spatial orientation, and memory.

BRAINSTEM AND CEREBELLUM

The brainstem consists of the midbrain, pons, and medulla, with various cranial nerve nuclei, tracts, and relay nuclei that connect the cerebral hemispheres, extrapyramidal system, and thalamus with the spinal cord (Fig. 2.8A,B). The cerebellar hemispheres coordinate movement through their interconnections with the frontal lobes, thalamus, spinal cord, and brainstem nuclei. Strategic lesions may cause a variety of syndromes that are discussed in subsequent chapters.

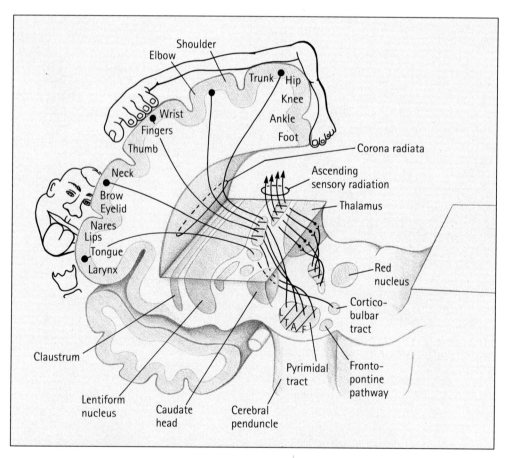

FIGURE 2.7 → A homuncular view of the basal ganglia and the thalamus. The relationship of the long tracts with the basal ganglia are also shown. (L=leg; T=trunk; A=arm; F=face)

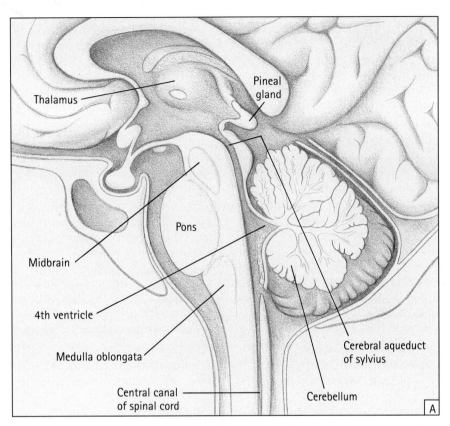

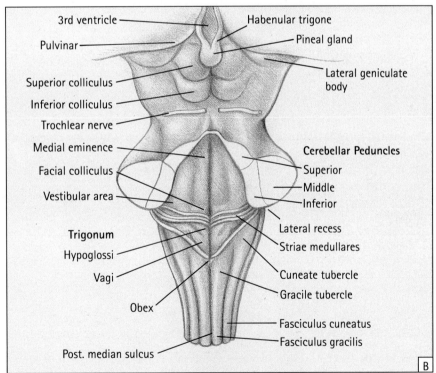

FIGURE 2.8 → **A,** Brainstem and cerebellum, lateral view.
B, Brainstem, posterior surface.

CLASSIFICATION OF STROKE SUBTYPES

Stroke is characterized by the abrupt or ictal onset of neurologic symptoms. By conventional definition, neurologic symptoms that continue for more than 24 hours are diagnosed as stroke; anything less is considered a transient ischemic attack (TIA). Many TIA patients are actually found to have a stroke if a brain image is performed at an appropriate time. Therefore, shorter symptom durations (e.g., 1 hr or 15 min) may be more pertinent for distinguishing between TIA and stroke. Stroke is also classified by the type of pathology (infarction or hemorrhage), although overlap does occur with hemorrhagic infarction. Intracranial hemorrhage can be subdivided into either subarachnoid or intracerebral, depending on the site and origin of the blood. Ischemic infarction can be classified by the mechanism of ischemia (hemodynamic or thromboembolic) and the pathology of the vascular lesion: atherosclerotic, lacunar, cardioembolic, or indeterminate, as outlined below. The various stroke subtypes differ in etiology, frequency, clinical signs, outcome, and treatment.

Overall, ischemic stroke is 3 to 4 times as frequent as hemorrhagic stroke types, accounting for 70% to 80% of all strokes (Fig. 2.9). Subarachnoid hemorrhage (SAH) occurs 33% to 60% less frequently than intracerebral hemorrhage (IH), except in the population-based cohort of Framingham, where SAH is more frequent than IH. Depending on the geographic origin of the patients, IH usually accounts for 10% to 30% of cases. Greater relative frequencies are reported in Chinese and Japanese series. The relative frequencies of the infarct subtypes vary from study to study. Cardioembolism ranges from 15% to 30% of cases, atherosclerotic infarction varies from 14% to 40%, and lacunar infarcts account for 15% to 30%. Stroke from other determined causes, such as arteritis or dissection, usually accounts for less than 5% of cases. Infarcts of undetermined cause may account for as many as 40% of ischemic infarcts (Fig. 2.10).

DISCREPANCIES IN STROKE SUBTYPE FREQUENCIES

The frequency of the different stroke subtypes varies depending on the basis of diagnosis. Pathologic series are biased toward fatal stroke cases and,

FIGURE 2.9 → FREQUENCY AND DISTRIBUTION OF STROKE TYPES

STUDY	N	SUBARACHNOID HEMORRHAGE (%)	INTRACEREBRAL HEMORRHAGE (%)	CEREBRAL INFARCTION (%)	ILL-DEFINED STROKE/OTHER (%)
Community-based, USA					
Framingham, MA	353	11	5	84	–
Rochester, MN	993	6	10	79	5
South Alabama	160	6	8	86	–
Lehigh Valley, PA*	1026	3	8	89	–
Northern Manhattan, NY*	1034	3	9	88	–
Hospital-based, USA					
Stroke Data Bank	1805	13	13	71	3
Community Stroke Program	4125	4	6	60	30
Harvard Stroke Registry	694	6	10	84	–
Outside USA					
Oxfordshire, UK	675	6	8	76	10
Dijon, France	418	5	15	80	–
Akita, Japan	2168	14	30	56	–
People's Republic of China	115	2	44	51	3
Shibata, Japan	415	8	23	58	11

*Community wide, hospital based
N=number of patients

therefore, have a disproportionate number of hemorrhages. Diagnoses in pre-CT series were based chiefly on clinical grounds, with heavy reliance on clinical syndrome, neurological examination, and coexisting risk factors. Before the advent of CT, normal cerebrospinal fluid and angiogram would have led to a diagnosis of ischemic stroke. CT distinguished between hemorrhage and infarction, resulting in the correct classification of up to 25% of IHs that were formerly classified as infarction. With the widespread application of CT, MRI, duplex as well as transcranial Doppler, SPECT, and other diagnostic studies, diagnostic stroke subtypes have been refined and supported by laboratory confirmation. Stroke subtype frequencies, however, still differ depending on the sample from which cases are drawn (hospital or population-based) and the design of investigator-driven algorithms. The presence or absence of an indeterminate stroke category also impacts diagnostic classification. When present, it insures that the defined stroke subtype categories are more homogeneous, while in the absence of an indeterminate category, ambiguous cases will be classified as determined subtypes. The latter practice can lead to overestimations of the relative stroke subtype frequencies and alteration of subgroup characteristics through misclassification.

SUBARACHNOID HEMORRHAGE

SAH occurs when the blood is localized to the surrounding membranes and cerebrospinal fluid. It is usually caused by blood leaking from a cerebral aneurysm. The combination of congenital and acquired factors (berry aneurysms, hypertension, smoking) leads to a degeneration of the arterial wall as well as the release of blood under arterial pressures into the subarachnoid space and cerebrospinal fluid. Aneurysms are distributed at different sites throughout the base of the brain, particularly at the origin or bifurcations of arteries. Other conditions that may lead to SAH include arteriovenous malformations, bleeding disorders or anticoagulation, trauma, amyloid angiopathy, or central sinus thrombosis. Signs and symptoms, which often occur in the absence of focal localizing signs, include the abrupt onset of severe headache, vomiting, altered consciousness, and sometimes coma.

FIGURE 2.10 → DISTRIBUTION OF STROKE SUBTYPES IN THE NINDS STROKE DATA BANK

Subtype	No. of Cases	Total Strokes (%)	Infarcts (%)
Infarction (N=1273)			
Atherosclerosis	113	6.3	8.9
Lacunar	337	18.7	26.5
Cardioembolic	246	13.6	19.3
Tandem arterial pathology	69	3.8	5.4
Infarct of undetermined cause	508	28.1	39.9
Hemorrhage (N=532)			
Parenchymatous hemorrhage	237	13.1	
Subarachnoid hemorrhage	243	13.5	
Other	52	2.9	
Total	1805	100.0	100.0

NINDS = National Institute of Neurological Disorders and Stroke.
N = Number of patients
Adapted from Sacco RL, et al. 1989

SAH tends to afflict younger patients and women. Hypertension, high-dosage oral contraceptives, and cigarette smoking are some of the factors that have been associated with it. Fatalities are high, ranging from 30% to 70%, depending on the severity of the initial presentation (Fig. 2.11). Among survivors, early rebleeding and delayed ischemic neurologic deficits from vasospasm can cause serious morbidity.

INTRACEREBRAL HEMORRHAGE

Characterized by bleeding into the substance of the brain, IH is usually the result of a small penetrating artery bleeding in the putamen, caudate, pons, cerebellum, thalamus, or deep white matter (Fig. 2.12). Hypertension has been implicated as weakening the walls of arterioles and in forming Charcot-Bouchard microaneurysms. Among elderly, nonhypertensive patients with recurrent lobar hemorrhages, amyloid angiopathy has been implicated as an important cause. Other causes include arteriovenous malforma-tions, aneurysms, moyamoya disease, bleeding disorders or anticoagulation, trauma, tumors, cavernous angiomas, and illicit drug abuse.

The clinical picture, dictated by the location and size of the hematoma, is characterized by headache, vomiting, and the evolution of focal motor or sensory signs over minutes to hours. Consciousness is rarely impaired at the start, but often becomes a prominent feature in the first 24 to 48 hours among the moderate and large hematomas. IH is associated with the greatest case-fatality rates.

CEREBRAL INFARCTION

When perfusion pressure falls to critical levels, ischemia develops, progressing to infarction if the effect persists long enough. Ischemic infarction can be either bland or hemorrhagic. Bland infarction results when thrombus prevents reperfusion of the infarcted region. Hemorrhagic infarction is less common, with hemorrhagic foci ranging from a few petechiae scattered through the infarct to a mass of

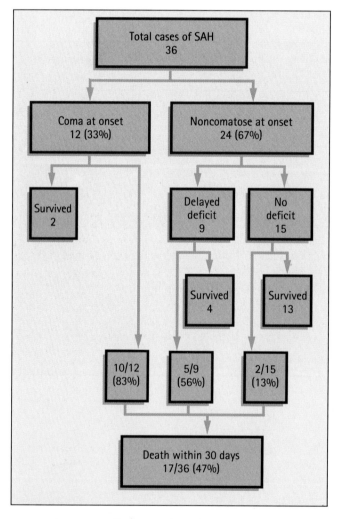

FIGURE 2.11 → Outcome after subarachnoid hemorrhage (SAH). (Adapted from Sacco RL, et al. 1984)

confluent petechial foci that resembles frank hematoma.

Classifying ischemic stroke into subtype, for instance separating embolism from thrombosis, is far from precise. Clinical grounds alone (age, risk factors, etc.) are the time-honored means of determining subtype, but they are often not distinctive enough to infer the cause of infarction. A thorough diagnostic work-up is required. However, even duplex Doppler, MRA, and conventional angiography often fail to show either the expected arterial stenosis or occlusion; acute findings on the brain image simply rule out acute hemorrhage. If a significant carotid stenosis is found, judging whether the clinical syndrome arose from an embolic or hemodynamic mechanism is often still difficult.

In the Stroke Data Bank, patients were deliberately classified into distinct categories, creating new subsets based on the presumed mechanism of infarction. The *atherothrombotic group* was divided into two subgroups: large artery thrombosis with no evidence of embolic infarction, and a form of artery-to-artery embolism arising from an atherosclerotic source. *Cardioembolism* and *lacunar* infarction were diagnosed based on the results of the evaluation. A separate category, *infarct of undetermined cause,* was created to help insure the homogeneity of the other subtypes. Distinguishing the infarct subtype is the first step toward directed therapeutic interventions (Fig. 2.13).

SUBTYPES OF ISCHEMIC STROKE

INFARCT WITH LARGE-ARTERY THROMBOSIS
In earlier studies, thrombosis was often a diagnosis of exclusion. The gradual decline in large-artery thrombosis as a leading diagnosis has resulted from several factors: 1) the more frequent use of duplex and transcranial Doppler; 2) the recognition of several clinical subtypes of thrombosis, especially lacunes; 3) the documentation that some ischemic strokes associated with large-artery atherothrombosis are produced by artery-to-artery (local) embolism; and 4)

FIGURE 2.12 → LOCATIONS OF INTRACEREBRAL HEMORRHAGES, STROKE DATA BANK

LOBAR HEMORRHAGE (N = 65)

1 LOBE		2 LOBES		3 LOBES	
Frontal	17%	Parieto-temporal	14%	Fronto-parieto-temporal	6%
Parietal	11%	Parieto-occipital	14%	Parieto-temporo-occipital	6%
Temporal	9%	Fronto-parietal	9%		
Occipital	9%	Temporo-occipital	3%		
		Fronto-temporal	2%		
Total:	46%		42%		12%

DEEP SUPRATENTORIAL HEMORRHAGE (N = 107)

Putamen	48%	Thalamus	43%	Caudate	9%

DEEP INFRATENTORIAL HEMORRHAGE (N = 37)

Cerebellum	70%	Pons	30%

Adapted from Massaro AR, et al. 1991

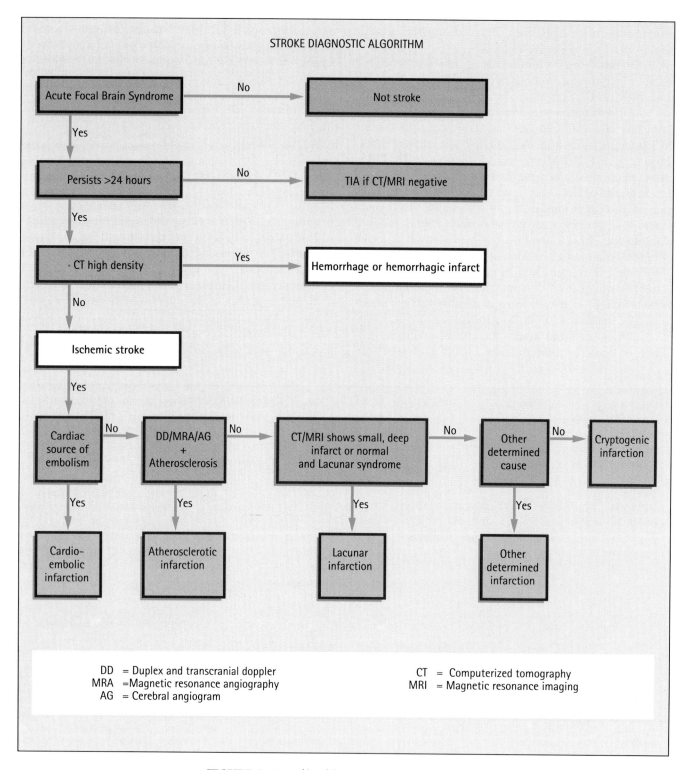

FIGURE 2.13 → Algorithm to classify stroke subtype.

the replacement of the casual stroke "atherothrombotic" classification by the category of "undetermined" cause.

The usual etiology for this subtype stems from atherosclerotic plaque at a bifurcation or curve in one of the larger vessels, leading to progressive stenosis. The final large-artery occlusion is due to thrombosis of the narrowed lumen. Intraplaque hemorrhage sometimes accelerates occlusion, although the frequency of this process is more often a matter of speculation, rather than a fact based on pathologic specimens. The mechanism for stroke in atherothrombus was initially attributed to perfusion failure distal to the site of severe stenosis or occlusion of the major vessel. The infarction site depends on the collateral flow, but is usually in the distal fields or border zones. The development of border-zone ischemia probably depends on many factors, not just the degree of stenosis.

Focal cortical syndromes are usually found in this group, but syndromes often attributed to lacunar disease, such as pure motor or sensorimotor stroke, can easily represent the first sign of impending flow failure. Discriminating between infarct subtypes on clinical grounds alone is difficult. In the Stroke Data Bank, patients with fractional arm weakness (shoulder different from the hand), hypertension, diabetes, and male sex were more

frequently found in the atherosclerotic category (Fig. 2.14). Clinical features that are observed at stroke onset can help distinguish cerebral infarction subtypes, but are not reliable enough to lead to a definite determination of infarct subtype without laboratory data.

In the clinical setting, a diagnosis of large-artery atherosclerotic occlusive disease is supported by MRI and CT findings and confirmed by the duplex Doppler, cerebral angiogram, or MRA. A "distal field" infarct along the border-zone territories can help suggest the diagnosis. Specifying the degree of stenosis that will lead to perfusion failure depends on multiple factors and is often not easily defined. Classification schemes have relied on stenoses greater than 70% to 80% as more predictive of impending hemodynamic compromise. Intracranial atherosclerotic artery stem stenoses or occlusions may also be due to arteriosclerotic thrombosis, but are often difficult to distinguish from embolism. Newer blood flow techniques have also helped confirm the perfusion failure mechanism in cases with atherosclerotic stenosis or occlusive disease through SPECT, xenon CT, regional cerebral blood flow, MRI, and positron emission tomography (PET). The increased use of these techniques should allow a more accurate distinction between embolism and perfusion failure.

FIGURE 2.14 → CLINICAL DISCRIMINATORS OF CARDIOEMBOLIC AND ATHEROSCLEROTIC INFARCTION, STROKE DATA BANK

VARIABLES FAVORING DIAGNOSIS OF CARDIOEMBOLIC INFARCT	ODDS RATIO*	VARIABLES FAVORING DIAGNOSIS OF ATHEROSCLEROTIC INFARCT	ODDS RATIO*
Decreased consciousness	4.0	Hypertension	2.4
Language deficit	4.4	Male gender	2.6
Cardiac disease history	16.6	Prior Stroke	2.6
		Diabetes	3.9
		Transient ischemic attack	4.1
		Fractional arm weakness (hand≠shoulder)	5.3

*Odds ratios are estimated from multivariate logistic regression adjusting for all variables listed in table. Odds of one diagnosis over the other.
Adapted from Timsit S et al. 1992

INFARCT WITH TANDEM ARTERIAL PATHOLOGY

Infarcts are also produced by emboli that travel from the proximally-situated atheromatous lesions to otherwise healthy branches located more distal in the arterial tree (artery-to-artery embolization). Nowadays, embolism from a carotid source has become recognized as another, perhaps more common, cause of stroke in a setting of proximal arterial stenosis. This mechanism of infarction cuts across most attempts to distinguish thrombus from embolus and has earned its own category—tandem arterial pathology. Embolic fragments may arise from extracranial arteries affected by stenosis or ulcer, stenosis of any major cerebral artery stem, the stump of the occluded ICA, and even from an intracranial tail of the anterograde thrombus atop an occluded carotid.

No satisfactory criteria have yet been developed to certify that a stroke is caused by extracranial arterial disease leading to artery-to-artery embolization. The mechanism is inferred when the clinical syndrome suggests a cortical branch territory, there is no obvious cardioembolic source, and the degree of stenosis is insufficient to explain the stroke on the grounds of hemodynamic insufficiency, or there is an ulcerative plaque imaged by noninvasive duplex Doppler, MRA, or cerebral angiogram. CT and MRI scans are helpful only in supporting a diagnosis of embolism, not in inferring its source from the neck. Angiographic evidence of branch occlusion above a carotid stenosis or ulcer is not proof of the source, but can classify this type of stroke as an infarct with tandem arterial pathology.

In the Stroke Data Bank, after controlling for differences in the frequency of cardiac disease, TIAs, and carotid bruits, the probability of an artery-to-artery embolism was increased by the finding of a superficial infarct, or by a higher hematocrit. The probability of cardiac embolism was greater with initial decreased consciousness or with an abnormal first CT (Fig. 2.15). Such findings suggest that these two embolic infarct subtypes differ in the location and extent of cortical infarction. Smaller and more distal infarction in embolism from an arterial source compared with cardiogenic embolism suggests a smaller embolic particle size.

CARDIAC EMBOLISM

Cardiac embolism accounts for between 15% and 30% of strokes, most of which occur from embolism into the territory of the MCA. The complexities of the embolic process make it difficult to account for on a case-by-case basis. Identifying the sources of occlusion is particularly problematic (Fig. 2.16). Recent improvements in the sensitivities of cardiac imaging have lead to better detection of sources of thrombus. This important stroke subtype is covered in depth in Chapter Seven, Cardioembolic Stroke.

LACUNAR (SMALL-VESSEL, DEEP) INFARCTION

In lacunar stroke, the zone of ischemia is confined to the territory of a single vessel, usually quite small. Lacunes are understood to reflect arterial disease of the vessels penetrating the brain to supply the capsule, basal ganglia, thalamus, and paramedian regions of the brainstem. Specific clinical syndromes are classified as pure motor, sensorimotor, ataxic hemiparesis, pure sensory, and dysarthria–clumsy hand (Fig. 2.17). Only a handful have been studied by autopsy technique, and an even smaller number have been subjected to serial section to document the lesion. Rare causes include stenosis of the MCA stem or micro-

---

FIGURE 2.15 → CLINICAL DISCRIMINATORS OF CARDIOEMBOLIC AND ARTERY-TO-ARTERY EMBOLISM, STROKE DATA BANK

Variables Favoring Diagnosis of Artery to Artery Embolism	Odds Ratio*	Variables Favoring Diagnosis of Cardiac Embolism	Odds Ratio*
Hematocrit	1.1	Abnormal initial CT	3.2
Transient ischemic attack	3.9	Cardiac disease history	20.5
Superficial infarction on CT	4.6	Decreased consciousness	39.3
Neck bruit	11.9		

*Odds ratios are estimated from multivariate logistic regression adjusting for all variables listed in table. Odds of one diagnosis over the other.

embolization to penetrant arterial territories. Lacunes were slow to gain clinical acceptance, but they are now considered to account for between 15% and 20% of all stroke cases. This special stroke subtype is described in detail in Chapter Eight, Lacunar Stroke.

INFARCT OF UNDETERMINED CAUSE, OR CRYPTOGENIC INFARCTION

Despite efforts to arrive at a diagnosis, the cause of infarction in a discouragingly large number of cases remains undetermined. The first of three major reasons for this failure is easily understood: no appropriate laboratory studies are performed. Advanced age, coexisting severe disease with a poor prognosis, patient or physician unwillingness, are only a few of the many problems that can defer a workup. A second reason is improper timing of appropriate laboratory studies. Imaging performed only once within a

few hours of onset has a low yield. The third reason, which occurs most frequently, is that normal or ambiguous findings are reached despite appropriate laboratory studies performed at the correct time. It would be comforting if most of these cases represented milder deficits, which could be easily missed due to the relative insensitivity of laboratory studies to smaller lesions. However, the scanty data available indicates that they are not. They are roughly as severe as ischemic strokes for which a cause is found.

Efforts to establish the subtype of infarction proved remarkably difficult in a high percentage of Stroke Data Bank cases. Despite the use of CT or angiogram, the basis for the diagnosis in many cases was still a "best clinical guess." What laboratory data was available indicated that large-artery atherosclerotic occlusive disease was a less frequent cause of stroke. Small-vessel or lacunar and cardioembolic

---

FIGURE 2.16 → POTENTIAL SOURCES OF CARDIAC EMBOLISM

HIGH CARDIOEMBOLIC RISK	MEDIUM CARDIOEMBOLIC RISK
Valvular surgery	Myocardial infarction within 6 months
Atrial fibrillation (AF), atrial flutter, or sick sinus syndrome (SSS) with valvular heart disease	Valvular heart disease without AF, atrial flutter, or SSS
AF, atrial flutter, or SSS without valvular heart disease	Congestive heart failure
Ventricular aneurysm by echocardiogram	Decreased left ventricular function by echocardiogram
Mural thrombus by echocardiogram	Hypokinetic segment by echocardiogram
Cardiomyopathy or left ventricular hypokinesis by echocardiogram	Mitral valve prolapse by history or echocardiogram
Akinetic region by echocardiogram	Mitral annular calcification by echocardiogram
Bacterial Endocarditis	
Atrial Myxoma	

Modified from Kittner SJ, et al. 1990.

FIGURE 2.17 → SYNDROMES AMONG 316 LACUNAR INFARCTS IN THE STROKE DATA BANK

LACUNAR SYNDROME	N	PERCENT
Pure motor hemiparesis	181	57
Sensorimotor	63	20
Ataxic hemiparesis	33	10
Pure sensory	21	7
Dysarthria–clumsy hand	18	6

infarction were relatively frequent, but the cause for the majority of cases could not be classified into these traditional categories. This forced the creation of a separate diagnostic category, known as "infarct of undetermined cause" or "cryptogenic infarction." Apart from a few common features, this category of infarction remains poorly understood and has not been successfully characterized as a clinical group.

In the Stroke Data Bank, cases categorized as ischemic stroke of undetermined cause showed no bruit or TIA ipsilateral to the hemisphere affected by stroke, and had no obvious source of embolism. In short, they did not have the risk factors or prior history that suggested a cardiac embolus or large-artery thrombosis. Among those cryptogenic infarcts studied with angiography, 27% worsened in the hospital and 41% had a moderate to severe weakness score. Hemispheral syndromes predominated in 66%; basilar syndromes occurred in 15%.

The CT or MRI performed within seven days may either be normal, show an infarct limited to a surface branch territory, or show a large zone of infarction affecting regions larger than that accounted for by a single penetrant arterial territory. Noninvasive vascular imaging fails to demonstrate an underlying large-vessel occlusion or stenosis. No cardiac source of embolism is uncovered by echocardiography, electrocardiography, or Holter monitor. If an angiogram is performed, the study may be normal or may show that a distal branch, a major cerebral artery stem, or the top of the BA is occluded. Because these latter foci of occlusion can be from thrombotic or embolic cause, their demonstration does not determine the mechanism; only if repeat angiography reveals that the occlusion is gone can a diagnosis of embolism be made.

Some examples of stroke attributed to meningitis, migraine, lupus anticoagulant, arteritis, dissection, hypercoagulable states, etc. may be represented in the cryptogenic subgroup. Efforts should be made in each case to establish the existence of these unusual causes, and all such instances should be classified as cerebral infarction from *other determined cause*. Adding together all the estimated frequencies of such unusual causes without accompanying evidence of the underlying disease cannot remotely approach the frequency of the cryptogenic subgroup of stroke.

One approach to dealing with this large cohort is by forcing reclassification into the traditional categories of atherothrombosis, embolism, or lacune. The presentation of a hemispheral syndrome, a sur-

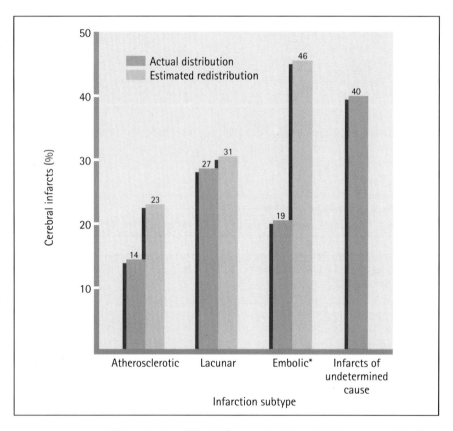

FIGURE 2.18 → Effect of reclassifying infarcts of undetermined causes on the distribution of cerebral infarction subtype. For embolic, the actual distribution represents cardioembolism. The estimated redistribution represents cardioembolism combined with embolism from undetermined cause.

face infarction by CT, and a corresponding branch occlusion documented by angiography or normal angiogram has long been considered suggestive of embolism. Nonthrombotic ischemia has been used to describe those cases with normal angiograms. Such findings could be inferred to represent emboli, despite the lack of documented cardiac source. Ample evidence exists for many occult sources of emboli, but it is difficult to prove their existence or to establish their roles in the first or succeeding ischemic strokes. Reclassifying such cases and others with limited cerebral infarction on CT scan as "embolism with inobvious source" would make embolism from all sources the largest stroke subtype (Fig. 2.18).

Emerging technologies have led to the suggestion that some strokes may be explained by hematologic disorders causing hypercoagulable states from protein C, free protein S, lupus anticoagulant, or anticardiolipin antibody abnormalities. Others have implicated paradoxical emboli through a patent foramen ovale or ulcerated aortic arch plaque. Rather than reclassifying these cases into embolism as the inferred mechanism, we suggest their continued separation as cryptogenic because they represent a sizable cohort of acute strokes for which no mechanism has yet been proven. Classifying as cryptogenic such cases where an embolic source or proof of the occlusion's nature is absent may eventually help determine if they differ in some way from those in which the mechanism of stroke is better defined, and will encourage the continued search for causes of brain infarction and precipitants of thromboembolism.

REFERENCES

Adams RD, Victor M. *Principles of Neurology*. New York: McGraw-Hill Book Co., 1981.

Bamford J, Sandercock P, Dennis M, et al. A prospective study of acute cerebrovascular disease in the community: the Oxfordshire Community Stroke Project—1981–86. *J Neurol Neurosurg Psychiatry*. 1990; 53:16–22.

Bogousslavsky J, Van Melle G, Regli F. The Lausanne Stroke Registry: analysis of 1000 consecutive patients with first stroke. *Stroke*. 1988; 19:1083–1092.

Carpenter MB. *Core Text of Neuroanatomy*. Baltimore: Williams and Wilkins, 1979.

Chamorro AM, Sacco RL, Mohr JP, et al. Lacunar infarction: clinical-CT correlations in the Stroke Data Bank. *Stroke*. 1991; 22:175–181.

Foulkes MA, Wolf PA, Price TR, et al. The Stroke Data Bank: design, methods, and baseline characteristics. *Stroke*. 1988; 19:547–554.

Kittner SJ, Sharkness CM, Price TR, et al. Infarcts with a cardiac source of embolism in the NINCDS Stroke Data Bank: historical features. *Neurology*. 1990; 40:281–284.

Li S, Shoenberg BS, Wang C, et al. Cerebrovascular disease in the People's Republic of China: epidemiologic and clinical features. *Neurology*. 1985; 35:1708–1713.

Massaro AR, Sacco RL, Mohr JP, et al. Clinical discriminators between lobar and subcortical hemorrhage. *Neurology*. 1991; 41:1881–1885.

Mohr JP, Sacco RL. Classification of ischemic strokes. In: Barnett HJM, Mohr JP, Stein BM, Yatsu FM (eds). *Stroke: Pathophysiology, Diagnosis, and Management*. New York: Churchill Livingstone, 1992.

Sacco RL, Ellenberg JA, Mohr JP, et al. Infarction of undetermined cause: the NINCDS Stroke Data Bank. *Ann Neurol*. 1989; 25:382–390.

Sacco RL, Wolf PA, Bharucha NE, et al. Subarachnoid and intracerebral hemorrhage: natural history, prognosis, and precursive factors in the Framingham Study. *Neurology*. 1984; 34:847–854.

Sheldon JJ. Blood Vessels of the scalp and brain. *Clin Symp*. 1981; 33:1–36.

Timsit S, Sacco RL, Mohr JP, et al. Early clinical differentiation of atherosclerotic and cardioembolic infarction: Stroke Data Bank. *Stroke*. 1992; 23:486–491

Wolf PA, Cobb JL, D'Agostino RB. Epidemiology of Stroke. In: Barnett HJM, Mohr JP, Stein BM, Yatsu FM (eds). Stroke: Pathophysiology, Diagnosis, and Management. New York: Churchill Livingstone, 1992.

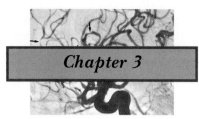

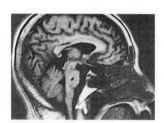

Chapter 3

MARC FISHER

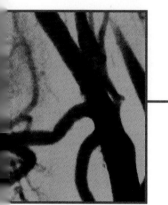

The Pathophysiology of Ischemic Stroke

UNDERSTANDING HOW STROKE-RELATED INJURY occurs is essential to developing fruitful preventive and therapeutic interventions. Research on the pathophysiologic basis for central nervous system injury secondary to stroke has begun to illuminate the cellular consequences of ischemic injury. A deeper comprehension of ischemic cellular injury has, in turn, provided important concepts upon which therapy can be designed. The underlying vascular causes of acute stroke, such as large- and small-vessel atherosclerosis, have been widely studied with a focus on their evolution at both the macroscopic and microscopic levels. Attention has also been turned to the pathophysiology of cardiac and hematologic disorders that predispose to local clot formation and cranial arterial embolization.

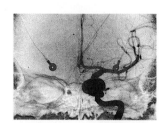

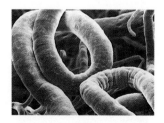

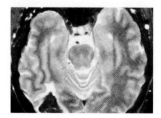

NORMAL PHYSIOLOGY

Before the effects of ischemia can be appreciated, the normal metabolic and perfusion activities of the brain need to be outlined. The brain must receive adequate and continuous supplies of oxygenated blood and glucose because there are few energy reserves within this metabolically active organ (Fig. 3.1). Normal oxygen consumption in the cerebral cortex averages approximately 6 mL/100 g/min in the gray matter and 2 mL/100 g/min in the white matter. Glucose consumption averages 4.5 to 7 mg/100 g/min, with widespread regional variation. Oxidative glucose metabolism, primarily in the mitochondria, leads to the formation of high-energy phosphates such as adenosine triphosphate (ATP) and adenosine diphosphate (ADP) via the citric acid cycle and mitochondrial electron transport chain (Fig. 3.2). Under normal oxygenation, anaerobic glucose metabolism via the glycolytic pathway contributes little to the brain's energy requirements.

A consistently high level of perfusion is required to supply the brain's constant demand for oxygen and glucose. The brain receives approximately 800 mL of blood per minute; normal regional cerebral blood flow (rCBF) is 40 to 60 mL/100 g/min. Cerebral perfusion or microcirculatory flow is influenced by both neurogenic and chemical factors that are related to systemic and local metabolic conditions (Fig. 3.3). Local rCBF is maintained at a fairly

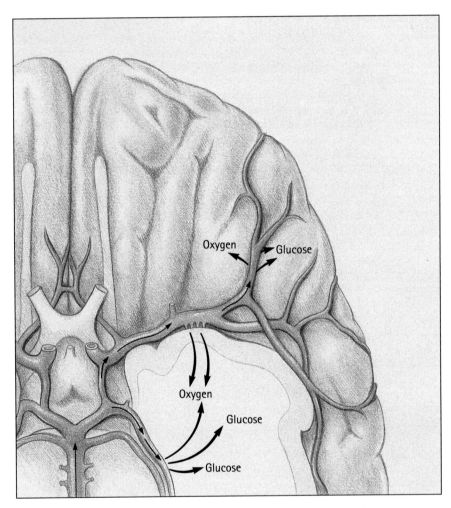

FIGURE 3.1 → The brain requires a constant supply of blood containing glucose and oxygen.

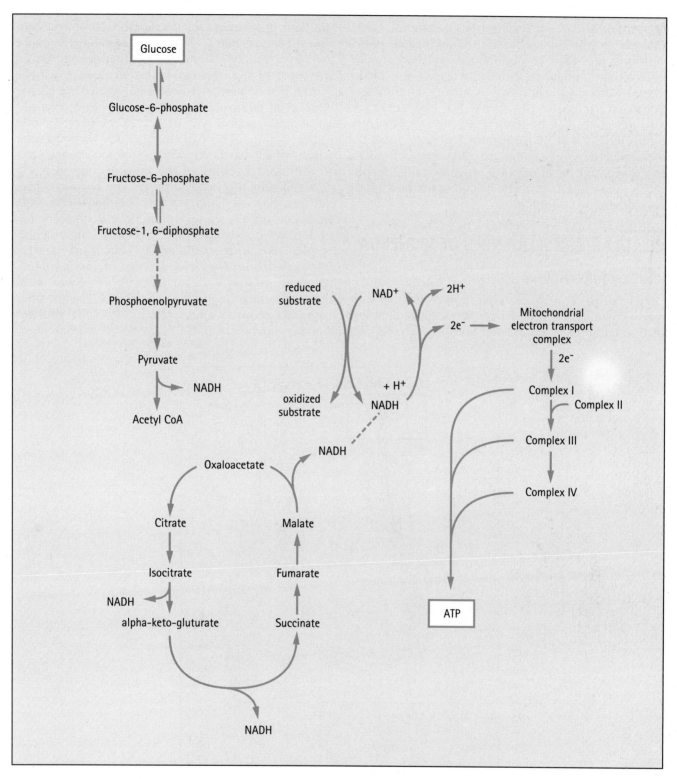

FIGURE 3.2 → Glucose is metabolised to yield NADH and ATP.

constant level over a wide range of systemic blood pressure by the brain's ability to autoregulate perfusion pressure. Flow can be influenced by local cerebral activity and, for example, will increase in the visual cortex in response to visual stimulation. Temperature, blood pH, blood PO_2 and PCO_2 will also affect CBF. A hematocrit of 30% to 31% promotes maximal rCBF. Intracranial pressure and the autonomic nervous system are additional influences. In general, the level of rCBF remains stable despite many physiologic variables, changing markedly only under extreme conditions.

CELLULAR CONSEQUENCES OF ISCHEMIA

IONIC DISTURBANCES

Under normal conditions, ionic homeostasis of neurons is maintained with a large intracellular gradient of potassium (K^+), contrasted with an extracellular gradient of sodium (Na^+), calcium (Ca^{++}), and chloride (Cl^-) ions (Fig. 3.4). This ionic gradient is generated by a variety of ionic pumps that depend on the presence of high-energy metabolites such as ATP. Almost immediately after ischemia begins, these energy-dependent pumps fail, leading to the rapid intracellular accumulation of Na^+ and Cl^-, accompanied by the inflow of water. This early intracellular water accumulation, which has been called cytotoxic edema, leads to the rapid swelling of the neurons and glia (Fig. 3.5). Calcium also begins to enter the cell via voltage and receptor-mediated calcium channels (Fig. 3.6). Intracellular Ca^{++}, released from the mitochondria and endoplasmic reticulum after ischemia, causes a substantial rise in free Ca^{++} levels, which may lead to irreversible injury by a variety of mechanisms. Another important cellular metabolic event is the development of lactic acidosis, which occurs when ischemia induces anaerobic glucose metabolism. Animal experiments have suggested that preischemic

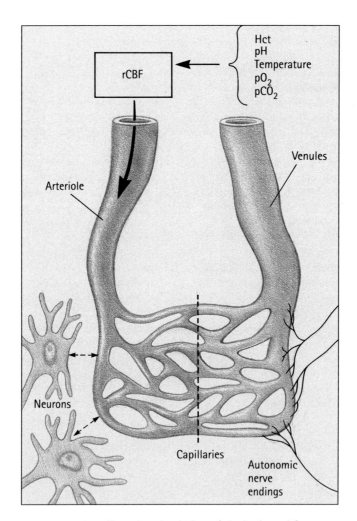

FIGURE 3.3 → The microcirculation of the brain and factors that influence it.

glucose levels can influence the extent of lactic acidosis; higher glucose levels appear to predispose to worse clinical outcomes. The reduction in high-energy substrates that occurs in ischemia influences ionic pump function. Interestingly, the degree of energy depletion does not correlate with the extent of cellular injury, suggesting that other influences on ionic concentration and pump function may promote irreversible cellular damage.

EXCITOTOXIC MEDIATION OF ISCHEMIC INJURY

Another consequence of ischemia is the excessive release of neurotransmitters such as glutamate and aspartate into the extracellular space. Because ischemic cells cannot adequately clear these excitatory transmitters, they are free to bind with receptors, particularly the NMDA receptor. Activation of the NMDA receptors leads to a further intracellular accumulation of Na^+, Ca^{++}, and water that may exceed accumula-

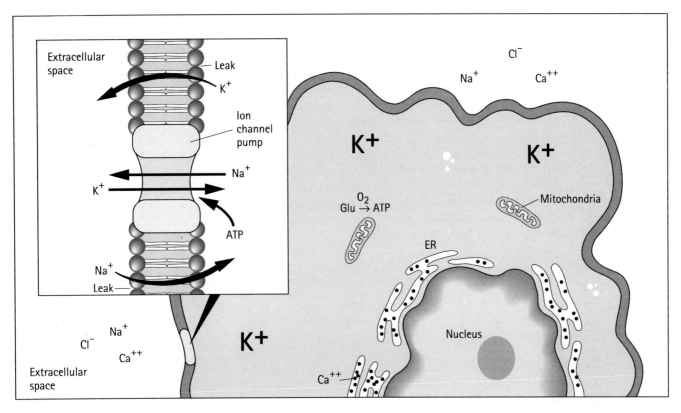

FIGURE 3.4 → Ionic gradients in the nonischemic neuron and an associated ionic pump.

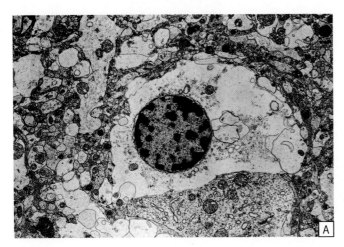

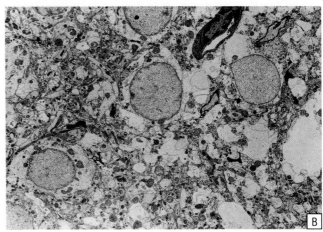

FIGURE 3.5 → **A,** Astroglial swelling indicative of cytotoxic edema demonstrated by electron microscopy, magnified 2000 X. **B,** A higher magnification (4500 X) showing a markedly enlarged, lucent cytoplasm and intact mitochondria. (**A,B:** Courtesy of Drs. J.H. Garcia and Y. Yoshida)

tion related to failure of the ionic pumps. Enhanced intracellular Ca^{++} due to NMDA channel activation by glutamate appears to induce neuronal death (Fig. 3.7), probably because Ca^{++} activates enzymes that can destroy nucleic acids, proteins, and lipids. Membrane phospholipids are particularly vulnerable targets; their destruction liberates arachidonic acid. Metabolizing arachidonic acid leads to the formation of toxic oxygen intermediates (free radicals) as well as eicosanoids and leukotrienes, promoters of platelet aggregation, leukocyte recruitment, and vasoconstriction. Thus, glutamate/aspartate release in ischemic brain regions can lead to a cascade of injurious biochemical events that amplify and promote a greater degree of neuronal injury than ischemia might have induced directly.

The excitotoxic-glutamate hypothesis of ischemic injury amplification suggests an important role for the NMDA channel and its receptors. Although the structure of the NMDA receptor-complex is complicated, understanding it is key to comprehending how the NMDA channel might be inhibited (Fig. 3.8). A glutamate binding site directly activates the NMDA complex to open the Ca^{++}/Na^{+} channel. Two additional receptor sites, the glycine and polyamine sites,

modulate the responses of the glutamate site. Within the channel are divalent cation binding sites, as well as binding sites recognized by dissociative anesthetics such as ketamine and phencyclidine (PCP). At normal resting membrane potentials, the channel is rigidly gated by magnesium ions related to the divalent cation binding site in the channel. Drugs that bind to all of these receptor sites can inhibit NMDA complex activity, potentially interrupting the NMDA-mediated excitotoxic cascade.

PENUMBRA

Numerous experiments have shown that the initial injury produced by focal brain ischemia produces a gradation of injury. The most severely injured areas, which receive little or no blood flow, are irreversibly damaged within minutes. The tissues surrounding the ischemic core have varying degrees of injury, but potentially can be salvaged if flow is restored or cytoprotective drugs are employed. This peri-infarct zone, or ischemia penumbra, has traditionally been defined as the moderately ischemic area where electrical function has been lost, but ionic pumps have not yet failed (Fig. 3.9). Blood flow in the range of 10 to 20 mL/100 g/min can lead to this dichotomy. Recent

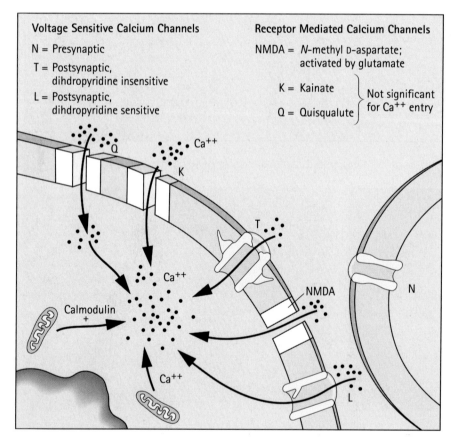

Voltage Sensitive Calcium Channels

N = Presynaptic

T = Postsynaptic, dihdropyridine insensitive

L = Postsynaptic, dihdropyridine sensitive

Receptor Mediated Calcium Channels

NMDA = *N*-methyl D-aspartate; activated by glutamate

K = Kainate

Q = Quisqualate

} Not significant for Ca^{++} entry

FIGURE 3.7 → EFFECTS OF CA^{++} THAT MEDIATE CELL DEATH

Triggering of intracellular proteases and lipases

Activation of phospholipase A$_2$, causing arachidonic acid synthesis

Secondary generation of free radicals and prostaglandins

Mitochondrial proteolysis and uncoupling of oxidative phosphorylation

FIGURE 3.6 → Postsynaptic calcium channels of both the voltage-regulated and receptor-mediated varieties are seen on this diagram.

data suggest that although the penumbra may have ionic disturbances and intracellular water accumulation, injury can still be reversed at least several hours after the onset of ischemia (Fig. 3.10). Defining the penumbra's extent and the amount of time before the injury becomes irreversible can help establish how long after stroke onset treatments will be effective and how much ischemic tissue can be salvaged.

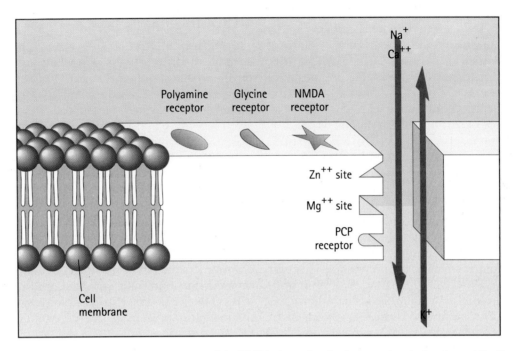

FIGURE 3.8 → Various receptor sites of the NMDA channel and other receptors in the channel itself.

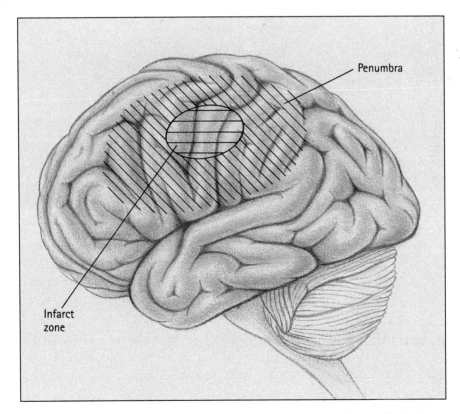

FIGURE 3.9 → An early ischemic stroke demonstrating a central area of infarction and surrounding ischemic penumbra.

BRAIN EDEMA

Brain edema is defined as an accumulation of fluid in the brain parenchyma that increases its volume. Edema related to ischemia can be classified into two types—cytotoxic and vasogenic—based on mechanism. As mentioned, cytotoxic edema begins rapidly after the ischemic insult and is caused by failure of energy metabolism. Cytotoxic edema formation, which has been detected as early as five minutes after ischemia, represents a shift of water from the extracellular space to the intracellular compartment (Fig. 3.11). It does not occur in totally ischemic tissue; it is more prominent in gray matter than white matter. Tissue that develops cytotoxic edema can be salvaged to some extent with early reperfusion or cytoprotective therapy.

Vasogenic brain edema develops hours after ischemia. It is caused by enhanced vascular permeability that allows the entrance of serum proteins and fluid. Elevated blood pressure directly influences vasogenic edema formation by increasing vascular permeability and parenchymal fluid accumulation. Disruption of the normally tight blood-brain barrier is also an important contributor to the development of vasogenic edema. The accumulation of substantial quantities of edema in the peri-infarct zone can further reduce rCBF, leading to secondary extension of irreversible injury (Fig. 3.12).

THROMBOSIS

Thrombosis related to stenotic cerebral arteries or cardiac disorders is an important substrate for the development of ischemic stroke. Platelet-fibrin thrombi develop because both the clotting cascade and blood platelets are activated. Hemostasis can prevent excessive bleeding when vascular injury occurs, but thrombosis represents inappropriate, perhaps excessive, hemostasis. Under normal conditions, blood flow and vessel patency persist because of an intact endothelium as well as the presence of antithrombotic molecules.

The coagulation cascade may be activated in areas of vascular injury, endothelial disruption, disturbances of flow, or abnormalities of the clotting/anticlotting systems. The blood coagulation cascade is divided into extrinsic, intrinsic, and common pathways (Fig. 3.13). The extrinsic pathway is activated by tissue factors present on both endothelial and suben-

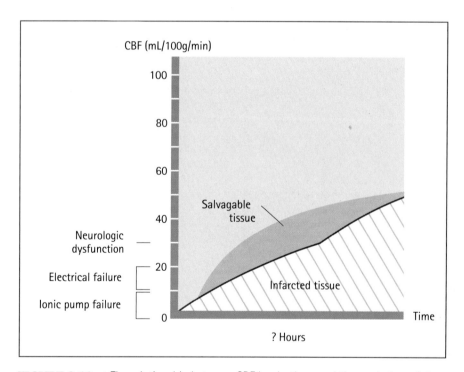

FIGURE 3.10 → The relationship between CBF levels, time, and the evolution of the ischemic penumbra to infarction.

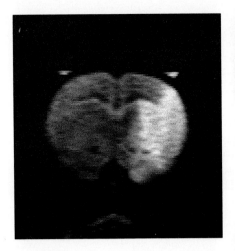

FIGURE 3.11 → A diffusion-weighted MRI study taken 30 minutes after the onset of middle cerebral occlusion in a rat. The hyperintense region represents early intracellular water accumulation (cytotoxic edema).

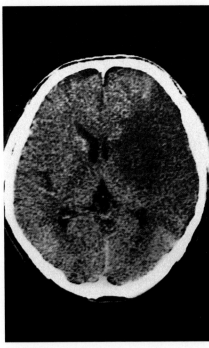

FIGURE 3.12 → A CT scan showing a large left middle cerebral area territory infarction with associated delayed edema (vasogenic edema).

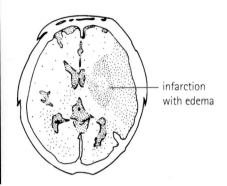

infarction with edema

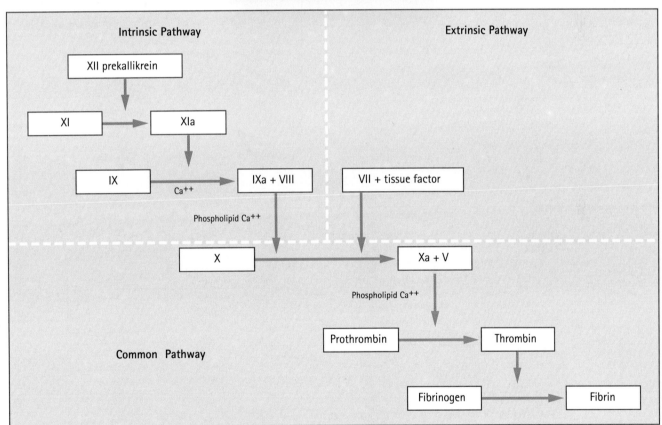

Intrinsic Pathway

Extrinsic Pathway

XII prekallikrein

XI → XIa

IX →(Ca++)→ IXa + VIII   VII + tissue factor

Phospholipid Ca++

Common Pathway

X → Xa + V

Phospholipid Ca++

Prothrombin → Thrombin

Fibrinogen → Fibrin

FIGURE 3.13 → The clotting cascade.

dothelial cells as well as inflammatory cells. The intrinsic system may respond more rapidly to vascular injury than the extrinsic clotting system.

The final step in the coagulation cascade is thrombin-mediated conversion of fibrinogen to fibrin. Platelet activation, which also occurs in response to vascular injury, appears to be mutually interdependent with the coagulation cascade (Fig. 3.14). Platelets adhere primarily at sites of arterial injury, leading to platelet activation and granular release. Inducers of platelet recruitment and further aggregation are also released, which causes the platelet plug to form. This platelet plug is stabilized by fibrin, which develops concurrently.

A variety of anticoagulant and platelet inhibitory mechanisms can reduce and modify the formation of the platelet-fibrin clot (Fig. 3.15). Antithrombin III is a potent inhibitor of thrombin associated with endothelial cells. Heparin amplifies the ability of antithrombin III thrombin neutralization; this interaction probably allows heparin infusions to exert their anticoagulant effects. Protein C is another potent naturally occurring anticoagulant. It is converted to its active form (protein Ca) by interacting with thrombin that is bound to the endothelial cell surface receptor known as the thrombomodulin. Protein Ca, along with its cofactor protein S, destroys several intrinsic coagulation cascade clotting factors

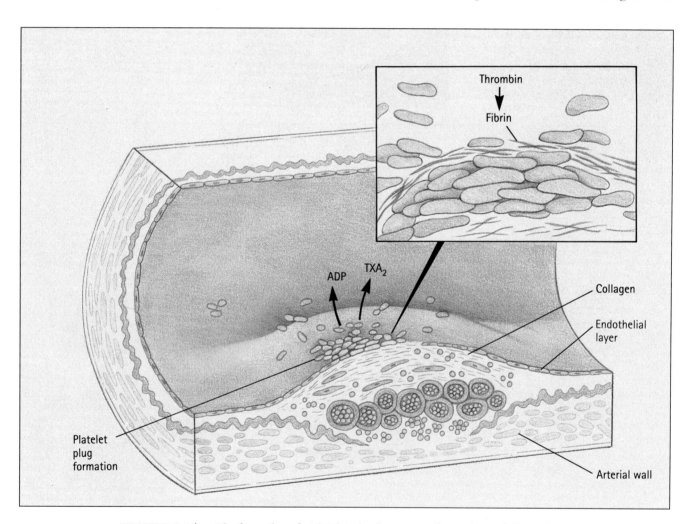

FIGURE 3.14 → The formation of a platelet plug in an area of vascular wall disruption.

(e.g., Va and VIIIa) and may also enhance fibrinolysis. Prostacyclin is a potent platelet antiaggregant and vasodilator produced by endothelial cells from arachidonic acid.

Normal endothelial cell function is obviously an important contributor to inhibiting platelet-fibrin clot formation. Fibrinolysis is the last defense mechanism available to prevent excessive clot formation. Tissue plasminogen activator (TPA) is released by endothelial cells in response to thrombin, converting plasminogen to plasmin. Plasmin digests fibrin and interferes with platelet activation. Tissue plasminogen activator's great affinity for fibrin makes it a relatively clot-specific activator of plasminogen, as compared to streptokinase and urokinase, which are not fibrin-specific (Fig. 3.16). Thus, the formation, inhibition, and digestion of platelet-fibrin clots represent a complex interplay of events with multiple interactions and modifications.

ATHEROSCLEROSIS

The development of atherosclerotic compromise in medium to large diameter cranial arteries and degenerative changes in small vessels are important substrates for the occurrence of ischemic stroke. Understanding how atherogenesis progresses at a cellular level, identifying risk factors that promote atherogen-

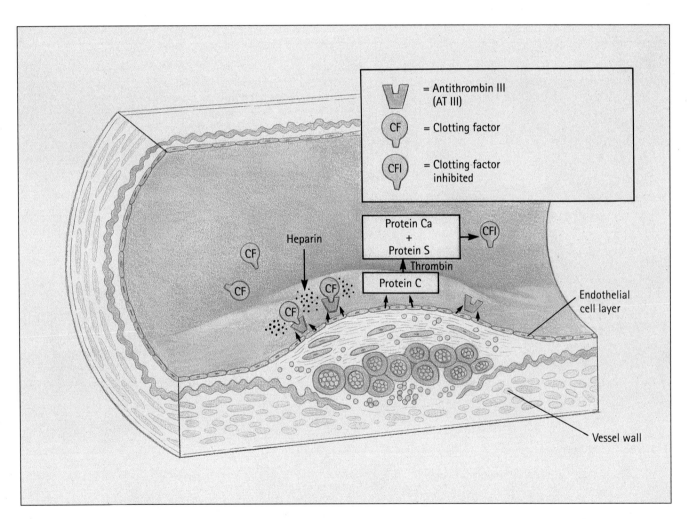

FIGURE 3.15 → The AT-III–heparin interaction speeds clotting factor inactivation; the protein C and S combination destroys clotting factors.

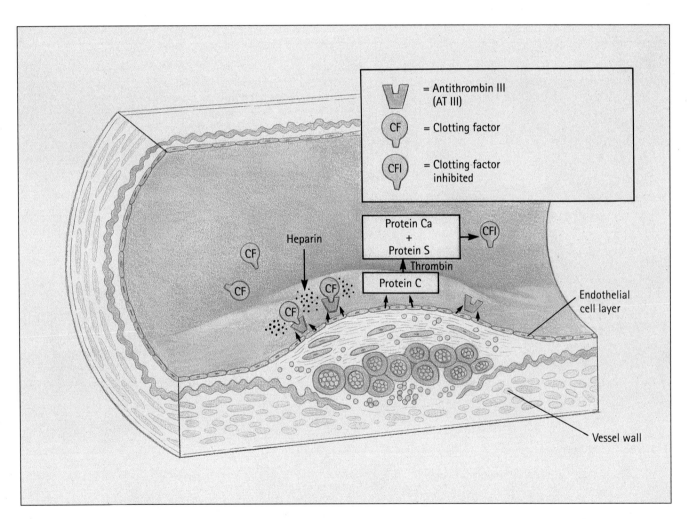

esis and, ultimately, determining how symptoms develop are essential concepts for clinicians interested in stroke. Therapies directed at risk-factor modification, and perhaps even at the cellular events of atherogenesis, can then be developed.

ATHEROSCLEROTIC PLAQUE DEVELOPMENT

Atherosclerosis in the carotid and vertebrobasilar arterial systems is an insidious disease that slowly progresses over decades (Fig. 3.17). Plaques usually develop at the bifurcation of the common carotid artery (CCA) where the internal carotid artery (ICA) originates. In the vertebrobasilar system, plaques are most commonly found at the origin of the vertebral arteries (VAs) and in the basilar artery (BA) at the ori-

gin of branch vessels. Isolated intracranial atherosclerosis in larger vessels often afflicts Asians and blacks, but is rarely observed in whites.

Hemodynamic factors appear to influence where plaques develop and may contribute to their eventual destabilization. At the carotid bifurcation, normal laminar blood flow is disturbed. Along the outer wall of the carotid artery, flow is nonlaminar, causing development of turbulence and eddy currents (Fig. 3.18). These flow disturbances promote an increased contact time between blood elements and toxins with vessel wall constituents. A micro-environment that promotes atherosclerotic plaque growth is created.

Atherosclerotic plaque development appears to be progressive, with well recognized pathologic

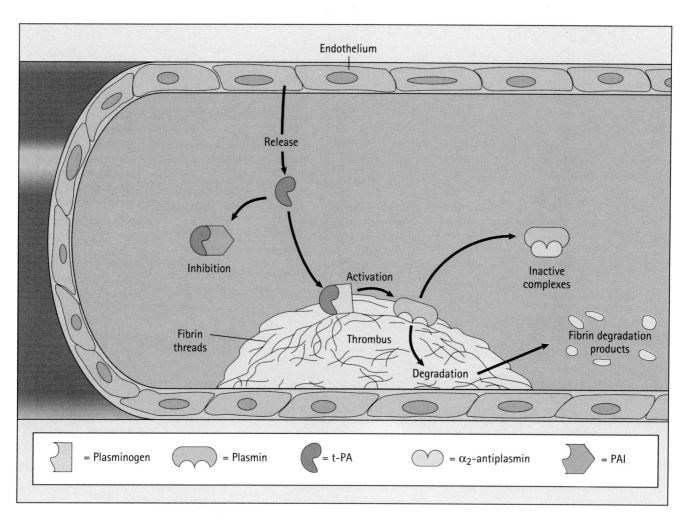

FIGURE 3.16 → Fibrinolysis induced by exogenous and intrinsic mechanisms.

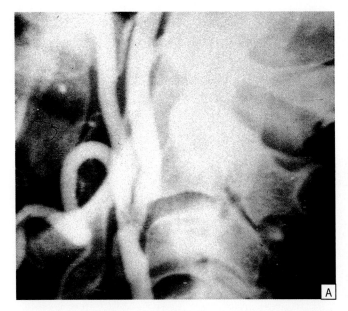

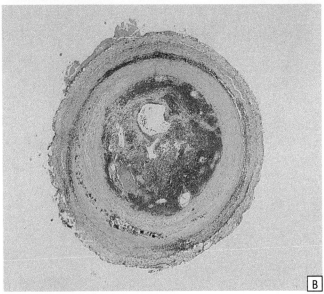

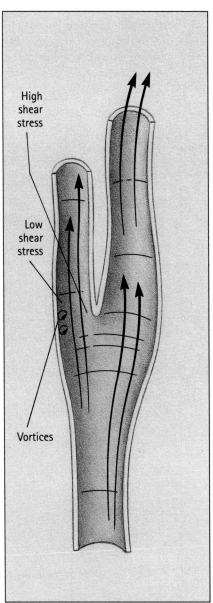

FIGURE 3.17 → **A,** Angiograph demonstrating a carotid artery plaque. **B,** Photomicrograph of extensive basilar artery narrowing by atherosclerosis.

FIGURE 3.18 → Laminar flow is disturbed opposite the carotid artery bifurcation, causing eddy currents and changes in wall shear stress on the outer arterial wall.

High shear stress

Low shear stress

Vortices

lesions that develop in a continuum (Fig. 3.19). The earliest lesion of atherosclerosis is the fatty streak, which may be widely distributed throughout the arterial vasculature. These yellowish areas in the arterial intima begin to develop as early as adolescence and consist primarily of lipid-filled foam cells. Fibrous plaques are more advanced atherosclerotic lesions that develop preferentially at arterial branch points and at the origins of smaller arteries. The fibrous plaque consists of a cap that overlies foam cells,

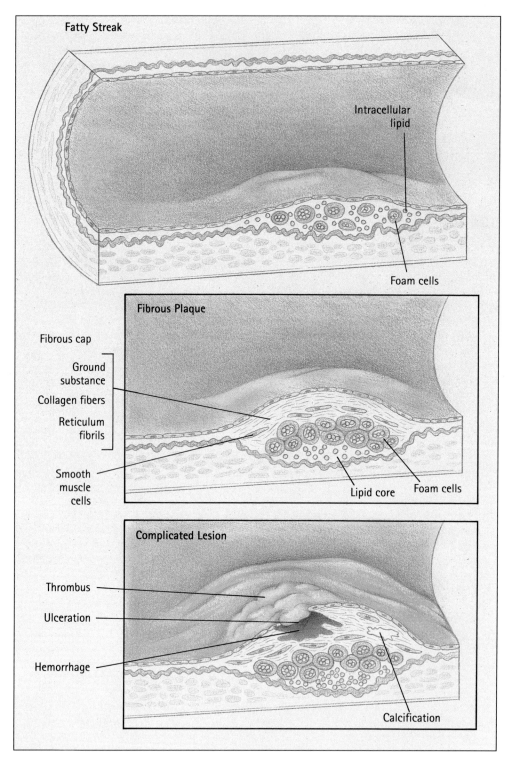

FIGURE 3.19 → Progression of atherosclerosis from the fatty streak to the fibrous plaque. A complicated lesion typically develops over decades. (Adapted from Grundy S, 1990)

macrophages, smooth muscle cells, and lymphocytes, as well as a central necrotic core composed of cellular debris, extracellular lipid, and cholesterol crystals. The most advanced stage of atherosclerosis is the complicated lesion, which is similar to the fibrous plaque, but contains evidence of calcification, hemosiderin deposition, and luminal surface disruption. The evolution of atherosclerotic plaques is a slowly progressive complex interaction of cellular events, intercellular messengers, hemodynamic factors, and vascular risk factors.

The three major cellular contributors to the atherosclerotic process are monocytes/macrophages, endothelial cells, and smooth muscle cells. Circulating monocytes are recruited at a very early stage, enter the arterial wall, and become macrophages. Macrophages imbibe lipid, primarily LDL-cholesterol, to form foam cells, a hallmark of early plaque formation (Fig. 3.20).

The complex relationship between the cellular components of atherosclerosis and intercellular

messengers has been incorporated into the "response to injury" hypothesis of atherogenesis (Fig. 3.21). This proposal by Dr. Russell Ross and colleagues has been supported and updated by widespread observations derived from animal atherosclerotic models as well as human pathologic material. According to this hypothesis, the initiating event for early plaque formation is functional or morphologic endothelial injury, induced by a variety of mechanical, biochemical or physical stimuli. Monocytes/macrophages are then recruited, collecting in the arterial wall. Lipids accumulate, growth factors and cytokines are released, smooth muscle cells and lymphocytes are recruited. As the process continues unimpeded, plaque slowly grows and matures. Platelets may gather at sites of endothelial disruption. As lipid-filled cells die, a central core is formed, leading to plaque remodeling and fibrosis. This complex process is not fully understood, but its slow evolution implies that intervention at a cellular or messenger level is possible.

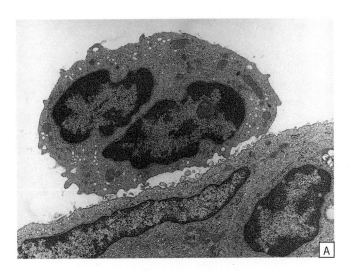 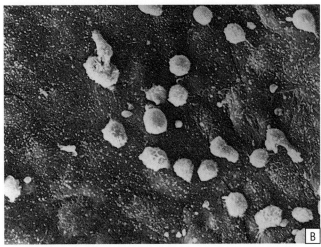

FIGURE 3.20 → **A,** Electron micrograph of a monocyte adhering to an endothelial cell. **B,** At a later point, monocytes and platelets adhere to the vessel wall at points of endothelial lining disruption. (**A,B**: Courtesy of J. Nunnari, Worcester, Massachusetts)

FIGURE 3.21 → FUNCTIONAL ACTIVITIES OF ENDOTHELIAL CELLS

Active and passive transport
Receptor binding: lipoproteins, clotting factors, growth factors
Synthesize many important molecules: connective tissue, enzymes, clotting and anticlotting factors, cytokines, nitric oxide, growth factors
Procoagulant and anticoagulant properties
Interact with circulating blood cells
Affect vascular tone

Macrophages release cytokines and growth factors that promote cellular recruitment and transformation. Oxygen free radicals are also produced by macrophages, which use them to oxidize LDL-cholesterol. Endothelial cells maintain the integrity of the arterial lumen, but are involved in the transport of plasma constituents into the arterial wall, along with many other activities (Fig. 3.22). Endothelial cells actively transport LDL-cholesterol and may modify it to allow for enhanced uptake by macrophages.

Growth factors, particularly platelet-derived growth factor (PDGF), are released by endothelial cells and other cellular plaque constituents. PDGF promotes smooth muscle cell migration from the media to the developing plaque in the subintima. It also induces smooth muscle cell transformation and induction. The transformation of smooth muscle cells from a contractile to a more synthetic state leads to their ability to uptake lipid and contributes to plaque growth (Fig. 3.23). Smooth muscle cells form much of the connec-

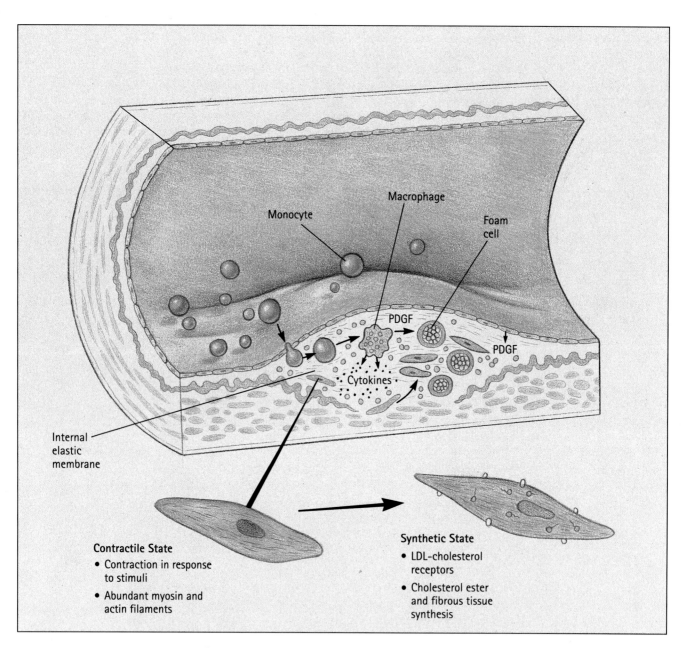

FIGURE 3.22 → Smooth muscle cells migrate into the developing plaque, transforming into a synthetic cell from a primarily contractile state.

tive tissue matrix contained within plaque. They also release PDGF and oxygen free radicals.

T-lymphocytes are observed within developing plaques, but their precise function remains unclear. Platelets do not appear to directly influence early plaque development. They are recruited later, after disruption of the luminal surface. Platelets do release PDGF, which can contribute to plaque growth. Growth factors appear to play an important role in intercellular communication and plaque development. PDGF has been the most widely studied growth factor, but others, such as fibroblast, epidermal, and transforming growth factors, may also contribute to plaque development. Cytokines, including interleukin-1, tumor necrosis factor, leukotriene B_4, and granulocyte-macrophage colony–stimulating factor are released by cellular plaque constituents, possibly contributing to cellular recruitment and activation.

RISK FACTORS

The most important risk factors for atherogenesis are elevated lipoprotein levels, hypertension, cigarette smoking, and diabetes mellitus. Elevated levels of total and LDL-cholesterol have been conclusively established as risk factors for coronary atherosclerosis. Recent studies have established their relationship with carotid atherosclerosis. Because HDL-cholesterol promotes the removal of cholesterol from lipid-laden cells, low HDL levels heighten the risk for atherosclerosis. Lipoprotein-a appears to be an independent risk factor for atherosclerosis.

Hypertension can promote atherogenesis by affecting hemodynamics and promoting endothelial injury. It is a well recognized risk factor for coronary and cerebral arterial atherosclerosis. Another risk factor is cigarette smoking, which can injure endothelial cells and cause thrombogenesis. Diabetes mellitus is associated with many cellular and lipid abnormalities that favor atherosclerotic plaque development.

LIPID-CELLULAR INTERACTIONS

Elevation of total and LDL-cholesterol must interact with the cellular cascade in order to promote plaque development. LDL-cholesterol is imbibed by foam cells, but native unmodified LDL-cholesterol is taken up at a relatively slow rate. Modified LDL-cholesterol

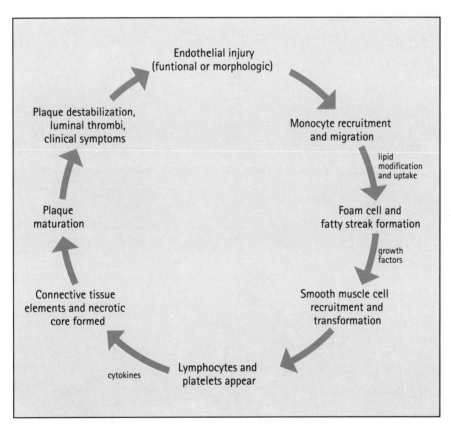

FIGURE 3.23 → The "response to injury" cycle leads to plaque growth. (Adapted from Fisher M, 1991)

is recognized by the so-called scavenger receptor at a much more rapid rate (Fig. 3.24). Oxidation of LDL-cholesterol is apparently the most important mechanism for modification and is promoted by oxygen free radicals, which are believed to be released primarily by monocytes/macrophages, endothelial cells, and smooth muscle cells. Oxidized LDL-cholesterol has been identified in both experimental and human plaques. In addition to rapid uptake by foam cells, oxidized LDL-cholesterol can favorably influence plaque development by several other mechanisms (Fig. 3.25). Oxidized LDL-cholesterol can attract circulating blood monocytes to developing plaques, paradoxically inhibiting their egress once they become vessel-wall macrophages. Oxidized LDL-cholesterol is also cytotoxic. It can therefore induce and maintain endothelial cell injury, an important promoter of atherogenesis. The apparent key contribution of oxidized LDL-cholesterol to atherogenesis suggests that inhibiting LDL oxidation could be a novel method for slowing early plaque development and subsequent maturation. Several naturally occurring and pharma-cologic antioxidants are presently being evaluated as potential antiatherogenic therapies.

DEVELOPMENT OF SYMPTOMS

Atherosclerotic plaques usually enlarge slowly over decades without any symptomatic manifestations. In some cases, the carotid artery can totally occlude but remain asymptomatic. Typically, symptoms develop acutely, suggesting an abrupt change in the characteristics of plaque as well as its relationship to blood elements. In the coronary arteries, myocardial infarction is almost always associated with arterial thrombosis. Coronary artery thrombi are commonly associated with disruption or ulceration of the luminal lining of underlying plaques, exposing blood clotting proteins and platelets to thrombogenic material in the subintima. Blood may secondarily dissect into the arterial wall, generating intraplaque hemorrhages. The primary event, however, is destabilization of the endothelial layer. In the carotid and intracranial arteries, the cause of symptom development is less clear because pathologic studies are more limited. Luminal

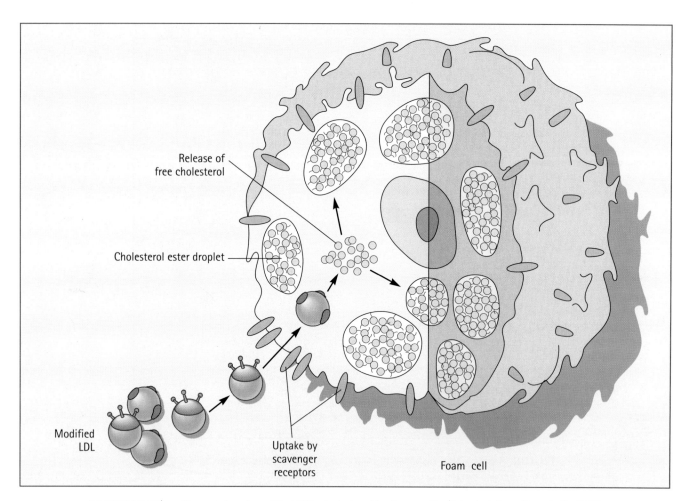

FIGURE 3.24 → The uptake of modified LDL-cholesterol by foam cells. (Adapted from Grundy S, 1990)

surface disruption is probably the primary event in most cases, and leads to local thrombus formation (Fig. 3.26). These thrombi may then embolize more distally to cause a particular stroke syndrome related to the occluded vascular territory. Alternatively, the compromised vessel could cause ischemia to develop distally because of hemodynamic compromise. Primary intraplaque hemorrhage may cause symptom development related to acute plaque expansion and rupture of blood from the plaque into the lumen. It is

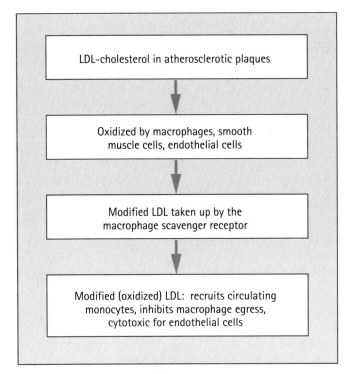

FIGURE 3.25 → Oxidized LDL-cholesterol promotes plaque development by several mechanisms.

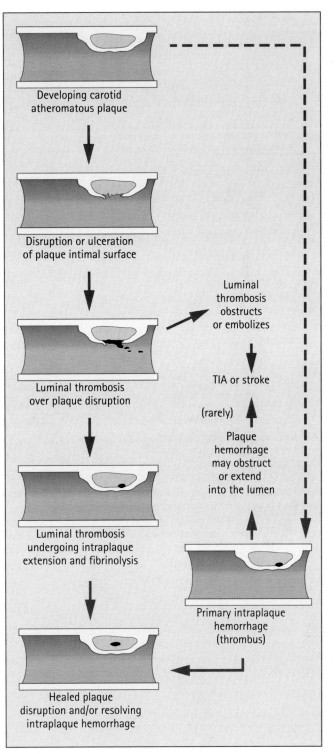

FIGURE 3.26 → Artery-to-artery embolization or hemodynamic compromise in plaque destabilization leads to stroke or transient ischemic attack (TIA) symptoms.

unlikely that primary plaque hemorrhage often causes ischemic cerebral vascular symptoms.

SMALL-VESSEL ARTERIOPATHY

The arteriopathy associated with small-vessel lacunar strokes has not been widely studied, but it appears to differ from large-artery atherosclerosis (Fig. 3.27). The small penetrating arteries involved in lacunar infarcts are much less muscular than larger arteries. Originally lipohyalinosis, an intermediate stage between fibrinoid necrosis and microatheromata, was described in small arteries associated with lacunar infarctions. Subsequently, microatheromata that consisted of lipid-laden macrophages were observed. Sclerosis and fibrohyaline changes have also been observed in small penetrating arteries. Features associated with fibrohyaline degeneration include proliferation of collagen fibers, appearance of cellular debris, and deposition of amorphous material in the subadventitia. It is uncertain how long these changes take to develop. Also unclear is whether the cellular participants notably differ from those associated with large-artery atherogenesis. Small-vessel arteriopathy is commonly linked with hypertension and diabetes mellitus. Acute symptoms are assumed to develop because of plaque destabilization and luminal thrombus formation, but there is no conclusive proof. Beyond risk factor modification, uncertainty also remains about therapeutic approaches to this condition.

THERAPY FOR ATHEROSCLEROSIS

Risk factor modification has been the traditional therapy for preventing atherosclerotic progression. Lowering elevated total and LDL-cholesterol levels, either by dietary modification or pharmacologic intervention, reduces the risk for ischemic vascular symptoms and continuing atherosclerotic plaque development, possibly promoting regression (Fig. 3.28). The cessation of smoking and the lowering of elevated blood pressure reduce the risk for clinical symptom occurrence, but it is uncertain whether these interventions affect the atherosclerotic process.

FIGURE 3.27 → Small-vessel arteriopathy with a microaneurysm.

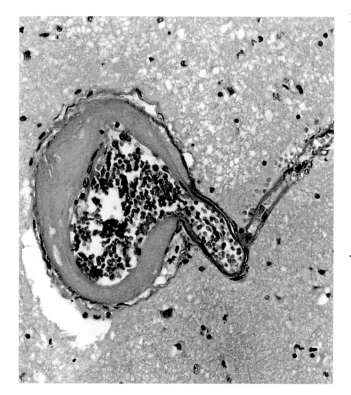

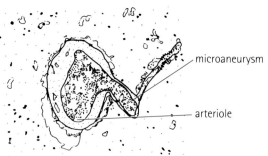

microaneurysm

arteriole

FIGURE 3.28A → INDICATIONS FOR LIPID-LOWERING DRUG THERAPY

SEVERE HYPERLIPIDEMIA

MODERATE HYPERCHOLESTEROLEMIA
In patients at high risk for CHD from other causes
In patients unresponsive to dietary therapy

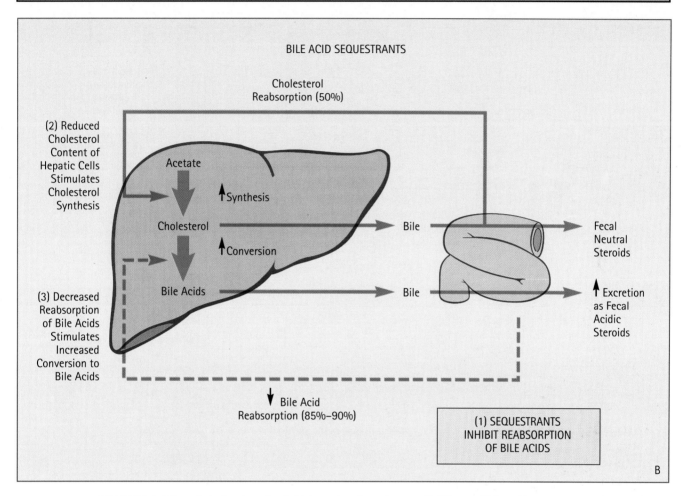

BILE ACID SEQUESTRANTS

Cholesterol
Reabsorption (50%)

(2) Reduced
Cholesterol
Content of
Hepatic Cells
Stimulates
Cholesterol
Synthesis

Acetate

↑Synthesis

Cholesterol

↑Conversion

Bile Acids

(3) Decreased
Reabsorption
of Bile Acids
Stimulates
Increased
Conversion to
Bile Acids

Bile

Bile

Fecal
Neutral
Steroids

↑ Excretion
as Fecal
Acidic
Steroids

↓ Bile Acid
Reabsorption (85%–90%)

(1) SEQUESTRANTS
INHIBIT REABSORPTION
OF BILE ACIDS

B

FIGURE 3.28 → **A,** Indications for lipid-lowering drug therapy. **B,** Effects of bile acid sequestrants on bile-acid and cholesterol metabolism. (Figure 3.28 is continued on page 3.22)

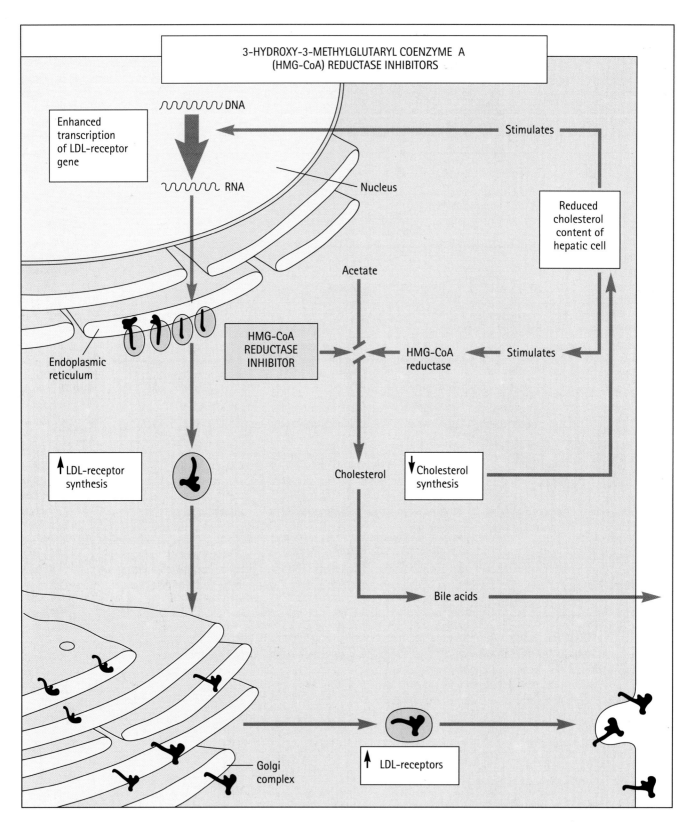

FIGURE 3.28 → C, Effects of HMG-CoA reductase inhibitors on the synthesis of cholesterol and LDL receptors. (Adapted from Grundy S, 1990.)

A variety of novel therapies directed primarily at the cellular events associated with atherogenesis are being explored (Fig. 3.29). As mentioned, antioxidants are being evaluated in experimental atherosclerotic models and humans because inhibiting the oxidation of LDL-cholesterol might retard early plaque development. The preliminary results in animals have been promising. The results in humans are eagerly awaited. Diets containing substantial amounts of marine fish oils, rich in n-3 fatty acids, are associated with a reduced incidence of ischemic coronary artery disease and, perhaps, ischemic stroke. In animal atherosclerotic models, n-3 fatty acids retard the development of coronary and carotid atherosclerosis without substantially lowering lipid levels. These fatty acids have many salutatory effects at cellular and cytokine levels, which may explain how they could inhibit atherogenesis. Current trials are attempting to inhibit restenosis with n-3 fatty acids in patients who have undergone coronary angioplasty. Voltage-sensitive calcium channel antagonists have also been extensively studied in animal atherosclerotic models, with predominantly positive results. One large human trial observed that formation of new coronary plaques was inhibited by a calcium channel antagonist, but progression in preexistent lesions was unaffected.

If a safe, effective inhibitor of atherogenesis can be developed, the incidence of clinically related symptoms such as ischemic stroke and myocardial infarction should be reduced. Evaluating the effects of pharmacologic interventions directed at inhibiting atherogenesis can probably be performed more easily in carotid arteries than in coronary arteries. The carotid arteries can be evaluated by noninvasive testing to document the extent of stenosis prior to treatment, then serially reevaluated at regular intervals to assess the effect of therapy on plaque progression. Such studies are eagerly anticipated.

FIGURE 3.29 → POTENTIAL MEDICAL THERAPY FOR ATHEROSCLEROSIS

Antioxidants	Monoclonal antibodies
Calcium channel blockers	Heparin derivatives
n-3 Fatty acids	

REFERENCES

Auer RN, Siesjö BK. Biological differences between ischemia, hypoglycemia and epilepsy. *Ann Neurol.* 1988; 24:699–707.

Choi DW. Methods for antagonizing glutamate neurotoxicity. *Cerebrovasc Brain Metab Rev.* 1990; 2:105–147.

Esmon CT. The regulation of natural anticoagulant pathways. *Science.* 1987; 235:1348–1351.

Fisher M. Atherosclerosis: cellular aspects and potential interventions. *Cerebrovasc Brain Metab Rev.* 1991; 3:114–133.

Fisher CM. Capsular infarcts: the underlying vascular lesions. *Arch Neurol.* 1979; 36:65–73.

Grundy S. *Cholesterol and Atherosclerosis.* New York: Gower Medical Publishing. 1990.

High KA. Antithrombin III, protein C, and protein S. *Arch Pathol Lab Med.* 1988; 112:28–36.

Klatzo I. Pathophysiological aspects of brain edema. *Acta Neuropathol.* 1987; 72:236–239.

Masuda J, Ross R. Atherogenesis during low level hypercholesterolemia in the non-human primate. *Atherosclerosis.* 1990; 10:178–187.

Proctor AW. Can we reverse ischemic penumbra? Some mechanisms in the pathophysiology of energy-compromised brain tissue. *Clin Neuropharm.* 1990; 13(Suppl 3):534–549.

Raichle MD. The pathophysiology of brain ischemia. *Ann Neurol.* 1983; 13:2–10.

Ross R. Platelet-derived growth factor. *Lancet.* 1989; 1:1179–1182.

Schafer AI. The hypercoagulable state. *Ann Intern Med.* 1985; 102:813–828.

Steinberg D, Parthasarathy S, Caren TE, Khoo JC, Witzum JL. Beyond cholesterol: modification of low density lipoprotein that increases its atherogenecity. *N Engl J Med.* 1989; 320:915–924.

Superko HR. Drug therapy and the prevention of atherosclerosis in humans. *Am J Cardiol.* 1989; 64:31G–38G.

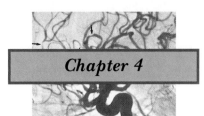

Chapter 4

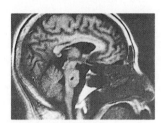

J.W. NORRIS

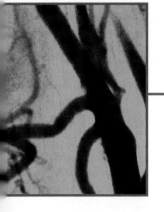

Transient Ischemic Attacks and Predictors of Stroke

TRANSIENT ISCHEMIC ATTACKS (TIAS) are abrupt, rapidly fading episodes of neurologic deficits of vascular origin. Defined as lasting less than 24 hours, their usual duration is less than 2 to 3 hours, and often only 5 to 10 minutes. TIAs of the retina, termed amaurosis fugax or transient monocular blindness, may last as little as 10 seconds. Since elderly, forgetful patients often have difficulty remembering or describing their symptoms, the observation of 10 seconds of total monocular blindness by an intelligent observer can be considerably more accurate than a confused patient's recollection of the event.

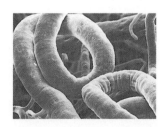

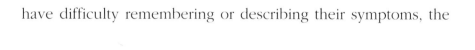

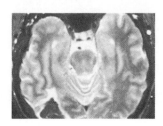

CLINICAL DIAGNOSIS

The symptom complex of TIAs is broad, and depends on whether the episodes take place in the carotid or vertebrobasilar territories. Frequently encountered carotid TIAs are transient monocular blindness, and paresis or paresthesia of a limb; commonly observed vertebrobasilar symptoms are diplopia, dysarthria, or vertigo, although rarely in isolation. Part of the problem of predicting outcome in these patients is incorrect diagnosis. TIAs do not produce unconsciousness or seizures, and are almost never the cause of acute confusional states or vertigo alone. Early published outcome data are undoubtedly contaminated by the inclusion of wrong diagnoses.

One of the most common misdiagnoses is post-ictal monoparesis (Todd's paralysis), especially when the focal seizure is due to a previous stroke (Fig. 4.1). A less common error is hypoglycemia following an insulin reaction in diabetics, which exactly mimics the temporal profile of a TIA. In less than 1% of cases, occult brain tumors may produce transient neurologic symptoms that are indistinguishable from a TIA.

In prospectively gathered data on asymptomatic populations, the most common TIA is transient monocular blindness, yet on retrospective questioning of patients following ischemic carotid strokes, this symptom is found in only a very small percentage. Fleeting monocular blindness is easily dismissed or forgotten by both patient and physician, or treated with oral antiplatelet therapy without further investigation.

Solitary transient symptoms in the vertebrobasilar system also make diagnosis difficult. Solitary vertigo or diplopia, which has a variety of benign causes, may occur in normal people. Neither can constitute a diagnosis of TIA by itself. There is usually no satisfactory laboratory test to prove or disprove the suspicion of TIA.

PATHOGENESIS

The outcome of TIAs, like that of stroke, relates closely to pathogenesis. Earlier observations of populations documenting stroke and death rate assumed that patients with TIAs have similar outcomes. Sophisticated data derived from medical and surgical trials have since indicated that outcomes vary depending on the cause and the patient's age. The outlook for a middle-aged man with a TIA secondary to hypotension due to acute myocardial infarction, for example, is different than an elderly woman experiencing TIAs from overzealous administration of antihypertensive drugs.

The two usual sources of transient cerebral ischemia are cerebral emboli from plaques in the extracranial arterial tree (carotid and vertebrobasilar), and cardiogenic embolism. Less often, hemodynamic factors produce transient ischemia in a cerebral arterial territory where there is already stenosis from atherosclerosis. For instance, transient hypotension may follow cardiac arrhythmias or hypotensive drugs, causing transient focal neurologic symptoms.

The behavior of carotid plaques may even differ between patients. Plaques are not static accretions of lipids in the cell wall that slowly enlarge, but are in a dynamic state, fluctuating in association with factors such as luminal blood flow and intraplaque hemorrhage (Fig. 4.2). In the same patient, one plaque may slowly stenose over years, while the other rapidly evolves to occlusion within months, possibly causing a stroke.

Data from studies of conservative treatment versus surgical intervention for symptomatic carotid stenosis illustrate this point. The North American Symptomatic Carotid Endarterectomy Trial (*NASCET*) found a striking difference between surgically treated and medically treated patients (Fig. 4.3). In the conservative group, the stroke rate over 18 months was

---

FIGURE 4.1 → UNDERLYING LESION IN 108 CASES MISDIAGNOSED AS "STROKE"

PRIMARY DIAGNOSIS	SEIZURE GROUP	NONSEIZURE GROUP	TOTAL
Previous stroke	13	12	25
Senile dementia	7	4	11
Cerebral tumor	3	6	9
Alcohol or drug effect	4	7	11
Psychoneurosis	0	8	8
Subdural hematoma	0	3	3
Miscellaneous	15	26	41
TOTAL	42	66	108

Adapted from Norris JW, Hachinski VC, 1982.

25%, or 16% per year. Because these patients were all treated with aspirin, the untreated rate would be even higher, at least 20% per year. This is four times greater than most published rates from epidemiologic studies, indicating that the subgroup of TIAs associated with severe carotid stenosis has a substantially more serious prognosis than other groups.

Cardioembolic sources of TIAs and strokes have gained attention in recent years, partly due to observations derived from stroke data banks and

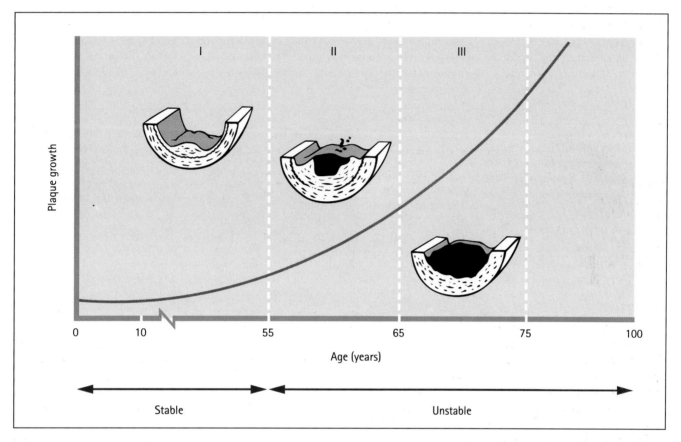

FIGURE 4.2 → Evolution of carotid plaque from a stable to an unstable condition. (Adapted from Bornstein NM, Norris JW, 1989)

FIGURE 4.3 → NORTH AMERICAN SYMPTOMATIC CAROTID ENDARTERECTOMY TRIAL IPSILATERAL STROKE RATE AT 18 MONTHS

% STENOSIS (# OF PATIENTS)	MEDICAL (N=295)	SURGICAL (N=300)	ABSOLUTE DIFFERENCE
90–99% (134)	33%	6%	27%
80–89% (214)	28%	8%	20%
70–79% (247)	19%	7%	12%
Total	25%	7%	18%

stroke units, and partly as a result of clinical trials (see Chapter 7). Although rheumatic valvular heart disease is a disappearing entity, mitral valve prolapse, prosthetic heart valves, and ischemic cardiac disease are common sources of cardioembolism (Fig. 4.4). Evidence from anticoagulant trials in patients with atrial fibrillation (AF) indicates at least a 5% stroke rate per year (Fig. 4.5).

The recurrence rate of TIAs and strokes also depends on the original etiology. Stroke data bank observations indicate a much lower rate of recurrence for lacunar infarctions than for cardioembolism (Fig. 4.6). The differing outcome data depend on laboratory facilities that were unavailable two decades ago, in particular, neurovascular scanning and cardiac imaging. Computed tomography (CT) scans may show small infarctions in as many as 50% of TIA patients, and in 20% of patients with asymptomatic carotid stenosis, thus affecting both the recurrence rate and type of future strokes (Fig. 4.7). The distinction of TIAs from strokes on duration alone is artificial. In reality, there is a continuous spectrum of

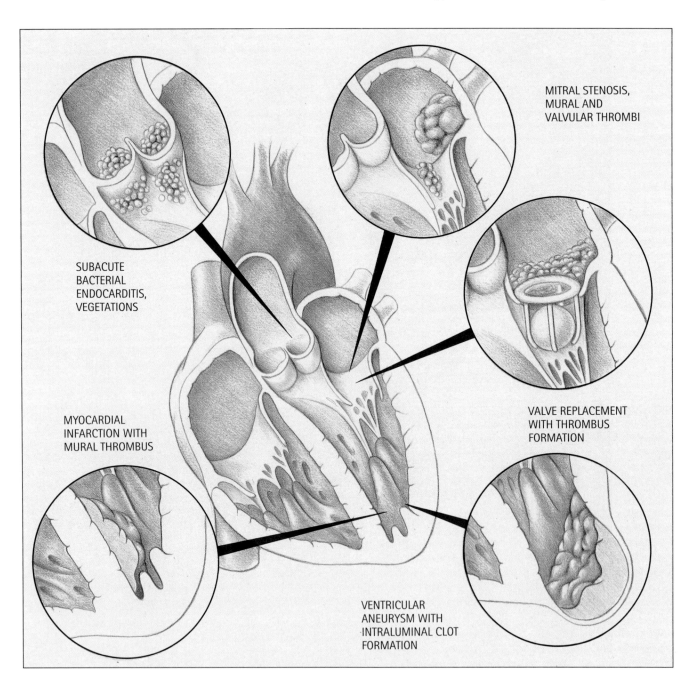

MITRAL STENOSIS, MURAL AND VALVULAR THROMBI

SUBACUTE BACTERIAL ENDOCARDITIS, VEGETATIONS

VALVE REPLACEMENT WITH THROMBUS FORMATION

MYOCARDIAL INFARCTION WITH MURAL THROMBUS

VENTRICULAR ANEURYSM WITH INTRALUMINAL CLOT FORMATION

FIGURE 4.4 → Cardiac sources of cerebral emboli.

increasingly severe neurologic deficits as well as positive laboratory findings. Magnetic resonance (MR) scanning, an extremely sensitive technique that detects tiny ischemic cerebral lesions, may bring even more accuracy in predicting outcome (Fig. 4.8).

RISK FACTORS IN TIAS AND STROKE

Risk factors for symptomatic atherosclerosis anywhere in the body are similar, but not identical, for different target sites. Hypertension is a major risk for TIAs and stroke, but a minor factor in ischemic cardiac disease, while cholesterol is just the opposite (Fig. 4.9). Smoking is a major risk factor for peripheral vascular disease, but is a minor factor for stroke. Although the role of cigarette smoking was once uncertain, there is now overwhelming evidence that it increases the risk of TIAs and stroke two to three times (Fig. 4.10).

The major factors in cerebrovascular disease are genetic, depending on race and family history. In Japan, stroke is the major cause of death, while it

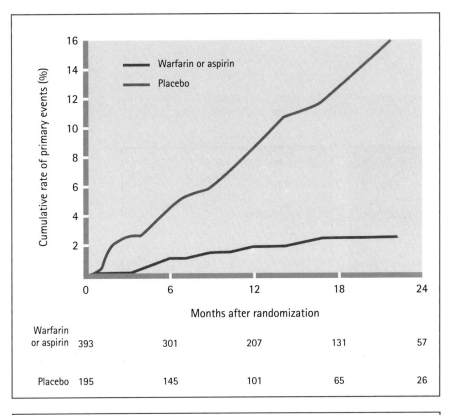

FIGURE 4.5 → Rates of stroke or systemic embolism (primary events) in patients with atrial fibrillation who were given active therapy (warfarin or aspirin) or placebo in Group 1. (Adapted from SPAF Report, 1990)

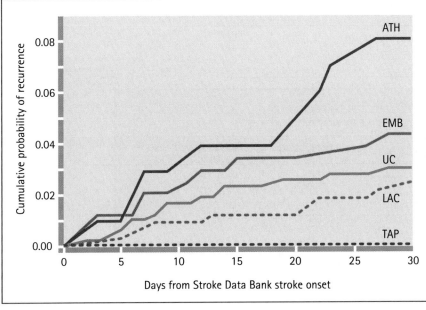

FIGURE 4.6 → Cumulative probability of stroke recurrence in the first month for patients with atherothrombotic stroke (ATH), embolic stroke (EMB), unknown cause (UC), lacunar stroke (LAC), or tandem arterial pathology (TAP). (Adapted from Sacco RL, et al. 1989)

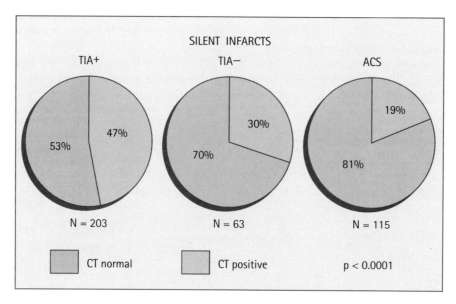

FIGURE 4.7 → Percentage of small infarcts found on CT in patients with transient ischemic attacks (TIAs) and carotid stenosis (TIA +), TIAs without carotid stenosis (TIA -), and asymptomatic carotid stenosis (ACS).

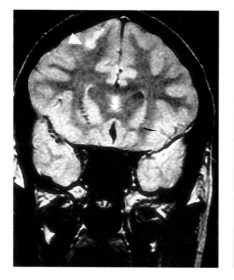

FIGURE 4.8 → Small lesion that was found in the right cerebral hemisphere (arrow) of a patient with a 10 minute TIA consisting of numbness in the left leg.

FIGURE 4.9 → RISK FACTORS FOR ATHEROSCLEROSIS*

1. Age and sex
2. Hypertension
3. Cardiac disease
4. TIAs
5. Blood lipids, diabetes, smoking, obesity
6. Neck bruits
7. Oral contraceptives

*In order of importance.

FIGURE 4.10 → SMOKING AND STROKE RISK		
No. CIGARETTES	RELATIVE RISK OF STROKE (%)	
SMOKED/D	MEN	WOMEN
10	1.17	1.19
20	1.38	1.40
30	1.62	1.67
40	1.90	1.97

ranks only third in the Western world. Male sex and increasing age are also important risk factors. The annual stroke incidence for females under age 35 is about 10 per 100,000, while for elderly males it approaches 600 to 700 per 100,000 (Figs. 4.11, 4.12).

Hypertension is a major contributor to many forms of acute and chronic cerebrovascular disease. It helps to account for plaque formation at arterial bifurcations (such as the carotids), for cerebral microaneurysms (a major cause of cerebral hemorrhage), and for many lacunar infarctions. Community screening programs have made possible the widespread

FIGURE 4.11 → INCIDENCE OF ATHEROTHROMBOSIS AND STROKE*

AGE**	ATHEROTHROMBOTIC BRAIN INFARCTION			STROKE—ALL TYPES		
	MEN	WOMEN	M/F RATIO	MEN	WOMEN	M/F RATIO
45–54	10	7	1.4	20	11	1.8
55–64	23	16	1.4	41	27	1.5
65–74	55	48	1.1	90	83	1.1
75–84	139	94	1.5	176	127	1.4

*Annual average per 10,000 **Age at biennal exam
Adapted from Wolf PA, et al. 1983.

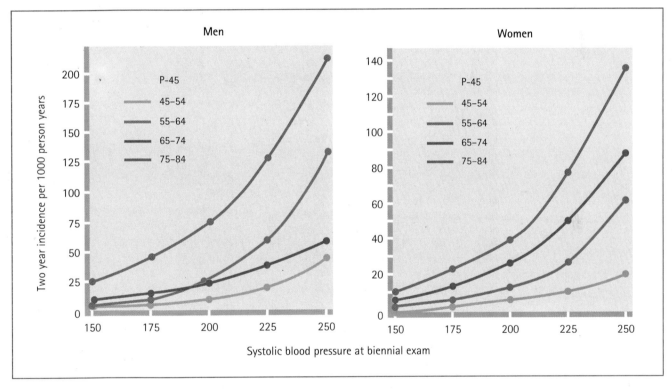

FIGURE 4.12 → Incidence of atherothrombotic brain infarction, according to systolic blood pressure and age, in a 24-year follow-up to the Framingham Study.

FIGURE 4.13 → ANNUAL PERCENTAGE OF VASCULAR EVENTS

DEGREE OF STENOSIS	TIA	STROKE	CARDIAC	VASCULAR DEATH
50% (mild)	1.0	1.3	2.7	1.8
50–70% (moderate)	3.0	1.3	6.6	3.3
75% (severe)	7.2	3.3	8.3	6.5

Adapted from Norris JW, et. al. 1991.

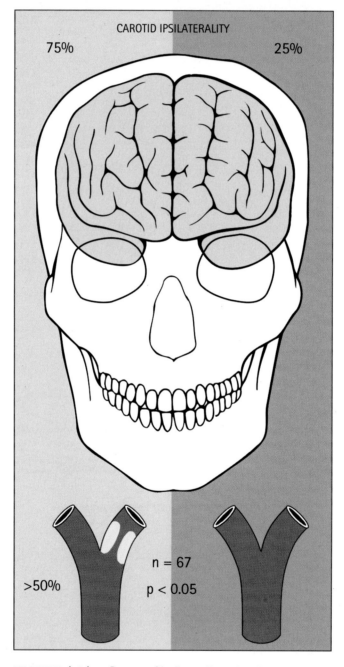

FIGURE 4.14 → Degree of ipsilaterality related to underlying carotid stenosis > 50% (by Duplex).

effective treatment of hypertension at earlier ages, thereby changing the outlook for patients who otherwise would have died prematurely from devastating brain hemorrhage or cerebral infarction.

The contraceptive pill has been implicated for decades as a major cause of stroke in young women, but the evidence is at best circumstantial. Most of the data, still quoted, were gathered 20 years ago when the estrogen content of the pill was much higher, the epidemiologic methodology poorer, and the diagnosis of stroke often made on flimsy evidence. Findings from the Royal College of General Practitioners in England (1968) are often quoted, but data from methodologic studies in stroke units indicate that diagnostic accuracy correlates highly with neurologic expertise, which was even more limited in the days before CT scanning.

TIA AND STROKE RISK IN ASYMPTOMATIC CAROTID STENOSIS

Asymptomatic patients with neck bruits that were discovered on routine medical examination have a greater incidence of cerebro- and cardiovascular disease (Fig. 4.13). Although neck bruits were originally thought to be simply markers of diffuse atherosclerosis, with the advent of noninvasive carotid imaging it

became clear that cerebral ischemic events were more likely to occur on the side of the carotid stenosis, if not on the side of the neck bruit (Fig. 4.14).

Neck bruits are poor localizers for the arterial lesion's site. Ipsilateral, severe carotid bifurcation stenosis may be "silent," while the diversion of blood up the contralateral carotid may produce turbulence as well as a bruit.

The incidence of TIA and stroke in patients with asymptomatic carotid disease depends on the severity of stenosis, but is variously estimated at 1% to 5% per year. The outcome of cardiac ischemic events relates similarly to the severity of the carotid lesion; the cardiac death rate is at least fourfold the stroke mortality (Fig. 4.15). This is an unfortunate correlation, since the patients who are most likely to benefit from carotid endarterectomy are also those most at risk of myocardial infarction, which can be caused by the stress of surgery.

LABORATORY DIAGNOSIS

BRAIN IMAGING
The advent of CT scans revealed that patients with TIAs often had structural cerebral lesions even though they had no clinical signs. Small infarcts or even brainstem hemorrhages produce transient symptoms

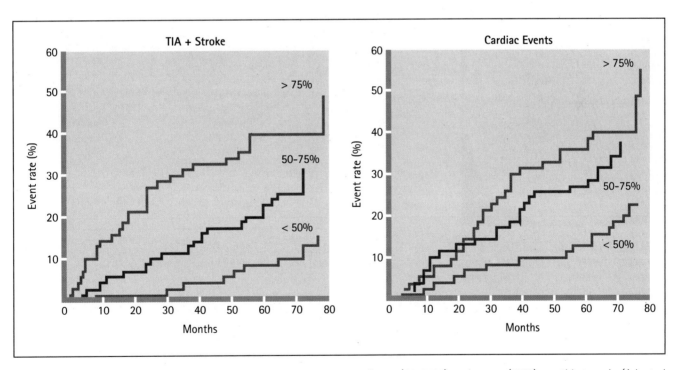

FIGURE 4.15→ Cumulative event rates of TIAs and strokes, as well as cardiac ischemic events, in patients with mild (50%),

moderate (50–75%), and severe (75%) carotid stenosis. (Adapted from Norris JW, et al. 1991)

and signs, while sometimes large lesions that displace brain (e.g., subdural hematoma or brain tumors) manifest with minimal clinical features (Fig. 4.16). Some transient "ischemic" attacks, therefore, are not really ischemic—a finding that clearly has major impli-cations for management.

MRI has added even more information about cerebral structural lesions in patients with TIAs. A temporary abnormality is often seen in patients with TIAs that last only a few days (see Fig. 4.8).

Single photon emission computerized tomography (SPECT) adds another dimension. SPECT imaging is a color-coded perfusion map of the brain superimposed on a CT template. A temporary perfusion deficit, which disappears in a few days, may appear on the scan.

VASCULAR IMAGING

Carotid Doppler (Duplex) imaging is a noninvasive, quick, inexpensive method of verifying an underlying carotid artery stenosis, the probable cause of the TIA due to artery-to-artery embolism. It should be per-formed in all patients early in the clinical evaluation, both to confirm the source of the TIA and to determine surgical or medical treatment. If a neck bruit is present, the TIA is more likely due to carotid stenosis; if absent, carotid disease is only a 1 in 5 probable cause (Fig. 4.17).

If Duplex imaging shows normal carotids, the TIA is more likely to be of cardioembolic origin. However, the "gold standard" of vascular imaging is cerebral angiography, which is performed if there is doubt, or if ultrasound indicates a surgically accessible carotid stenosis over 70%. Angiography confirms the presence and allows measurement of the stenosis (Fig. 4.18). It demonstrates whether carotid ulceration is present. It can also indicate whether intracranial "tandem" lesions negate prophylactic surgery of the extracranial carotid artery.

The hazards of cerebral angiography have been considerably reduced in recent years, with safer contrast agents and without direct carotid puncture. Computerized digital subtraction angiography (DSA) also avoids catheterization of individual vessels, such

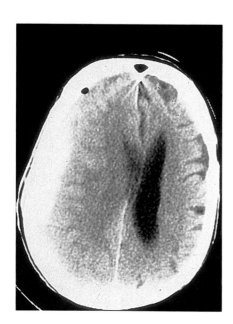

FIGURE 4.16→ Large right subdural hematoma displaces the brain, flattening the ipsilateral ventricle. This patient had only transient, though recurrent, left-sided symptoms.

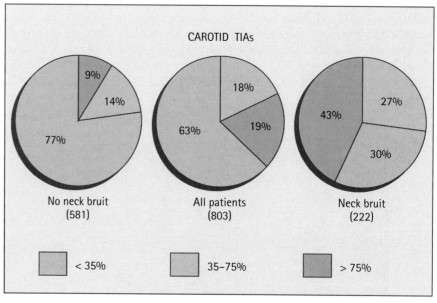

FIGURE 4.17→ The relationship of underlying carotid stenosis and neck bruits in 803 patients with TIAs.

as the carotids. The present techniques (e.g., inserting the catheter in the femoral artery, producing images of the vessels by computerized subtraction techniques) involve a 0.01% to 0.03% risk of stroke or death.

MR angiography is a promising, noninvasive technique with minimal hazards. As yet, images satisfactory enough to imbue confidence in surgical endarterectomy have not been consistently produced. "Standard" angiography using injection of contrast material remains the only gold standard (see Chapter 14).

CARDIAC INVESTIGATIONS

Cardiac investigations should be performed in patients with negative carotid Doppler or angiography, or if there is clinical uncertainty about the pathogenesis. Recent drug trial results indicate that AF, irrespective of its duration, is an important cause of systemic embolism. Age–sex-matched populations with AF have a stroke risk six times that of their controls.

Routine electrocardiograms (ECGs) to evaluate silent myocardial infarctions causing cardioem-

bolic TIAs, Holter monitoring to detect cardiac arrhythmias, and transthoracic echocardiography (TTE), may all be needed to find the source of cerebral emboli.

Transesophageal echocardiography (TEE) better defines the cardiac chambers and valves. Unfor-tunately, it is necessary to swallow an echo probe about the size of a finger. The probe slides down the esophagus to rest just behind the left atrium. It may reveal thrombi in the atrium that were missed on TTE.

OTHER TESTS

Lumbar puncture and radioisotope scanning are obsolete when modern imaging techniques are available. Skull x-rays play no diagnostic role; electroencephalography (EEG) is of limited value. The erythrocyte sedimentation rate may be raised in rare cases of vasculitis. Occasionally, hematologic causes of TIA include polycythemia (increased blood viscosity), sickle-cell disease, as well as protein C and protein S deficiencies. Thrombotic and thrombocytopenic pur-

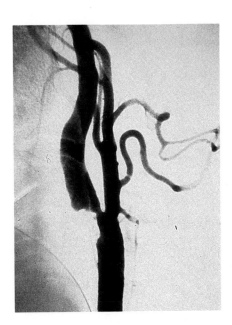

FIGURE 4.18→ This carotid angiogram shows large, severely stenosing irregular plaque at the origin of the internal carotid artery (ICA).

pura may also occasionally present with TIA or stroke due to intraarterial thrombosis. These are all rare causes and such hematologic tests should be left until more common causes of TIAs have been excluded.

MANAGING TIAS

There is no place for "catch-all" remedies, such as aspirin given without further evaluation. Omitting the small battery of tests that in most cases will reveal the cause of TIAs, providing a rational basis for therapy, is inexcusable. In patients with ipsilateral carotid artery stenosis over 70%, carotid endarterectomy is now the optimal treatment if they are fit enough and agreeable to surgery, as recent results from NASCET and the European Carotid Surgery Trial have demonstrated (see Fig. 4.3). Patients with stenoses less than 35% are, in most cases, inappropriate surgical candidates. Those with 35% to 70% stenoses are still under trial.

If no underlying carotid disease is demonstrated, a cardiac source should be sought. In most cases, cardioembolic TIAs are treated lifelong with anticoagulants such as warfarin.

In those patients with no demonstrated (or trivial) carotid or cardiac lesions, antiplatelet drugs are indicated. Although aspirin is the drug of choice, it is presently being challenged by a variety of newer antiplatelet aggregate drugs, such as ticlopidine, which has been demonstrated to be more effective (Fig. 4.19).

More specific measures are sometimes needed. In patients with TIAs, venesection for polycythemia, for example, invariably abolishes the cerebral symptoms.

CONCLUSION

The diagnosis of TIA is retrospective and clinical. It cannot be made by tests. When in doubt, carefully retaking the history is the best way to make an accurate diagnosis. This step has no laboratory substitute. Once the diagnosis is made, CT scanning and carotid Doppler or carotid angiography are the minimal laboratory aids for deciding on management. Untreated TIAs carry a 5% yearly risk of stroke, which, with surgical or medical treatment, can be reduced two- to threefold.

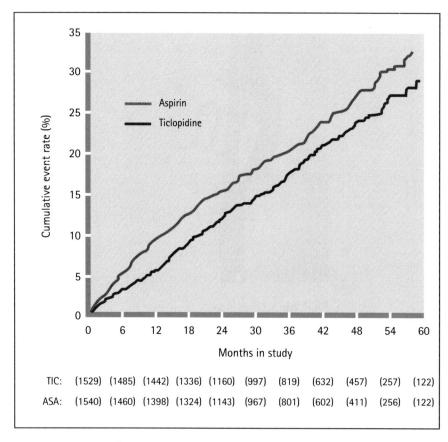

FIGURE 4.19→ Cumulative event-rate curves for death from any cause or nonfatal stroke. (Adapted from Hass WK, et al. 1989)

REFERENCES

Barnett HJM. Progress towards stroke prevention: Robert Wartenberg Lecture. *Neurology.* 1980; 30:1212–1225.

Bornstein NM, Norris JW. The unstable carotid plaque. *Stroke.* 1989; 20:1104–1106.

Hass WK, Easton JD, Adams HP, et al. A randomized trial comparing ticlopidine hydrochloride with aspirin for the prevention of stroke in high-risk patients. *N Engl J Med.* 1989; 321:501–507.

Norris JW, Hachinski VC. Misdiagnosis of stroke. *Lancet.* 1982; 1:328–331.

Norris JW, Hachinski VC. *Prevention of Stroke.* New York: Springer-Verlag. 1991.

Norris JW, Zhu CZ, Bornstein NM, et al. Vascular risks of asymptomatic carotid stenosis. *Stroke.* 1991; 22:1485–1490.

North American Symptomatic Carotid Endarterectomy Trial Collaborators: beneficial effect of carotid endarterectomy in symptomatic patients with high-grade stenosis. *N Engl J Med.* 1991; 325:445–453.

Preliminary Report of the Stroke Prevention in Atrial Fibrillation Study (SPAF). *N Engl J Med.* 1990; 322:863–868.

Sacco RL, Foulkes MA, Mohr JP, et al. Determinants of early recurrence of cerebral infarction. The Stroke Data Bank. *Stroke.* 1989; 20:983–989.

Ticlopidine (editorial). *Lancet.* 1991; 1:459–460.

Warlow C, Morris PJ. *Transient Ischemic Attacks.* New York: Marcel Dekker, Inc. 1982.

Wolf PA, D'Agostino RB, Kannel WB, et al. Cigarette smoking as a risk factor for stroke. *JAMA.* 1988; 259:1025–1029.

Wolf PA, Kannel WB, Verter J. Current status of risk factors for stroke. In: Barnett HJM (ed). *Neurologic Clinics.* Philadelphia: W.B. Saunders Company. 1983; 1:320–324.

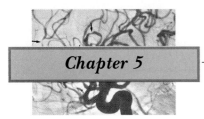

Chapter 5

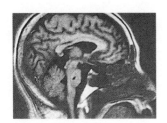

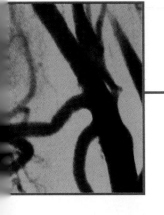

MICHAEL S. PESSIN

PHILIP A. TEAL

Carotid Territory Ischemic Stroke

THE IMPORTANCE of identifying extracranial internal carotid artery (ICA) occlusive disease has recently been highlighted by the scientifically proven benefits of carotid endarterectomy for symptomatic patients with high-grade stenosis. Surgical treatment of carotid disease had previously been a mere reflection of opinions marshalled from the anecdotal experiences of individual practitioners. The lack of scientific proof was related, in part, to a dearth of well designed studies and, more important, to the disease's variable natural history and clinical subtleties. This chapter will focus on the prevalence of carotid occlusive disease, its anatomic features, and the basic mechanisms underlying its many clinical expressions.

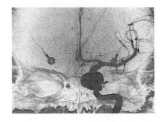

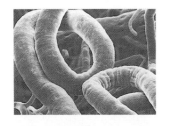

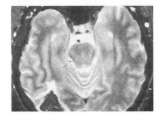

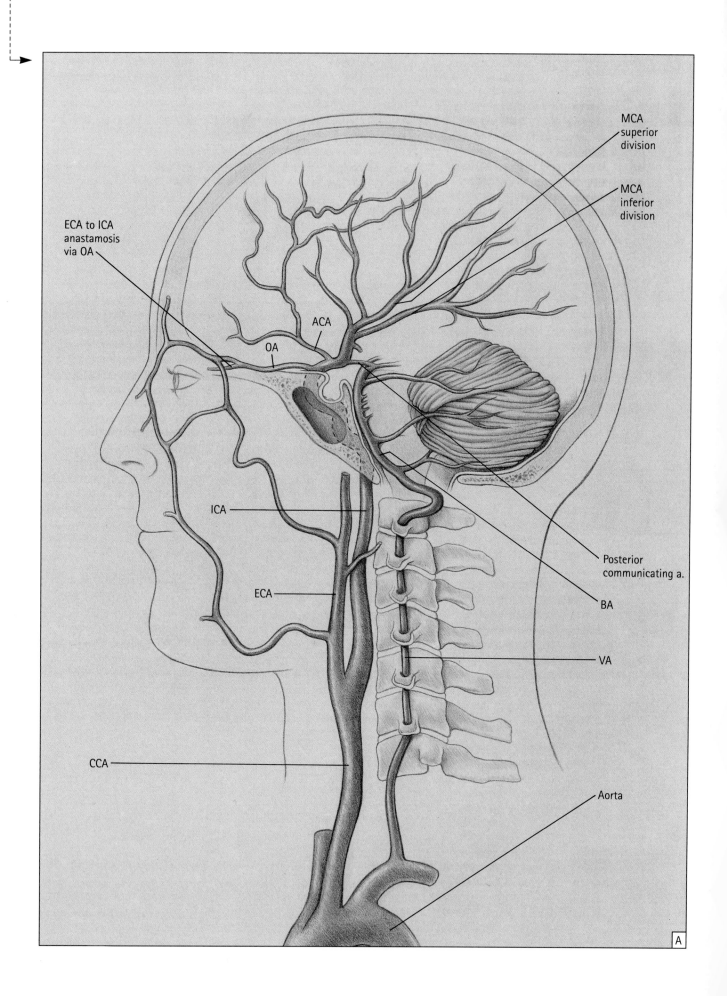

ECA to ICA
anastamosis
via OA

MCA
superior
division

MCA
inferior
division

ACA

OA

ICA

ECA

Posterior
communicating a.

BA

VA

CCA

Aorta

A

EPIDEMIOLOGY

Extracranial ICA occlusive disease has a significant impact on the 500,000 new strokes that occur in the United States each year. It may account for as few as 10% of new strokes in population-based studies (South Alabama Study), or up to as many as 25% to 35% recorded in stroke registries where specific referral patterns may influence the overall incidence.

Since carotid occlusive disease represents only one aspect of the general expression of atherosclerosis, patients often have associated coronary and peripheral vascular disease. Hypertension, cigarette smoking, diabetes mellitus, and hyperlipidemic states are important risk factors. Men are more often affected than women. Racial differences also influence the distribution of cerebrovascular atherosclerosis; compared to black or Asian patients, whites are more prone to extracranial vascular lesions in the ICA.

BLOOD SUPPLY, TARGET TERRITORIES, AND COLLATERAL CIRCULATION

The eyes and cerebral hemisphere are the principal recipients of the ICA circulation. The ICA originates where the common carotid artery bifurcates into internal and external carotid arteries, at the level of the thyroid cartilage in the cervical region, toward the angle of the mandible. The external carotid artery (ECA) is easily recognized by its principal branches: the ascending pharyngeal, superior thyroid, lingual, facial, occipital, posterior auricular, internal maxillary, and superficial temporal. In the presence of ICA and vertebral artery occlusion (Fig. 5.1), the ECA branches that surround the orbit and are present in the occipital area provide important anastomotic collateral

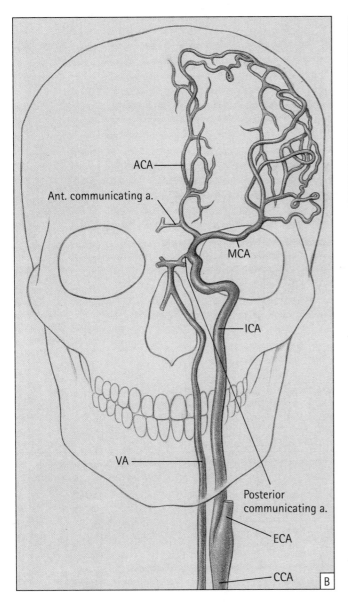

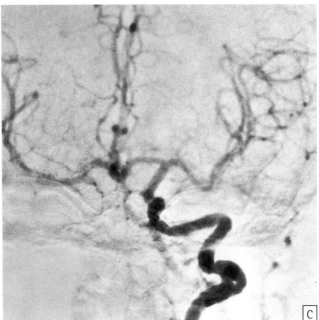

FIGURE 5.1 → Extracranial course and intracranial branches of the internal carotid artery (ICA). **A,** Lateral view demonstrates the bifurcation of the common carotid artery (CCA). The ICA terminates in the anterior and middle cerebral arteries (ACA, MCA). Also shown are important anastomotic collaterals from the external carotid artery (ECA) via the ophthalmic artery (OA), and from the vertebrobasilar system via the posterior communicating artery. **B,** Frontal view shows the bifurcation of the ICA into the ACA and MCA. The anterior communicating artery provides collateral flow from the opposite carotid system (VA = vertebral artery). **C,** Left carotid angiogram (AP view) demonstrates the filling of the left MCA and the ACA. Filling of the right MCA and ACA via the circle of Willis is also shown. The right ICA was occluded.

blood supply to the intracranial ICA (via the ophthalmic artery) and the vertebrobasilar circulation (via the vertebral artery).

The ICA ascends from its origin in the cervical region, giving rise to its three main segments—the petrous, cavernous, and supraclinoid portions. The petrous ICA runs through the petrous part of the temporal bone before entering the cranium at the carotid canal. The ICA then passes through the foramen lacerum, entering the cavernous sinus. Several small branches from these petrous and cavernous segments have no important stroke implications. The characteristic tortuosity of the S-shaped carotid siphon develops with advancing age.

The supraclinoid portion of the ICA pierces the dura mater medial to the anterior clinoid process, then produces several important branches that may be associated with ischemic syndromes. The first is the ophthalmic artery, which enters the orbit through the optic foramen. The ophthalmic artery gives rise to the central retinal artery and serves as a collateral conduit between the ECA's periorbital branches and the intracranial ICA. The posterior communicating artery arises next, coursing caudally and medially to join the posterior cerebral artery (PCA). The posterior communicating artery, depending on its size, can act as a collateral connection between the vertebrobasilar and carotid circulations. The anterior choroidal artery, which originates just distal to the posterior communicating artery, supplies the anterior choroid plexus, hippocampus, internal capsule, as well as the basal ganglia. The ICA finally terminates in the anterior cerebral artery (ACA) and the middle cerebral artery (MCA), which supply the major portion of the cere-

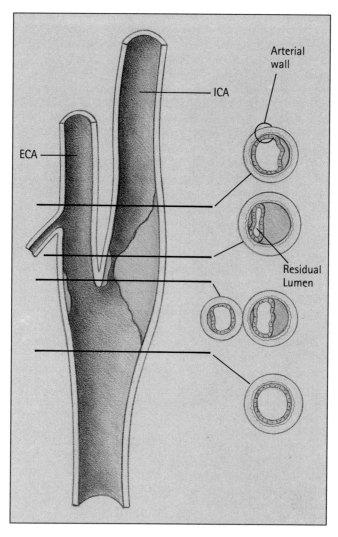

FIGURE 5.2 → Atherosclerotic plaque (yellow area) at the ICA origin causes a hemodynamically significant high-grade stenosis.

bral hemisphere. The important anastomotic collateral networks between the ACA, MCA, and PCA compose the so-called border zone or watershed regions.

CONDITIONS AFFECTING THE INTERNAL CAROTID ARTERY

ATHEROSCLEROSIS

Atherosclerosis is the most significant disease affecting the extracranial ICA (Fig. 5.2). In whites it has a predilection for the common carotid bifurcation, external carotid origin, and the first 2 cm of the ICA origin, sparing the remainder of the cervical ICA. The ICA has been called the artery of atherothrombosis because of its atherosclerotic propensity. Atherosclerosis may also affect the siphon region and the origins of the ACA and MCA stems, but to a lesser extent than the extracranial ICA. The pattern of atherosclerosis in Asians and blacks exhibits a preference for intracranial lesions rather than extracranial plaques (Fig. 5.3). Atherosclerosis is a progressive condition that is strongly influenced by genetic factors. Much attention has focused on modifiable or treatable risk factors such as hypertension, cigarette smoking, diabetes mellitus, and hyperlipidemic states, all of which accelerate the disease's progress.

ARTERIAL DISSECTIONS

The routine use of angiography has brought wide recognition to arterial dissection as a nonatherosclerotic cause of carotid disease. Dissection may occur spontaneously or may be related to minor, inobvious trauma such as vomiting, sneezing, coughing, neck move-

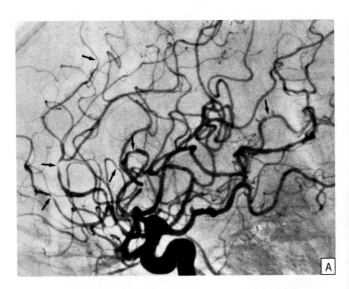
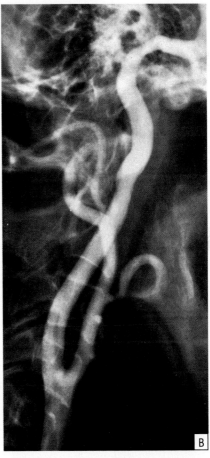

FIGURE 5.3 → A, Carotid angiogram of an Asian male presenting with transient ischemic attacks (TIAs) shows multiple areas of intracranial atherosclerosis with stenotic narrowing (arrows). **B,** Normal carotid bifurcation of the same patient.

ments, or other routine activities. The pathogenesis of dissection involves hematoma formation within the arterial wall. If the hematoma lies in a subintimal position, the arterial lumen will be compressed and may even be occluded over a long segment of the vessel, depending on the extent of the disruption (Fig. 5.4). When the hematoma extends toward the adventitial surface, aneurysmal formation occurs with a relatively patent lumen. Underlying structural defects in the vessel wall are a factor in some cases of dissection.

Angiography may establish the diagnosis based on characteristics such as contrast patterns and location. The so-called string sign depicts a thin tiny column of contrast extending over a long segment of the cervical carotid, reflecting luminal compromise by the subintimal hematoma. Aneurysmal outpouching appears as a pod and is due to ballooning of the weakened adventitial surface from the pressure of hematoma formation. Occasionally, both features may be present. Dissection is readily distinguishable from typical atheroma, except in cases of occlusion, which may not have any characteristic features. Ischemic symptoms can result from either a low-perfusion state due to luminal compromise, or thrombus dislodged as an embolic fragment occluding intracranial branches. The arterial injury in dissection may eventually heal with full restoration of the lumen and normal anatomy on angiography.

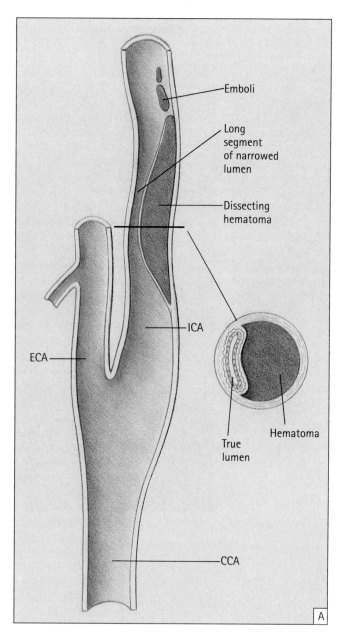

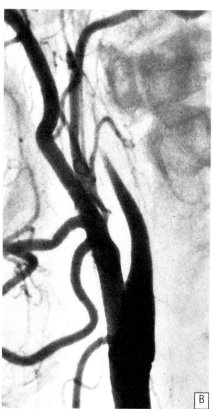

FIGURE 5.4 → **A,** Schematic depiction of a carotid dissection. The subintimal hemorrhage has produced a long region of stenosis. **B,** An angiogram of a carotid artery dissection that resulted in a long tapered occlusion starting distal to the origin of the ICA.

FIBROMUSCULAR DYSPLASIA

Fibromuscular dysplasia (FMD) is a rare arteriopathy that may affect the cervical ICA, but its relationship to clinical symptoms remains controversial. FMD is a widespread systemic vascular condition that is not restricted to the cerebrovasculature. Pathologic changes include an arterial wall disorganization characterized by smooth muscle hyperplasia or thinning, fibrous proliferation, and elastic fibroid disorganization. Based on the arterial wall structure most affected, angiographic patterns vary, but the "string of beads" configuration predominates, reflecting localized, concentric narrowing from media involvement (Fig. 5.5). Long segments of tubular narrowing or aneurysmal dilatation are less common patterns. Arterial kinking of the ICA involved by FMD may also create a stenosis.

OTHER DISORDERS

Less common, or even rare, conditions may also affect the extracranial ICA, giving rise to symptoms based on hemodynamic and embolic mechanisms similar to atherosclerosis. Intense vasospasm associated with migraine has occasionally been documented in the extracranial ICA. Such events may simulate a dissection on angiography because of the long segment of narrowing. As in dissection, this vasospastic narrowing is usually reversible. Stagnation thrombus may complicate the event, however, leading to infarction or, rarely, postvasospasm reperfusion may result in intracranial hemorrhage. Coagulation disorders may lead to in situ thrombus formation in any artery, even without underlying arterial disease. This has been demonstrated in the extracranial ICA circulation (Fig. 5.6). Finally, cardiac source embolism that is too

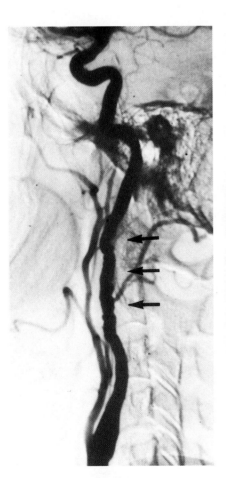

FIGURE 5.5 → Angiogram of common carotid shows the typical beaded appearance of multiple concentric areas of fibrostenosis (arrows) in fibromuscular dysplasia.

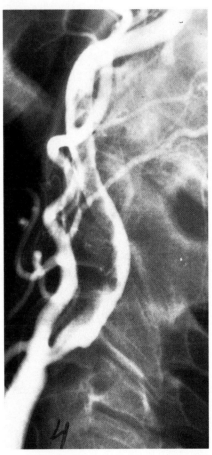

FIGURE 5.6 → Left carotid angiogram reveals a long intraluminal filling defect due to in situ thrombus formation in the ICA.

large to pass through the common carotid bifurcation may occlude the ICA and ECA.

MECHANISMS OF ISCHEMIA

Atherosclerosis at the ICA's origin is the principal underlying condition that leads to retinal and cerebral ischemia. Two basic mechanisms have been proposed to account for ischemic events: 1) intracranial embolism (Fig. 5.7), and 2) a low-perfusion state, also referred to as hemodynamic or distal insufficiency (Fig 5.8). These mechanisms may operate concomitantly or individually. Their impact varies based on the availability of effective collateral circulation. Understanding the inter-

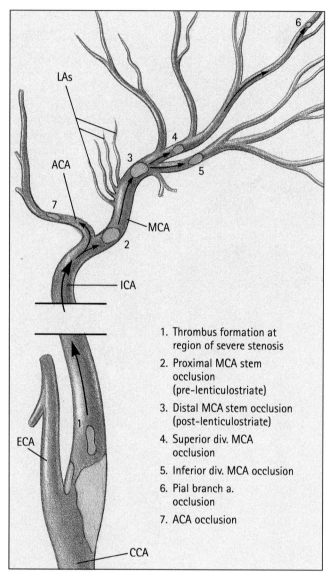

LAs
ACA
MCA
ICA
ECA
CCA

1. Thrombus formation at region of severe stenosis
2. Proximal MCA stem occlusion (pre-lenticulostriate)
3. Distal MCA stem occlusion (post-lenticulostriate)
4. Superior div. MCA occlusion
5. Inferior div. MCA occlusion
6. Pial branch a. occlusion
7. ACA occlusion

FIGURE 5.7 → Carotid stroke—embolic mechanism. Thrombus formation at the region of severe atherostenosis may embolize distally, most frequently to the MCA. An embolus often impacts at an arterial bifurcation but may later fragment and move distally. (LA=lenticulostriate artery)

play between these pathologic conditions provides a rationale for the evaluation and treatment of patients with carotid occlusive disease.

GENERAL FEATURES

The relationship between atherosclerosis of the extracranial ICA and clinical symptoms is complex. The facts suggest that atheroma develops progressively at a pace that varies from patient to patient due to genetics and factors that stimulate plaque growth, including hypertension, cigarette smoking, and hyperlipidemic states. The pathogenesis of the atheromatous plaque—the fundamental lesion of atherosclerosis—is reviewed in detail in Chapter 3. Suffice it to say

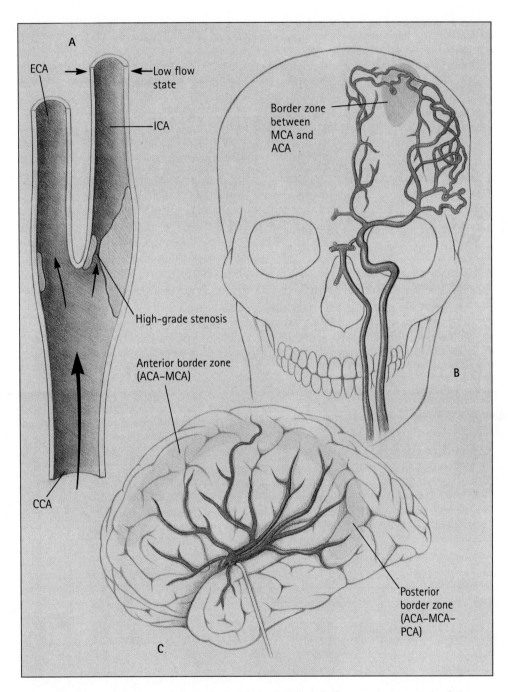

FIGURE 5.8 → Carotid stroke—low perfusion mechanism. **A,** Severe atherostenosis of the proximal ICA results in decreased distal blood flow. **B,** Frontal view of the ICA and the "border zone" between its ACA and MCA branches. Colored area represents low perfusion infarction. **C,** Lateral view of the brain depicts the anterior and posterior border zones between major arterial territories.

that the progression of atheroma eventually leads to high-grade stenosis or occlusion of the artery at a unifocal site, typically at the extracranial ICA origin. Less severe but potentially dangerous lesions such as irregular and ulcerative plaques may also occur. Platelet-fibrin thrombus, an important complication of the process, may adhere to the plaque surface either because of disruption and irregularity of the plaque, or because of stagnation from a critically narrowed lumen and impaired blood flow. Almost as soon as the platelet-fibrin thrombus forms it may be swept distally into the intracranial circulation as an embolic fragment, blocking vessels and causing ischemia. Alternatively, the thrombus may occlude the narrowed ICA, then propagate as an enlarging, solid coagulum into and beyond the circle of Willis, impairing intracranial blood flow. The final stage in ICA occlusion is the thrombotic event, which may remain localized without fragmentation and distal migration. This extracranial localized occlusion may cause ischemia in the eye and hemisphere beyond due to a low-perfusion state associated with inadequate collateral circulation.

EMBOLISM

Some of the first observations implicating local (arterial-to-arterial) embolism were made in the retinal circulation. Particulate material (platelet-fibrin) was occasionally seen on fundoscopic examination during episodes of transient monocular blindness (TMB),

establishing for the first time that emboli could cause transient events. This theory received further support when it was found that the atheromatous plaque removed at the time of carotid endarterectomy was more likely to be covered with platelet-fibrin debris if patients were recently symptomatic with transient ischemic attacks (TIAs) than if they had no symptoms in the 7 weeks preceding surgery. However, this observation leaves unsettled the role played by the stenosis itself in producing TIAs from a low-perfusion state and also the significance of less severe carotid lesions.

The type of carotid lesion and its role in symptom production continues to generate controversy. The embolic theory of ischemic symptoms in its simplest interpretation may lead to the uncritical conclusion that any degree of atheroma may stimulate thrombus deposition and result in local embolism. The disturbing implication is that small irregularities in the plaque architecture or even more definitive ulcerations may harbor thrombus and lead to symptoms, even in the absence of critical flow-reducing stenosis (Fig. 5.9). This view has been contested in a detailed serial section analysis of the atheromatous plaque removed at endarterectomy. Some instances of platelet-fibrin thrombi adherent to ulcerations were found, but the amount of material was tiny (less than 1 mm) compared to larger thrombi found at sites of severe narrowing. Furthermore, clinical studies of carotid territory ischemic events usually show a correlation with severe, not minor, lesions.

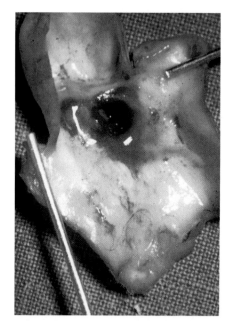

FIGURE 5.9 → Pathologic specimen of carotid artery showing thrombus formation within an ulcerated atherosclerotic plaque.

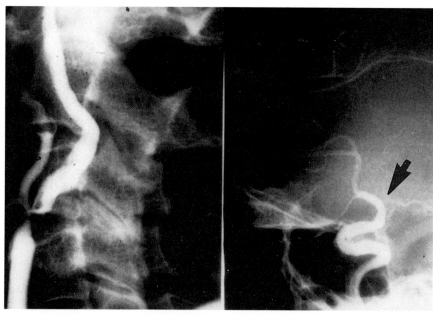

FIGURE 5.10 → Carotid angiogram demonstrates severe atherostenosis of the proximal ICA and thrombus formation as exhibited by the intraluminal filling defect (left). The intracranial view (right) shows complete occlusion of the MCA stem due to embolus (arrow). Flow is preserved through the ACA.

Embolic particle size is probably important in determining symptoms. The embolic material necessary to produce retinal ischemia or central retinal artery occlusion may be too small to block hemisphere vessels thought likely to produce symptoms. Material other than platelet-fibrin aggregates, such as cholesterol crystals, are frequently seen as asymptomatic curiosities in the retinal circulation, but only rarely have been documented to cause TIAs or stroke. The persistence of an occlusion and the absence of effective collateral circulation are essential to determining whether symptoms are transient or permanent.

The embolic theory of TIAs may account for solitary events or several different clinical events, reflecting a variable distribution of embolic material within the carotid territory. However, even the presumption that recurrent stereotyped TIAs are due to hemodynamic rather than embolic factors has been challenged by the observation that tiny stainless steel bearings injected into a dog's ICA may occasionally line up in one MCA branch due to a streamlining effect.

Embolism to the intracranial circulation from carotid origin disease disproportionally involves the MCA and its branches, partly because the MCA supplies such a large territory. It is also possible that the ACA is supplied from the other carotid, based on common anatomic variations. The particular portion of the MCA occluded by embolism is significantly related to thrombus size. Thrombus of 3 mm may easily block the MCA stem or division, whereas smaller material (approximately 1 mm) will occlude only pial branches. Contrary to the popular but unproven view, embolism released in the circulation does not spray the entire intracranial circulation. Rather, the common pattern is for a main trunk occlusion (Fig. 5.10) with several distal branches affected by fragmentation and migration of embolic material. The site of occlusion determines clinical symptoms, infarct location, and size.

LOW-PERFUSION STATE

A low-perfusion state is the other major mechanism accounting for distal ischemia to the retina or cerebral hemisphere. This condition implies a "distal insufficiency" to those regions furthest from the site of occlusion and susceptible to inadequate collateral circulation. Intracranial occlusive lesions are not necessary, as they are in embolism. In a profound low-perfusion state "stagnation thrombus" may develop in distal vessels, but the hemisphere vessels are often fully patent when angiography is performed shortly after the clinical event. Both the retina and cerebral hemisphere may be considered the distal fields of the carotid circulation.

Infarcts that develop in response to distal insufficiency follow a suprasylvian topography, occurring in the superior aspect of frontal, parieto-occipital and lateral occipital areas (Fig. 5.11). These are the so-called border zones or watershed regions between the ACA-MCA, MCA-posterior cerebral artery (PCA), and ACA-PCA. In these distal extremes of the major hemi-

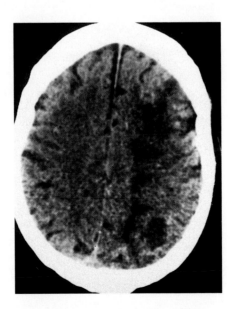

FIGURE 5.11 → CT scan shows a low attenuation area of infarction extending along the anterior and posterior border zones in a patient with internal carotid occlusion.

sphere blood supply, important anastomotic networks connect the vascular territories but often are not sufficient to prevent infarction. More proximal (sylvian) areas tolerate the perfusion failure due to the collateral flow across the circle of Willis and extracranial-intracranial collateral channels, such as retrograde ophthalmic artery flow from the ECA.

The nature of distal insufficiency implies a severe, hemodynamically significant carotid lesion, not a minor irregularity or ulceration that does not impair blood flow. The concept of a low-perfusion state more adequately accounts for patients with recurrent and similar (stereotyped) TIAs since the same brain region would be rendered ischemic on repeat insults, a situation not easily explained by random intracranial embolic occlusions.

CLINICAL MANIFESTATIONS OF INTERNAL CAROTID ARTERY OCCLUSIVE DISEASE

The clinical expression of extracranial ICA occlusive disease varies widely. Even patients with severe disease may be asymptomatic, seeking medical attention only because a bruit was incidentally detected on routine physical examination. In others, stroke with varying degrees of severity may be the initial presentation. Many patients have TIAs as their first symptoms.

Defined as reversible brief (<24 h, usually less than 15 min) episodes of focal retinal or cerebral ischemia that reflect underlying atherothrombotic disease, TIAs are a common warning symptom of carotid occlusive disease. In retrospective series of patients with carotid territory stroke and ICA occlusive disease, TIAs occurred in 54% to 64% of patients, a prevalence that emphasizes their importance. Prospectively studied patients with ICA occlusive disease provide a different picture, however; only approximately 10% of patients had TIAs and an annual stroke risk of 1.7%. Only 43 of 1617 patients (2.6%) had a stroke without warning TIAs. The discrepancy between these studies relates in part to the inclusion of patients with less than severe carotid disease and follow-up periods that may be insufficient to clarify the disease's natural history. The unexpected finding of infarction on CT or MRI in patients experiencing TIAs has been documented in several studies, indicating that some transient (although not necessarily brief) ischemic events may reflect infarction (Fig 5.12).

The two major types of TIAs that delineate the principal target areas of carotid territory ischemia—the retina and hemisphere—are transient monocular blindness (TMB) and transient hemispheral attacks (THA) (Fig. 5.13).

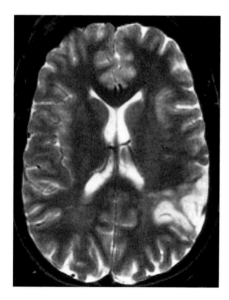

FIGURE 5.12 → Unexpected infarction in a patient with a TIA of transient aphasia. The T2-weighted MRI shows an area of high signal intensity representing an infarct in the left posterior temporal-parietal region.

FIGURE 5.13 → FEATURES OF CAROTID TIAS

TYPES:	Transient monocular blindness (TMB)
	Transient hemispheric attacks (THA)
	Limb-shaking spells
DURATION:	Usually less than 15 minutes
FREQUENCY:	Single or multiple
TIME COURSE:	May recur over weeks or months
PATTERNS (THA):	Motor and sensory, isolated motor, isolated sensory, dysphasia
(TMB):	Monocular visual loss, "fog," "curtain"
DISTRIBUTION:	Hand; distal arm and hand; hand and face; face; leg; retina
ASSOCIATED FINDINGS:	Focal carotid bruit often present
SIGNIFICANCE:	Associated with high grade stenosis
	Ominous if increasing in frequency, duration, or present on awakening

TRANSIENT MONOCULAR BLINDNESS

Also known as amaurosis fugax, TMB is a temporary monocular obscuration of vision described by patients as a gray or black fog, blur, mist, or cloud. In a minority of patients the visual interference is described as a "shade" or "curtain" effect involving either the entire monocular field or only the upper or lower half. Positive visual phenomena such as lights and scintillations are unusual manifestations that are more typical of migraine. The attacks are brief, lasting 1 to 15 minutes, usually with full restoration of vision. Visual loss due to retinal infarction has occasionally been reported. Most patients will have one to several attacks; others will have as many as a hundred over varying periods of time.

TMB bears a strong relationship to severe extracranial ICA occlusive disease in as many as 30% to 50% of patients. The relationship to lesser carotid lesions is unclear. Benign forms of TMB related to migraine, vasospasm, or other nonatherosclerotic processes are common, especially in younger patients.

TRANSIENT HEMISPHERAL ATTACKS

Hemisphere dysfunction, referred to as transient hemispheral attacks (THAs), is the other major manifestation of carotid territory ischemia. The usual features are motor and sensory dysfunction of the opposite limbs with dysphasia if the dominant hemisphere is involved, or behavioral disturbances of neglect due to impairment of the nondominant hemisphere. In one study of 52 patients, motor and sensory abnormalities were the most common THA manifestation, followed by motor alone, sensory alone, and isolated dysphasia. Involvement of the contralateral distal arm alone is common during an attack, presumably reflecting distal insufficiency that affects a restricted suprasylvian region of motor cortex. The restricted nature of the disability is often unanticipated as a symptom of carotid disease by clinicians expecting a larger deficit from hemisphere ischemia. Like TMB, THAs are brief, usually lasting less than 15 minutes (most last 1–10 min), and may occur over extended periods of time. THAs lasting one hour or more have been associated with a widely patent artery in one study and may have been the result of rapidly fading embolism.

THAs are strongly correlated with carotid occlusive disease in about 50% of patients, leaving the possibility that other mechanisms produce similar symptoms, such as small-vessel disease or cardiac embolism.

COMBINED TMB AND THA

Some patients will experience both eye and hemisphere attacks but rarely at the same time. In one study of 10 patients with nonsimultaneous occurrence of both events, a strong correlation (80%) with severe carotid disease was found. Usually the first attack was TMB followed later by THAs.

A rare form of carotid TIAs has been described as "limb shaking." These attacks are characterized by brief involuntary movements of either the arm and hand only, arm and leg, or leg only. The movements are coarse, irregular, and wavering, but not rhythmic or tonic–clonic as in epileptiform activity. Sometimes the limb movements are associated with other symptoms such as speech difficulty or weakness, but this is atypical. Since these spells are easily mistaken for seizure activity, many patients are initially evaluated and treated for epilepsy, without benefit, before their symptoms are recognized as carotid territory ischemic events. Many of the patients had more typical carotid TIAs at other times. Major extracranial carotid occlusive disease contralateral to the affected limbs is present in all patients reported with limb shaking. Distal field insufficiency from a low perfusion state is the presumed mechanism underlying the attacks. Revascularization procedures (endarterectomy, EC-IC bypass grafting) appear to be beneficial.

Extracranial carotid occlusive disease may be detected by simple auscultation on routine examination. Turbulent blood flow through a narrowed vessel produces a characteristic bruit along the course of the artery, usually maximal at the bifurcation region at the level of the superior thyroid cartilage. This is so common a finding in severe disease that its presence should be expected and sought. If the residual lumen narrows enough to hinder flow, the bruit may fade or disappear. Ocular bruits are also common manifestations of carotid occlusion when they occur over the contralateral eye, presumably reflecting increased flow through the patent carotid.

STROKE—HEMISPHERAL AND RETINAL INFARCTION

HEMISPHERAL INFARCTION

Hemispheral stroke from extracranial carotid occlusive disease varies in severity based on the infarct's size and location, both of which are partly influenced by whether the underlying mechanism is a local embolism or a low-perfusion state. Local embolism affecting the MCA and its branches accounts for the majority of hemisphere infarcts from extracranial carotid occlusive disease (Fig. 5.14A). This observation is reinforced by the fact that cardiac source embolism of the MCA is not, on clinical grounds alone, distinguishable from carotid source embolism. As in cardiac source embolism, any portion of the MCA circulation can be affected—stem,

CAROTID TERRITORY STROKES–EMBOLIC PATTERNS

Arterial Territory	CT Appearance	Motor	Sensory	Visual	Language	Behavior
MCA Complete Territory		Hemiplegia F-A-L Head and eye deviation	Hemianesthesia	Homonymous Hemianopia	Global aphasia	Neglect (ND > D)
MCA Superior Division		Hemiparesis F-A > L Head and eye deviation	Hemianesthesia F + A > L	—	Expressive aphasia ("Brocas") (D)	Neglect (ND)
MCA Inferior Division		Minimal weakness	Rapidly resolving hemisensory	Homonymous hemianopia or Upper quadrantanopia	Receptive aphasia ("Wernicke's") (D)	Behavioral disturbances: Constructional apraxia Delerium (ND)
ACA		Weakness in foot and leg > shoulder and arm	Mild sensory loss in leg	—	Transcortical motor aphasia (D)	± Abulia ± Incontinence ± Lt. limb apraxia ± Contralateral grasp reflex

F = Face   A = Arm   L = Leg   D = Dominant hemisphere   ND = Nondominant hemisphere

A

CAROTID TERRITORY STROKES-LOW PERFUSION PATTERNS

Arterial Territory	CT Appearance	Motor	Sensory	Visual	Language	Behavior
Anterior Watershed (ACA–MCA)		Crural or brachial paresis, face spared ± Impaired volitional eye movements	Sensory loss in hand and arm	—	± Transcortical motor aphasia (D)	± Mood disturbance Abulia Euphoria (ND)
Posterior Watershed		Minimal motor findings	± "Cortical" hemi-hypesthesia	Hemianopia or lower quadrant	Aphasia: Transcortical sensory or Wernicke's (D)	Constructional apraxia Neglect (ND) Dyslexia Dysgraphia Acalculia (D)

F = Face   A = Arm   L = Leg   D = Dominant hemisphere   ND = Nondominant hemisphere

B

FIGURE 5.14 → **A,** Embolic patterns of carotid territory strokes. **B,** Low-perfusion patterns of carotid territory strokes.

division, or cortical branches. Characteristic CT patterns of infarction occur based on the site of occlusion but the perisylvian region is hardest hit in contrast to the low-perfusion ischemic cases. The largest infarcts are those from proximal MCA occlusion, prelenticulostriate, which leaves a swath of infarct in the basal ganglia, the adjacent capsular region, as well as the extensive MCA cortical territories. If the occlusion is more distal (after the take-off of the lenticulostriate vessels) then the deep territory is spared and infarction is limited to the cortex and underlying white matter. Further parcelization of the MCA territory occurs if either the superior or inferior division is blocked. The impact in the former is on the posterior frontal-anterior parietal area. The temporal-parietal region is impacted in the latter case. Individual branches or a combination of one or more branches may lead to restricted infarcts. Sometimes the ACA territory may be affected as well as the MCA. If the PCA arises from a large, fetal posterior communicating artery it may be affected by embolism from a carotid source, but this is rare.

The large infarcts from proximal MCA occlusions, prelenticulostriate, produce maximal hemispheral deficits of hemiplegia (from capsular involvement), hemisensory loss, hemianopia, and global aphasia or nondominant behavior depending on the affected hemisphere. If the lenticulostriate territory is spared but the cortical regions are involved, similar widespread neurologic abnormalities may occur. However, when only the superior division is affected, the deficit is predominantly motor with expressive aphasia. Persistent sensory and visual field defects are uncommon. In contrast, inferior division infarcts spare motor function and produce a posterior type aphasia or nondominant behavior, hemianopic defects, and sensory loss. Individual branch syndromes have been described that reflect parts of larger territory deficits. Because the infarcts center around the perisylvian region, the motor deficits disproportionately affect the face and distal arm-hand with relative sparing of the leg unless the ACA has also been compromised.

In a low-perfusion condition, the patient may awaken from sleep with a mild neurologic deficit that progressively or intermittently worsens throughout the course of one to several days. The clinical signs are sensitive to blood pressure variations and may be exacerbated by position changes. Clinical deficits reflect the hemisphere region, which is underperfused and is usually in the distal field or border zone region between the MCA and ACA. Suprasylvian infarcts in the superior frontal region are considered anterior border zone infarcts; those in the parietal-

occipital area are posterior border zone infarcts. Positron emission tomography (PET) and cerebral blood flow (CBF) studies of patients with severe disease have supported the concept of hemodynamic insufficiency. CT and MRI have provided clear infarct localizations in the border zone regions (Fig. 5.14B).

Low-perfusion infarcts may produce a milder clinical deficit than that found with embolism. Often the arm is the main target, with face and leg relatively spared. If the border zone is higher on the convexity, the leg may exhibit the brunt of weakness. One interesting variation has been ipsilateral leg weakness due to the common anatomic variation of both ACAs filling from one carotid that has severe disease. Infarcts localized to the more posterior regions in the parietal-occipital areas give rise to visual-spatial and constructional abnormalities with a hemianopic field defect. Motor function is relatively unaffected.

Severe language disturbances are more often associated with perisylvian regions of destruction than with the suprasylvian areas described above. The key elements of language useful in analyzing aphasia at the bedside are fluency, repetition, comprehension, and naming, as well as reading and writing. Anterior perisylvian infarcts produce a Broca's type aphasia characterized by slow, effortful, agrammatic speech with impaired repetition but relatively preserved comprehension. A more limited anterior perisylvian infarct involving only Broca's area (Brodmann's area 44) produces a rapidly improving minor motor aphasia with reduced output and dyspraxic articulation. Posterior perisylvian infarcts commonly result in Wernicke's aphasia characterized by fluent, paraphasic speech with poor repetition, comprehension, and naming. Less frequently, a conduction aphasia is detected with severely impaired repetition and literal paraphasic speech, but with much better comprehension than found in Wernicke's. Large infarcts involving both anterior and posterior perisylvian regions produce a global aphasia with severe impairment of all language functions. The perisylvian aphasias are often due to embolism. The so-called transcortical aphasias are distinguished by their suprasylvian location. The principal feature is the preservation of repetition. Transcortical motor aphasias show nonfluent speech with reduced output but preserved comprehension. In contrast, although transcortical sensory aphasias exhibit fluency, content is often irrelevant and comprehension is poor. Transcortical aphasias are seen with both embolic and low perfusion stroke mechanisms (Fig. 5.15).

RETINAL INFARCTS

Although the retina and the hemisphere can be similarly compromised by the mechanisms underlying carotid disease, the retina is less frequently affected. Retinal infarcts from embolism may be partial, as in individual branch occlusion, or complete with central retinal artery occlusion (CRAO) (Fig. 5.16A). Many times embolic material in the form of cholesterol will be incidentally discovered on routine fundoscopic examination in an asymptomatic patient. With branch retinal artery occlusion (BRAO), an area of infarcted retina supplied by that branch will result in a persistent scotoma, but vision will otherwise be preserved (Fig. 5.16B). The embolic material is often visualized, appearing as white-gray (platelet-fibrin) or cholesterol material. In CRAO, sudden painless extensive visual loss occurs, leading to persistent blindness that may not resolve if the vascular obstruction persists beyond a short time. Unless partial fragmentation occurs, the embolus is usually not directly visualized since it lodges proximal to the point where the central retinal artery emerges from the disk. The fundic findings of ischemic retinal pallor, stringlike retinal arteries, and a cherry-red macular area (supplied by the intact ciliary artery) make the diagnosis easy on visual grounds alone.

FIGURE 5.15 → CLINICAL PATTERNS OF APHASIA

	SPONTANEOUS SPEECH	REPETITION	COMPREHENSION	NAMING	TYPICAL LOCALIZATION
BROCA'S APHASIA	Nonfluent*, agrammatic, meaningful content, telegraphic	Poor	Relatively preserved	Poor	Perisylvian, Broca's area (44) & adjacent prerolandic cortex & subcortex. "Minor motor aphasia" confined to Broca's area. (sup. div. branch, MCA)
WERNICKE'S	Fluent**, paraphasic+, meaningless	Poor	Poor	Poor, paraphasic	Posterior superior temporal plane (inf. div. MCA)
GLOBAL APHASIA	Nonfluent, mute, or stereotypic utterances	Poor	Poor	Poor	Large infarct involving both anterior & posterior perisylvian areas (MCA stem)
CONDUCTION	Fluent, word finding pauses, literal paraphasias	Disproportionately impaired	Relatively preserved	Paraphasic	Supramarginal gyrus, posterior temporal (inf. div. MCA)
TRANSCORTICAL MOTOR	Nonfluent, reduced output	Preserved	Good	Impaired	Supplementary motor area, or anterior, superior to Broca's. May be subcortical (ACA or MCA branches or anterior watershed)
TRANSCORTICAL SENSORY	Fluent, paraphasic, irrelevant	Preserved	Poor	Poor	Parietotemporal junction, posterior to Wernicke's (post-watershed or PCA)

* Slow, effortful, poorly articulated, reduced phrase length
** Effortless, normal output, well articulated
+ Verbal paraphasias are word substitutions; literal paraphasias are phonemic substitutions

Both BRAO and CRAO appear to have a significant association with extracranial carotid occlusive disease serving as the embolic source in 50% to 60% of cases studied.

A rare but serious condition of progressive visual loss, venous stasis retinopathy, develops from a low-retinal perfusion state caused by carotid occlusion. Chronic ocular ischemia leads to neovascularization of the iris, secondary glaucoma, and proliferative retinopathy with blot hemorrhages (Fig. 5.16C). Finally, the rare occurrence of simultaneous optic nerve and cerebral infarction has been reported in 3 out of 612 (.5%) patients on the basis of a low-perfusion state (the opticocerebral syndrome).

CONCLUSION

We have reviewed the spectrum of extracranial carotid occlusive disease from the asymptomatic carotid bruit to frank occlusion with accompanying stroke. Symptoms alerting the clinician to the condition in the prestroke phase include monocular and hemispheral TIAs. Carotid territory stroke may encompass a minor disability or major retinal or hemisphere infarction. The mechanisms underlying both carotid TIAs and stroke include local embolism to the retina or hemisphere and/or a low-perfusion state whose effects depend on the adequacy of the collateral circulation. Predicting the clinical outcome in individual patients with carotid disease has proven difficult, if not impossible, except in a statistical sense of a definite stroke risk per annum.

Treatment in the form of carotid endarterectomy has been established from recent multicenter, controlled studies for the subgroup of patients with symptomatic high-grade stenosis. The results for lesser symptomatic carotid lesions as well as asymptomatic disease promises to emerge from several ongoing trials.

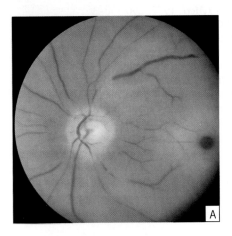 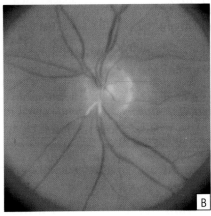 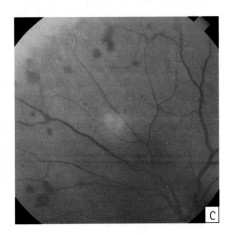

FIGURE 5.16 → Retinal manifestations of carotid disease. **A,** Central retinal artery occlusion demonstrates ischemic retinal whitening, attenuation of arterioles, and macula cherry-red spot. **B,** Branch retinal artery occlusion: saddle embolus of platelet-fibrin material in the inferior retinal artery. **C,** Venous stasis retinopathy: dot and blot hemorrhages in the mid-peripheral retina in a patient with ipsilateral high-grade carotid stenosis.

FIGURE 6.1 → SYMPTOMS THAT SUGGEST VERTEBROBASILAR LOCATION

- Dizziness, especially vertigo
- Diplopia or oscillopsia
- Staggering, veering, and ataxia
- Bilateral weakness and/or numbness
- Crossed numbness or weakness (1 side of face and opposite side of body)
- Hemianopia or bilateral visual field loss
- Headache or pain in the occiput, base of neck, or shoulder
- Acute onset of hearing loss or tinnitus
- Dysesthesias or burning on one side of the face

FIGURE 6.2 → SIGNS THAT SUGGEST VERTEBROBASILAR LOCATION

- Nystagmus—horizontal or vertical
- Third, fourth, and sixth cranial nerve paralysis
- Internuclear ophthalmoplegia
- Ocular skew
- Numbness of the face in fifth nerve distribution
- Peripheral facial nerve paralysis
- Gait or limb ataxia
- Hemianopia
- Bilateral visual field defects
- Bilateral or crossed motor or sensory signs
- Bilateral facial, pharyngeal, or lingual paralysis

FIGURE 6.3 → DISTINCTIVE FEATURES OF VERTEBROBASILAR ANATOMY

- Less blood flow (one fifth of CBF) compared to two fifths of flow for each carotid artery
- More territory fed by penetrating arteries (Fig. 6.4)
- Bilateral arteries (vertebral and anterior spinal) join to form larger single midline arteries (Fig. 6.5)
- Higher frequency of congenital anomalies, hypoplastic arteries, and adult retention of fetal arterial communications and patterns
- Geometry of the VA origin differs from the subclavian artery as compared to the carotid system. The VA has a nearly 90° take-off and is much smaller than the parent artery. The internal carotid artery (ICA) is nearly a 180° continuation of the common carotid artery (CCA) and is almost the same size (Fig. 6.6)
- Rich collaterals available in the neck from the thyrocervical and external carotid arteries (ECAs)

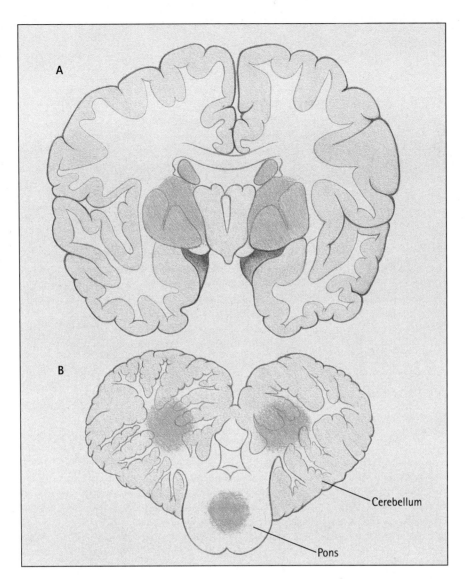

FIGURE 6.4 → A, The cerebral hemispheres supplied mostly by anterior circulation arteries. **B,** Cross-section of posterior circulation structures (through the pons and cerebellum). The regions supplied by penetrating arteries are shaded. Penetrating arteries supply a relatively larger proportion of the posterior circulation structures as compared to the anterior circulation.

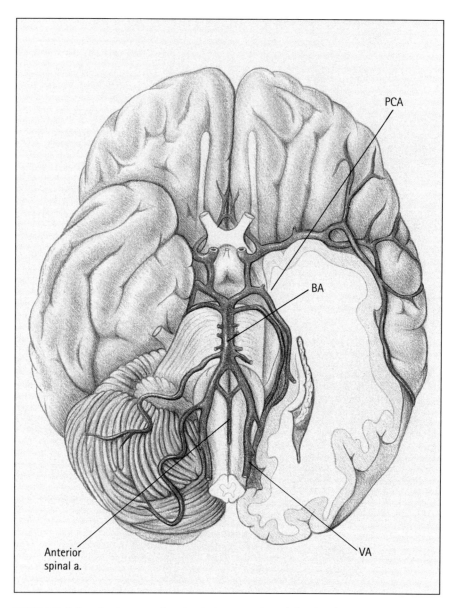

FIGURE 6.5 → In the posterior circulation, arteries originating from each side merge to form single midline arteries. The two vertebral arteries (VAs) merge at the medullopontine junction to form the basilar artery (BA). Anterior spinal artery branches originate from the distal intracranial VA. The anterior spinal artery descends in the anterior spinal sulcus into the cervical region.

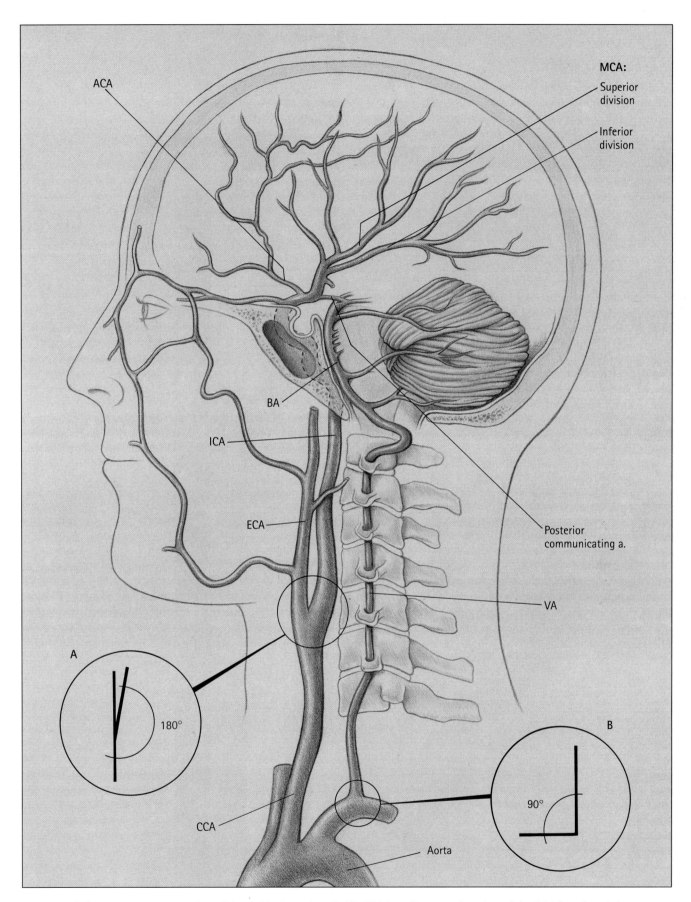

FIGURE 6.6 → The geometry of the CCA and its branches. **A,** The ICA is a direct continuation of the CCA (180°) and the two vessels are nearly the same size. **B,** In contrast, the VA is much smaller than its parent subclavian artery and arises at a nearly 90° angle. (ACA = anterior cerebral artery; MCA = middle cerebral artery)

COMMON VASCULAR PATHOLOGIES

ATHEROSCLEROSIS

Atherosclerosis is by far the most common disease affecting the posterior circulation arteries. Racial and sex differences are factors in the distribution of occlusive lesions. The usual sites of disease in white men are the vertebral artery (VA) origin, as well as the proximal subclavian, intracranial vertebral, and basilar arteries (Fig. 6.7A). There is a high incidence of accompanying coronary and peripheral vascular occlusive disease, as well as hypercholesterolemia. In contrast, premenopausal women, blacks, and Asians are prone to intracranial occlusive disease involving intracranial branches (long cerebellar and posterior cerebral arteries) in addition to the intracranial vertebral and basilar arteries, but have a low incidence of subclavian and vertebral artery disease in the neck (Fig. 6.7B).

Atherosclerotic lesions cause ischemia and infarction by intraarterial embolism, or by decreasing brain perfusion in the territory of the atherostenotic vessels. Since the VAs are paired, if one is diseased, the other often compensates. When the disease is bilateral, however, or when the critical midline basilar artery (BA) is occluded or severely stenosed, persistent and severe ischemia due to hypoperfusion often results. Proximity of the occlusive process to the brain increases the likelihood of persistent ischemia.

EMBOLISM

Embolism of cardiac origin and intraarterial embolism each accounts for about 20% of posterior circulation infarcts. Approximately 1 in 5 emboli from the heart reaches the vertebrobasilar system. This is in proportion to the amount of blood that supplies the posterior circulation. The most common arterial embolic donor sites are the VA origins in the neck and the intracranial VAs. Frequent recipient sites are the intracranial VAs and their posterior inferior cerebellar artery (PICA) branches, the superior cerebellar arteries, posterior cerebral arteries (PCAs), and the rostral end of the BA (Fig. 6.8).

DISSECTIONS

Dissections are tears within arterial walls that cause intramural hematomas. The tear is often due to trauma, but diseases of the arterial media, such as fibromuscular dysplasia and hereditable disorders of connective tissue, can predispose to dissections. Dissections are frequently located in the portion of the VA's distal extracranial segment that winds around the axis and atlas. Dissections sometimes affect the proximal VA above the origin, but before penetration into the vertebral foramina. Occasionally, they involve the intracranial VAs and BAs (Fig. 6.9).

PENETRATING ARTERY DISEASE

Occlusive disease of penetrating arteries often affects the paramedian branches of the BA that supply the pons (Fig. 6.10) as well as branches from the rostral basilar apex and PCAs that supply the thalamus (Fig. 6.11). Infiltration of the arterial walls with hyaline and lipid material ("lipohyalinosis") disorganizes the vessels with luminal encroachment (Fig. 6.12). Alternatively, plaques within the parent arteries block or extend into the penetrating artery branches or form microatheromas in the orifices of the branches (Fig. 6.13). Both lipohyalinosis and atheromatous branch disease cause focal infarcts in the territories of penetrating arteries, most often in the pons and thalami.

CLINICAL FEATURES, DIAGNOSIS, AND MANAGEMENT OF LESIONS IN VARIOUS LOCI

A tour through the posterior circulation beginning proximally and travelling distally is now in order. Vascular lesions at each site share common clinical features and evaluation strategies.

SUBCLAVIAN ARTERY/PROXIMAL VERTEBRAL ARTERY

Occlusive disease of the subclavian artery proximal to the VA origin diminishes anterograde flow into the VA (Fig. 6.14). Subclavian artery occlusive disease is most often detected during routine ultrasound testing of patients referred to the noninvasive laboratory for study of possible carotid artery disease. Most patients have no arm or posterior circulation symptoms, but when symptoms are present, they are usually described as discomfort, cramping, or coolness in the arm. Athletes may report lack of stamina, fatigue, and weakness of the arm after effort. Although neurologic symptoms are uncommon, transient spells of dizziness, loss of balance with veering and staggering, double vision, and blurred vision are sometimes reported. Attacks are usually brief, occasionally precipitated by exercising the ischemic arm. Strokes are rare.

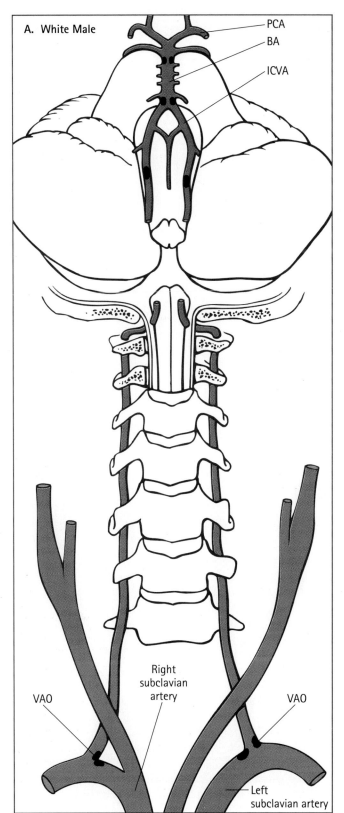

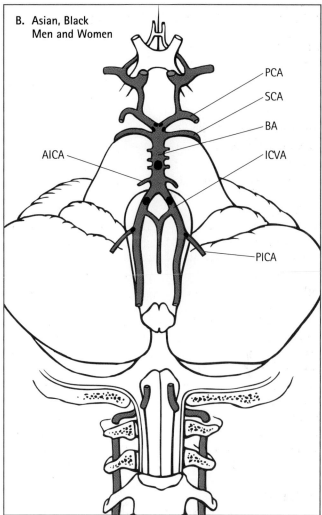

FIGURE 6.7 → Large extracranial and intracranial posterior circulation arteries. **A,** Shaded areas represent regions with a predilection for atherosclerotic narrowing in white men. The most frequent sites are the subclavian arteries, VA origins (VAO), the intracranial VAs (ICVA), and the proximal and distal BA. **B,** Shaded areas represent regions of predilection for atherosclerotic narrowing in black and Asian men and women. The ICVA and proximal BA are involved, as they are in white men. In addition, the branches [posterior inferior cerebellar arteries (PICA); anterior inferior cerebellar arteries (AICA); superior cerebellar arteries and posterior cerebral arteries (PCA)] are more involved than in white men.

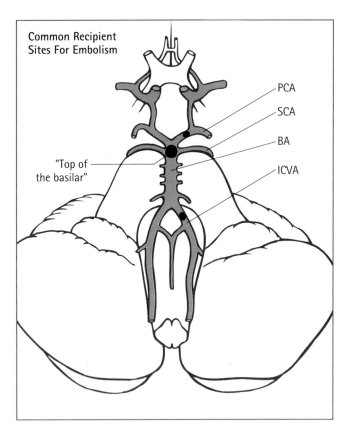

FIGURE 6.8 → Large posterior circulation arteries, showing most common recipient sites for embolism. The ICVAs and PICAs are often involved. If emboli pass through the ICVAs, they often lodge at the distal basilar bifurcation ("top of the basilar") or the superior cerebellar and PCA branches.

Common Recipient Sites For Embolism

PCA
SCA
BA
ICVA
"Top of the basilar"

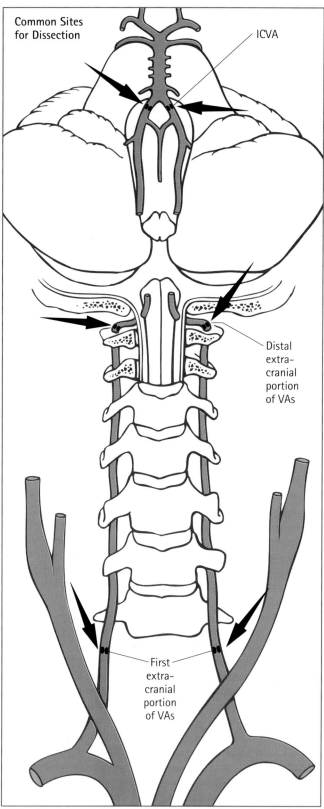

Common Sites for Dissection

ICVA
Distal extra-cranial portion of VAs
First extra-cranial portion of VAs

FIGURE 6.9 → Large posterior circulation arteries, showing sites of predilection for arterial dissection, including the first extra-cranial portion of the VAs between their origin and their penetration into the intravertebral foramina, the distal extracranial VAs, and the ICVAs.

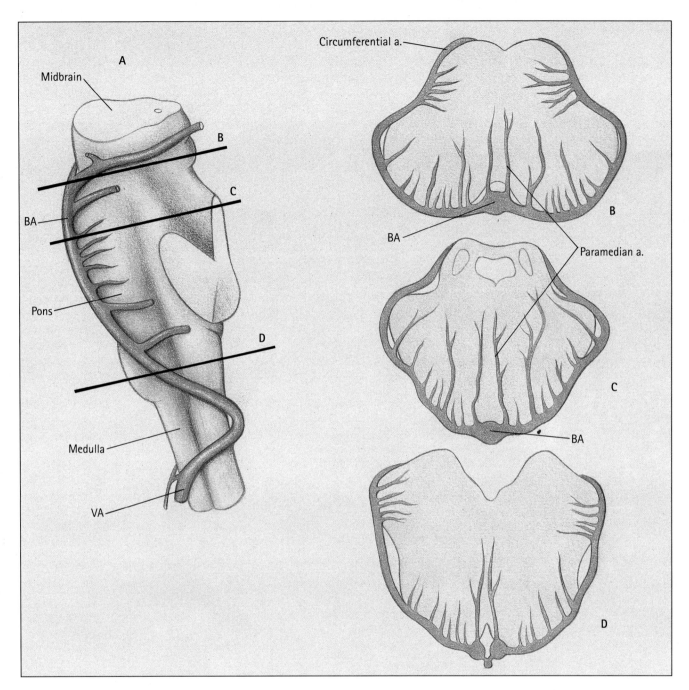

FIGURE 6.10 → The distribution of penetrating arteries supplying the brainstem. **A,** Longitudinal sagittal section shows the VAs, BAs, and brainstem. Horizontal lines represent planes of section for the cross-sections shown in B, C, and D. **B,** Section through the midbrain. **C,** Pontine section. **D,** Medulla.

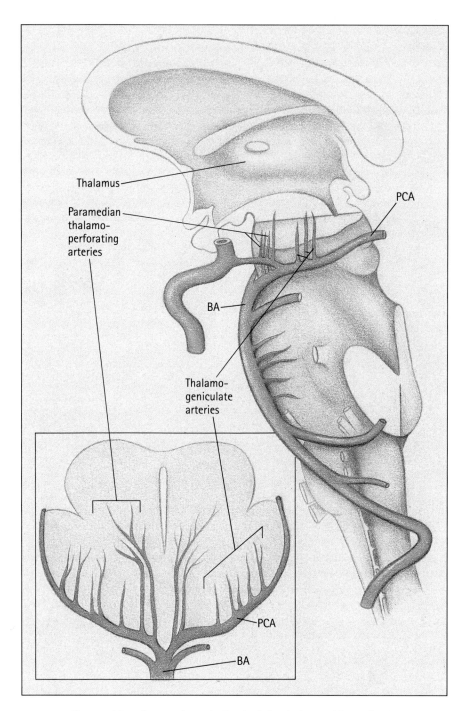

FIGURE 6.11 → Vascular supply at the level of the thalamus. The region is supplied by paramedian thalamoperforating arteries and more laterally placed thalamogeniculate arteries.

Cerebrovascular Disorders

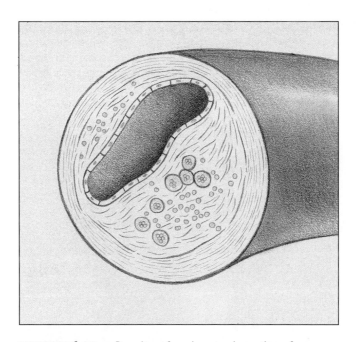

FIGURE 6.12 → Drawing of a microscopic section of a penetrating artery extensively damaged by lipohyalinosis. Fibrinoid material as well as lipid and connective tissue are deposited in the arterial wall, narrowing the lumen.

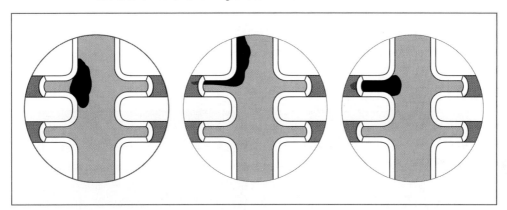

FIGURE 6.13 → Mechanisms of occlusion of BA branches. On the left, plaque in parent artery blocks branch. In the middle, plaque in parent artery extends into branch. On the right, the branch is blocked by a microatheroma forming within the branch.

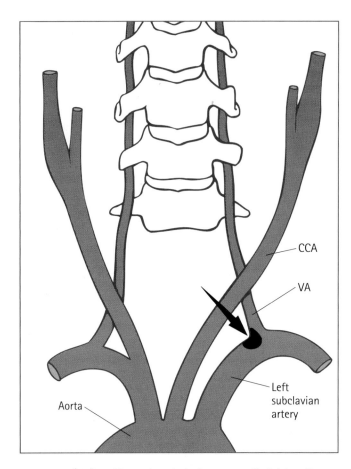

FIGURE 6.14 → Plaque in subclavian artery diminishes flow into the VA branch.

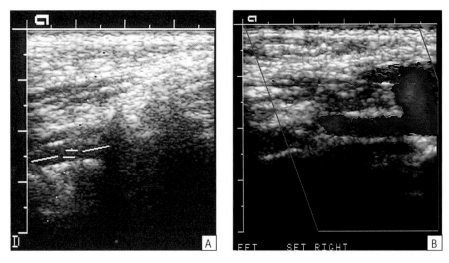

FIGURE 6.15 → **A,** Duplex scan of the VAO. On top is B-mode showing the artery (lines are in the lumen). Below is Doppler spectra from the VAO. **B,** Color-flow Doppler of normal subclavian-VAO region. The subclavian artery is to the right. The VA originates from it and goes to the left of the figure.

The left subclavian artery is involved in stroke much more often than the right. However, occlusions of the right subclavian artery or the innominate artery are more serious than disease of the left subclavian artery. Thrombi propagate from the right subclavian and innominate arteries into the carotid system and embolize intracranially, causing severe hemispheric stroke. On examination, the ischemic arm is usually cooler; the pulse is smaller in amplitude and may be delayed in comparison to the pulse in the opposite arm. Blood pressure in the ischemic arm is reduced, usually by more than 15 mm Hg.

Arm plethysmography, B-mode ultrasound, and Doppler can accurately detect significant subclavian artery occlusive lesions. Ultrasound and angiography often show poor anterograde flow through the ipsilateral VA. The delayed flow derived from the contralateral intracranial VA courses retrograde down the ipsilateral VA to supply the ischemic arm. This vascular pattern of flow has been called the "subclavian steal." Neurologic symptoms in patients with subclavian artery occlusion, with or without steal, are no different than for those with VA origin occlusions, indicating that the symptoms are caused by decreased anterograde flow through the ipsilateral VA.

Although the phenomenology of subclavian steal is intriguing, the syndrome is benign and self-limited unless the patient is a professional athlete who depends on the ischemic arm for a livelihood. Because the subclavian lesions are atheromatous, they are often accompanied by significant carotid artery occlusive disease. Strokes, especially those with hemiparesis, are invariably due to the concurrent carotid artery disease and are not attributable to the subclavian lesions. Controlling risk factors, therefore, is the primary treatment. Surgical repair should be undertaken only if the lesion is right sided or the patient is disabled by arm ischemia.

Atherosclerosis of the VA origin in the neck is very common. Plaques usually extend from the parent subclavian artery or develop at the VA origin. Patients with vertebral origin occlusive disease are predominantly white men who have a high incidence of accompanying coronary, carotid artery origin, and peripheral vascular occlusive disease. Common symptoms are transient attacks of dizziness, ataxia, diplopia, and blurred vision. Usually the attacks are brief and self-limited. Extensive potential neck collaterals from the ECA and the thyrocervical trunk branches invariably reconstitute the VA in the neck

when it occludes. Persistent ischemia due to brainstem and cerebellar hypoperfusion is unusual. As in the anterior circulation, however, white platelet-fibrin clumps and red fibrin-dependent thrombi can form on ulcerative or irregular plaques and embolize intracranially. When intraarterial embolism occurs, the most frequent recipient sites are the intracranial VA/PICA region (causing a lateral medullary syndrome or cerebellar infarct) and the distal BA or its SCA and PCA branches.

Duplex scans and color-flow Doppler imaging can show the VA origins (Fig. 6.15). Continuous wave (CW) Doppler with the probe held in the proximal neck and at the atlantoaxial region can define the direction and velocity of VA flow. Magnetic resonance angiography (MRA) and standard cerebral angiography also yield diagnostic images of arteries in the region.

Aspirin or other antiplatelet aggregates are advised for patients with VA plaque disease without severe stenosis or occlusion. Short-term warfarin anticoagulation (6–12 weeks) should be used for patients who have an acute recent VA symptomatic occlusion. In patients with severe stenosis, the choices are warfarin anticoagulation or surgical reconstruction. If anticoagulants are used, a prothrombin time of $1\frac{1}{2}$ times control (International Normalized Ratio [INR] of 1.3–1.5) is recommended. Treatment is continued until the artery has been shown by ultrasound testing to be occluded for more than a month.

DISTAL EXTRACRANIAL AND INTRACRANIAL VERTEBRAL ARTERY

Occlusive lesions of the interosseous portion of the VA in the neck are rare. Severe neck trauma with cervical vertebral fractures can injure the arteries within the transverse foramina, but severe atherostenosis rarely involves the interosseous or distal extracranial VA. Dissection—traumatic, related to neck manipulation, or spontaneous—most often affects the VAs after they emerge from the cervical vertebral foramina, but before dural penetration. Often the dissections are bilateral, presenting mainly with pain in the occiput, mastoid region, or neck. Dissections can extend into the intracranial VA (Fig. 6.16).

The most frequent sites of infarction and ischemia are identical to those found in disease of the intracranial VA—the lateral medulla and posterior inferior surface of the cerebellum. Infarction can be caused by one of two mechanisms: 1) spread of the

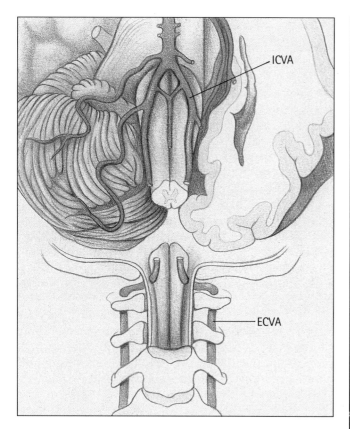

FIGURE 6.16 → Penetration of the extracranial VAs through the foramen magnum and their relation to the adjacent bony structures.

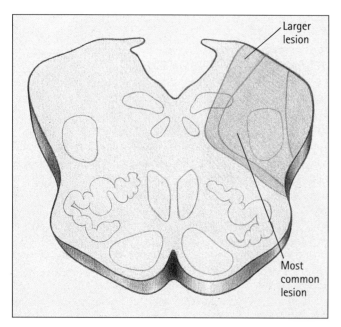

FIGURE 6.18 → Cross-section of the medulla. The shaded area represents the usual location of lateral medullary infarction.

Larger lesion

Most common lesion

FIGURE 6.17 → SYMPTOMS AND SIGNS IN LATERAL MEDULLARY SYNDROME

IPSILATERAL
• Pain in the eye or face
• Decreased pain and temperature sensation on the face
• Decreased corneal response
• Horner's syndrome
• Hoarseness and dysphagia due to pharyngeal and laryngeal paralysis
• Slight facial weakness
• Leaning to the side when sitting or standing

CONTRALATERAL
• Decreased pain and temperature sense on the limbs and trunk, sometimes with a sensory level

OTHER (NOT LATERALIZED)
• Nystagmus, generally horizontal or vertical, usually greater when looking to the side of the lesion
• Gait ataxia
• Tachycardia, blood pressure lability
• Decreased respiratory drive when sleeping
• Crowing cough to extricate food from the pyriform recess of the pharynx

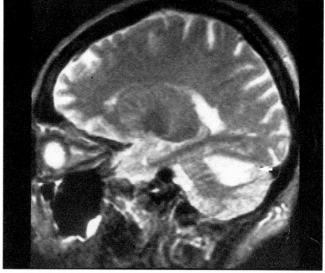

FIGURE 6.19 → T2-weighted MRI sagittal section through the cerebellum. White region (arrow) represents infarct in SCA territory in the superior portion of the cerebellum.

intramural thrombus into the lumen through a tear in the intima, or 2) formation of a thrombus in the lumen due to reduced flow and activation of the coagulation cascade by endothelial stimulation. Results of Doppler ultrasound (CW Doppler in the high neck, transcranial Doppler [TCD] intracranially) can suggest obstruction to distal cervical VA flow. MRA and standard angiography show tapered stringlike regions, sometimes with aneurysmal outpouchings. Magnetic resonance imaging (MRI) or CT with sections cut through the dissected artery can also suggest intramural blood. Temporal arteritis in the elderly can concentrically narrow the distal extracranial VAs just before they pierce the dura to enter the cranium.

Atherosclerosis usually involves the intracranial VAs before the PICA branches. Lateral medullary infarction results when the occlusive lesion blocks long circumferential medullary arteries that supply the dorsolateral medulla. The signs and symptoms of the lateral medullary syndrome are enumerated in Figure 6.17; the usual sites of infarction and the structures affected are shown in Figure 6.18.

Cerebellar infarction results when flow through the PICA branch of the intracranial VA is obstructed. The infarct involves the posterior portion of the cerebellum's undersurface. The distribution of infarction is best shown on T2-weighted sagittal section MRIs of the posterior fossa (Fig. 6.19). The most common symptoms of cerebellar infarction are dizziness, inability to stand or walk, veering and ataxia, and vomiting. Pain in the occiput or posterior neck is also common. Large cerebellar infarcts can cause mass effect with compression of the brainstem and the fourth ventricle. Ipsilateral conjugate gaze palsy, sixth nerve palsy, extensor plantar reflexes, stupor, and coma may develop. These large compressive lesions can be fatal unless they are treated effectively by medical decompression (corticosteroids, mannitol, glycerol, and hyperventilation), ventricular drainage, or surgical removal of the infarct.

Occasionally, the intracranial VA lesion extends into the most distal VA, blocking the branch to the anterior spinal artery. Infarction of the medial medulla or the medial and lateral medulla ("hemimedullary syndrome") develops (Fig. 6.20). Medial medullary infarction usually causes ipsilateral tongue paralysis, in addition to a hemiparesis and loss of position and vibration sense in the contralateral limbs. Other patients with intracranial VA stenosis or occlusion have 1) only transient ischemic attacks (TIAs)—the collateral circulation compensates well; 2) embolism to the distal BA, SCAs, or PCAs; or 3) spread of throm-

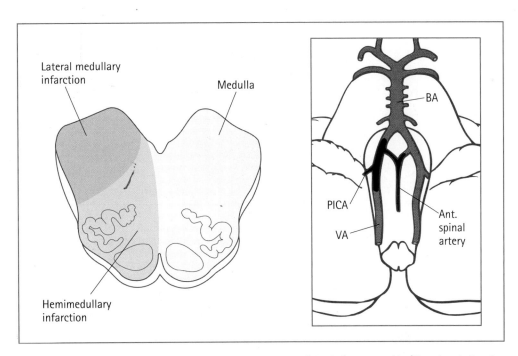

FIGURE 6.20 → Section of medulla showing infarct (shaded) on one side ("hemimedullary" infarct) caused by occlusion of the VA with blocking of both the PICA and anterior spinal artery branches (insert).

bus to the BA with pontine infarction (Fig. 6.21).

TCD ultrasound has a high sensitivity and specificity for detecting obstructive disease of the intracranial VAs. MRI accurately shows the distribution of medullary and cerebellar infarction. Both MRA and catheter angiography can precisely define the vascular lesions, as well as the adequacy of flow through the opposite vertebral and basilar arteries. Patients with unilateral intracranial VA occlusions and good contralateral flow should receive short-term anticoagulants for 6 to 12 weeks. Long-term anticoagulation is appropriate for severe intracranial VA stenosis.

Bilateral intracranial VA stenosis and occlusion is a potentially severe disorder that can result in progressive bilateral medullary and cerebellar ischemia. Especially common are position-related attacks of dizziness and weakness. Bilateral pyramidal and cerebellar signs develop, often progressing inexorably despite anticoagulants. Severe bilateral intracranial VA occlusive disease with persistent ischemic symptoms that do not resolve—despite anticoagulants and medical maximizing of intracranial blood flow—can be surgically treated with an extracranial–intracranial posterior circulation shunt.

BASILAR ARTERY—PROXIMAL AND MID PORTIONS

Severe stenosis or occlusion of this critical midline vessel compromises flow to the territories of the paramedian pontine penetrating arteries. Collateral circulation from the VA/PICA usually travels around the cerebellum to supply the anterior inferior cerebellar artery (AICA) or the SCA, which then supplies the BA beyond the block (Fig. 6.22). These vessels course laterally around the brainstem, allowing perfusion of the lateral base and tegmental regions. Blood also travels from the internal carotid circulation via the posterior communicating arteries to the PCAs, then to the rostral BA. The tegmentum of the pons is supplied mostly by the SCAs and other branches that arise near the basilar apex. Figure 6.23, modelled after the diagrams from

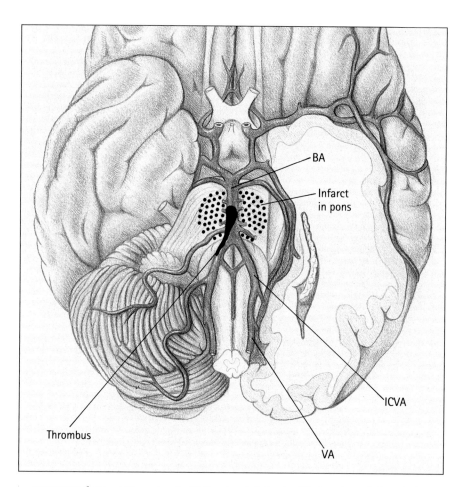

FIGURE 6.21 → Thrombus in ICVA extends into the BA. Resultant infarct is in the pons.

Kubik and Adams's original description of BA occlusion, illustrates the vascular and brainstem findings in a typical patient. The paramedian pontine base and tegmentum are most often involved. When the BA occlusion extends to the distal segments and blocks the SCA origins, fatal tegmental pontine and midbrain infarction usually occurs.

The main clinical findings are *motor* and *oculomotor*. Bilateral limb paralysis is often accompanied by some degree of limb ataxia. Some patients have a hemiparesis with minor abnormalities on the contralateral side, such as increased reflexes, slight weakness, and an extensor plantar reflex. Paralysis also often includes bulbar muscles, causing dysarthria or complete inability to speak, dysphagia, and inability to handle secretions in the pharynx. Bilateral facial, pharyngeal, and laryngeal weaknesses are found on examination. Diplopia and oscillopsia are related to dysfunction of the vestibular and oculomotor systems in the pontine tegmentum. Sixth nerve palsy, conjugate gaze palsy ipsilateral or bilateral to the lesion, and unilateral or bilateral internuclear ophthalmoplegia (INO) are often present. Both horizontal and vertical nystagmus are common findings. Sensory functions are usually spared because the spinothalamic tract and the descending tract of V are each laterally placed. When ischemia involves the paramedian pontine tegmentum bilaterally, patients are comatose. When paralysis is extreme, involving both limb and bulbar muscles bilaterally, patients may be awake and alert but unable to communicate, except by signalling with their eyes. This state has been called the locked-in syndrome and must be differentiated from coma.

Survival of brainstem tissue depends on optimal perfusion through collaterals. The patient should be kept supine during the initial days, maintaining optimal blood pressure, intravascular volume, and cardiac output. Heparin is given to prevent formation of a BA thrombus in the case of stenosis, and prevent propagation of thrombus when occlusion has already

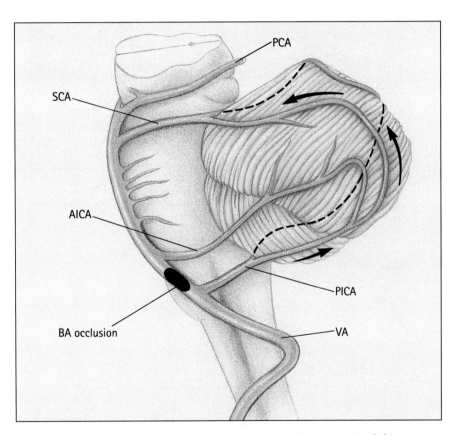

FIGURE 6.22 → BA occlusion. Collateral supply goes from the VA to PICA around the cerebellum (arrows) to the SCA, and finally to the distal BA beyond the region of the occlusion.

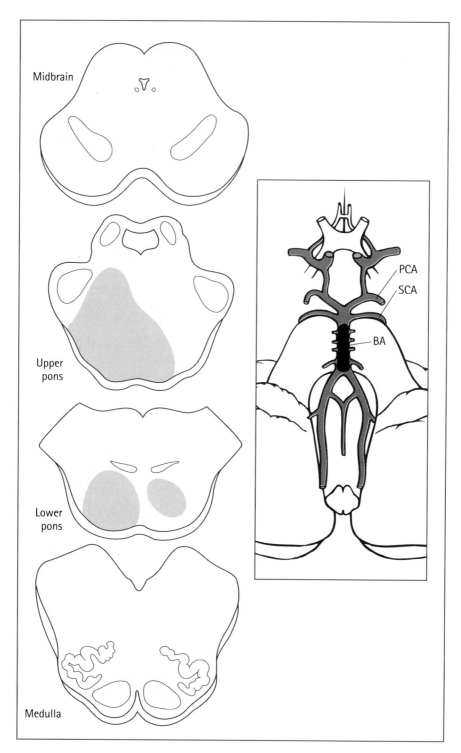

FIGURE 6.23 → On the right, the occlusion of the BA is seen. The sections on the left show the resultant infarct in the paramedian pontine base and tegmentum. (Adapted from Kubik C, Adams RD. 1946)

occurred. Treatment is first guided by the clinical signs and symptoms, the distribution of infarction on MRI, the patency of the vertebral and basilar arteries on MRI or MRA, and the findings from TCD. After the patient's condition has stabilized, angiography can help guide long-term treatment. If standard catheter angiography, or MRA of sufficient quality, shows a severe BA stenosis, long-term warfarin is prescribed, followed by TCD or MRA. If the BA occludes without symptoms during follow-up, warfarin can be stopped 1 month after the occlusion is identified. In patients with angiographically documented BA occlusion, warfarin is recommended for 6 to 8 weeks. By that time, the thrombus has organized and become adherent to the arterial wall, collateral circulation has been established, and anticoagulants need no longer be given.

Penetrating Artery Disease

The most frequent sites of disease are the paramedian pons, and the medial and ventrolateral portions of the thalami (see Figs. 6.10, 6.11). Paramedian pontine infarcts cause three recognizable clinical syndromes: 1) *pure motor hemiplegia*—paralysis of the arm, leg, and sometimes face on one side of the body without sensory, visual, or cognitive abnormalities. An ipsilateral INO, sixth nerve palsy, or conjugate gaze palsy may accompany the contralateral hemiparesis; 2) *ataxic hemiparesis*—some degree of weakness accompanied by ataxia in the arm and leg on one side of the body; and 3) *dysarthria–clumsy hand syndrome*—facial and lingual weakness on one side with minor clumsiness of the hand on the same side and thickened, slurred speech. MRI often can confirm the presence of a paramedian pontine infarct.

In the thalamus, penetrating artery lesions most often involve the thalamogeniculate artery and its branches. The predominant resulting syndrome has been dubbed *pure sensory stroke* by Miller Fisher. In this syndrome, paresthesiae or numbness is noted in the face, arm, trunk, and lower extremity on one side of the body without other symptoms or signs. In some patients, the area of ischemia extends beyond the somatosensory thalamic nuclei (VPL and VPM), involving the motor connections from the striatum and cerebellum to the lateral thalamus. These patients have some ataxia and dystonic posturing or choreic movements on the same side as the sensory symptoms. When the adjacent posterior limb of the internal capsule is involved, a *sensory-motor stroke* results, with combined paresis and sensory loss without other findings. In patients with thalamogeniculate territory lateral thalamic infarcts, CT or MRI shows an infarct in the ventrolateral thalamus.

Occasionally, lipohyalinosis or atheromatous branch disease involves the polar (tuberothalamic) artery, which supplies the anterior and anterolateral portions of the thalamus. Infarction in this region causes a predominantly behavioral syndrome. Patients are apathetic, inert, and abulic. Usually there are no major motor, visual, or sensory abnormalities. Slight dysarthria may be present. There may be minor nonpyramidal motor abnormalities, such as decreased arm swing, in the contralateral limb. MRI shows infarction in the anterior portion of the thalamus (Fig. 6.24).

Patients with penetrating artery disease usually have predisposing conditions, such as hypertension or diabetes mellitus. The temporal profile may include stereotyped TIAs, sudden onset strokes, fluctuating signs, or stepwise accumulation of the deficit, but the full clinical syndrome usually evolves in less

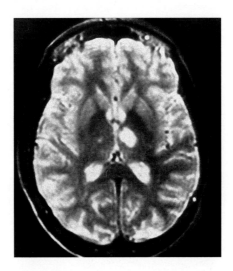

FIGURE 6.24 → MRI through thalamus shows infarct on right of section in the contralateral thalamus in the territory of the polar artery.

than 1 week. The symptoms, signs, and neuro-imaging abnormalities should be compatible with occlusion of a single penetrating artery branch. Extracranial and transcranial Doppler as well as MR angiography may help exclude occlusive disease of the parent vertebral, basilar, and posterior cerebral arteries in uncertain cases. Treatment consists of risk factor control. Some physicians also prescribe aspirin, although there is little theoretical or practical evidence that it prevents new lacunar infarcts.

TOP OF THE BASILAR ARTERY

The PCAs and penetrating arteries to the paramedian midbrain and thalamus arise from the BA apex (Fig. 6.25). Emboli to this site—either from the heart or the proximal vertebrobasilar arterial system—and less frequently, thrombosis engrafted upon previous athero-stenosis, produce characteristic neuroimaging and clinical findings. Midbrain, thalamic, and bilateral PCA territory infarction results (Fig. 6.26).

Bilateral rostral brainstem infarction affects alertness, behavior, memory, and oculomotor functions. Patients may initially be comatose or hyper-somnolent. When aroused or awakened, they are often confused and disoriented, and may have visual, auditory, and tactile hallucinations, especially in the evening or during the night. Memory is poor. Even when awake, patients are usually apathetic, with diminished spontaneous speech and behavior. The pupils may be small and poorly reactive. Vertical gaze paresis and hyperadduction of one or both eyes may be present, mimicking the well-known oculomotor abnormalities in patients with thalamic hemorrhages.

Bilateral PCA territory infarction may accompany the rostral brainstem ischemia, or may occur in isolation when an embolus blocks the distal BA. Bilateral PCA territory temporo-occipital lobe ischemia causes cortical blindness, amnesia, and a hyperactive, agitated state. The visual loss results from infarction of the striate cortex. The visual symptoms may be limited to one visual field (hemianopia) or may be bilateral but patchy. Often the infarction seems to emphasize the lower bank of the calcarine cortex bilaterally, causing an altitudinal loss of vision in the upper fields, as well as a loss of color perception and difficulty recognizing faces. Memory dysfunction results from infarction of the medial thalamus, the hippocampus, and adjacent medial temporal lobe structures.

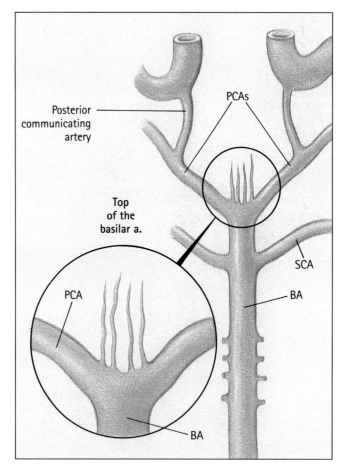

FIGURE 6.25 → Arteries arising from the BA apex to supply the midbrain and thalami.

Clinically, the memory loss produces a Korsakoff-like syndrome with inability to produce new memories, plus amnesia for recent events. Agitation and restlessness are due to involvement of limbic cortex in the fusiform and lingual gyri. The hyperactivity and delirium are often so severe that they overshadow the visual loss and amnesia, leading to a wrong diagnosis of an acute psychiatric or toxic disorder.

Usually the signs develop suddenly. CT and MRI show infarction in the rostral brainstem and bilateral PCA hemispheral territories. The PCA infarction can be unilateral; in some cases the infarct is limited to the upper brainstem. The most common etiology by far is embolism. Heparin should be administered. Cardiac evaluation, including electrocardiogram (ECG), echocardiography, and rhythm monitoring, should be performed. The proximal vertebrobasilar system is also evaluated using extracranial and transcranial ultrasound and, sometimes, MRA. Because the thalamic-subthalamic arteries that supply the posterior paramedian regions of the thalami sometimes originate from a single artery or an arterial ring (Fig. 6.27), bilateral thalamic infarction can occasionally be caused by atheromatous branch disease. Treatment depends on the nature of the vascular disease and the source of embolism.

POSTERIOR CEREBRAL ARTERY

The PCAs supply the occipital lobes, also the medial and inferior portions of the temporal lobes (Fig. 6.28). Unilateral infarction most often causes a hemianopia or a quadrantanopsia. Patients usually realize that they can't see to one side and are very much aware of the visual loss. The hemianopia usually spares the macular region. Despite the hemianopia, patients usually do not neglect objects in their blind fields. They read whole paragraphs, see features on both sides of pictures, and cross off or bisect lines on both sides of a page. Optokinetic nystagmus is usually preserved. When right PCA infarction is extensive, involving both the temporal and lower parietal lobes, left visual neglect is present in addition to the hemianopia. When infarction involves the left occipital lobe, including the white matter adjacent to the corpus callosum, the syndrome of alexia without agraphia is present. Although able to speak, spell, and write normally, the patients cannot read. They also are unable to name colors shown to them, but can match colors

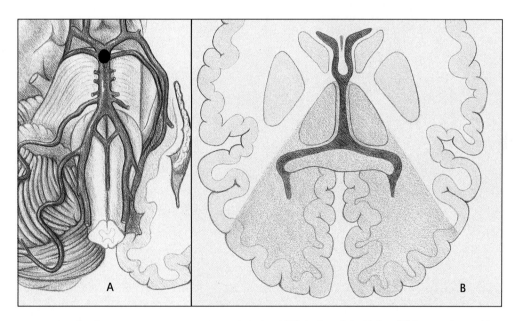

FIGURE 6.26 → Infarction in the bilateral thalami (**A**) and occipital lobes (**B**) in a patient with embolic occlusion of the distal BA.

and describe the colors of familiar objects. Patients with left PCA territory infarction involving the medial temporal lobe are often amnesic and cannot form new memories. The memory dysfunction usually subsides after about 6 months.

After visual loss, the most common symptoms are somatosensory. Paresthesiae and numbness usually involve the face, arm, leg, and trunk on the contralateral side of the body. On examination, various degrees of touch, pain, temperature, vibration, and position-sense loss are found. At times the sensory loss is severe. In some patients, the involved arm seems to have a mind of its own and levitates or moves by itself, sometimes getting caught or trapped in odd circumstances. The sensory dysfunction is due to involvement of the main sensory nuclei in the lateral thalamus, or to the thalamoparietal radiations from the medial and lateral thalamus travelling to the synapse in the postcentral gyrus and the sensory II area in the parietal operculum.

Unilateral PCA territory infarction is most often caused by embolism from the heart, aorta, or proximal vertebrobasilar system. Evaluation of the heart and proximal posterior circulation arteries is mandatory in all patients with PCA territory infarction. Treatment will depend on the location and nature of the embolic source. Occasionally, the proximal PCA is the site of intrinsic atherostenosis, especially in diabetics, blacks, Asians, and individuals with extensive atherosclerosis of the more proximal extracranial and intracranial arteries. When PCA infarction is caused by intrinsic PCA stenosis, spells of hemianopic visual loss

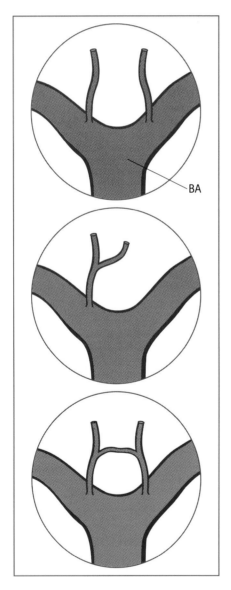

BA

FIGURE 6.27 → Diagrams showing the various types of thalamosubthalamic artery branching from the BA. In the top figure, one artery rises from each side. In the middle, an artery from one side branches to supply each side. On the bottom, branches from each side form an arcade artery that supplies both sides.

and transient hemisensory symptoms commonly precede the stroke. MRA or standard angiography are usually needed to define the lesion. Aspirin is given for minor degrees of stenosis. Warfarin is employed for severe stenosis if important at-risk tissue remains uninfarcted, but is almost useless if a severe hemianopia is already present. Migraine can also lead to PCA territory infarction, often in association with thrombosis within the PCA.

CONCLUSION

Vascular lesions at various sites within the posterior circulation cause recognizable clinical syndromes. Neuroimaging tests, especially MRI, help localize the process within the brain. Cardiac evaluation, including ECG, echocardiography, and rhythm monitoring, is important in nearly all patients with posterior circulation disease. The heart is a common donor source for embolism. Atherosclerosis within the major vertebrobasilar arteries is often associated with coronary and peripheral vascular occlusive disease. Ultrasound of the extracranial subclavian and vertebral arteries, as well as TCD of the intracranial vertebral and basilar arteries and the PCAs, helps define stenosis, occlusion, and patterns of collateral flow in the posterior circulation. MRA and standard angiography usually allow definition of the occlusive vascular lesions. Medical and surgical management consists of risk factor control and treating the specific stroke mechanism found in the individual patient.

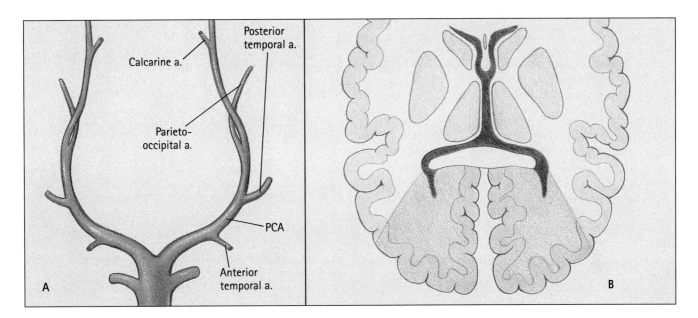

FIGURE 6.28 → **A,** PCA branches. **B,** Regions that the PCAs supply (shaded).

REFERENCES

Caplan LR. The 1991 E Graeme Robertson lecture: verte-brobasilar embolism. *Clin Exp Neurol.* 1991.

Caplan LR. Top of the basilar syndrome: selected clinical aspects. *Neurology.* 1980; 30:72–79.

Caplan LR. Vertebrobasilar occlusive disease. In: Barnett HJ, Mohr JP, Stein B, Yatsu F (eds). *Stroke: Pathophysiology, Diagnosis, and Management.* New York: Churchill-Livingstone, 1985; 549–620.

Caplan LR. Vertebrobasilar systems syndromes. In: Vinken P, Bruyn G, Klawans H (eds). *Handbook of Clinical Neurology* (revised series) Toole J, Ed. Cerebrovascular Disease (part 1), Amsterdam: North Amsterdam Publishing Co., 1989; 53:371–408.

Caplan LR, Amarenco P, Rosengart A, et al. Embolism from vertebral artery origin occlusive disease. *Neurology.* 1992; 42:1505-1512.

Caplan LR, Baquis GD, Pessin MS, et al. Dissection of the intracranial vertebral artery. *Neurology.* 1988; 38:867–877.

Caplan LR, Tettenborn B. Vertebrobasilar occlusive disease: review of selected aspects. Part 1: Spontaneous dissec-tion of extracranial and intracranial posterior circulation arteries. *Cerebrovasc Dis.* 1992; 2:256–265.

Caplan LR, Zarins C, Hemmatti M. Spontaneous dissection of the extracranial vertebral artery. *Stroke.* 1985; 16:1030–1038.

Gorelick PB, Caplan LR, Hier DB, et al. Racial differences in the distribution of posterior circulation occlusive dis-ease. *Stroke.* 1985; 16:785–790.

Hennerici M, Klemm C, Rautenberg W. The subclavian steal phenomenon: a common vascular disorder with rare neurologic deficits. *Neurology.* 1988; 38:669–673.

Koroshetz WJ, Ropper AH. Artery-to-artery embolism caus-ing stroke in the posterior circulation. *Neurology.* 1987; 37:292–296.

Kubik C, Adams RD. Occlusion of the basilar artery: a clini-cal and pathological study. *Brain.* 1946; 69:73–121.

Pelouze GA. Plaque ulcerie de l'ostium de l'artere verte-brale. *Rev Neurol* (Paris). 1989; 145:478–481.

Pessin MS, Kwan E, DeWitt LD, et al. Posterior cerebral artery stenosis. *Ann Neurol.* 1987; 21:85–89.

Pessin MS, Lathi E, Cohen MB, et al. Clinical features and mechanisms of occipital infarction in the posterior cerebral artery territory. *Ann Neurol.* 1987; 21:290–299.

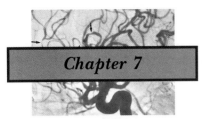

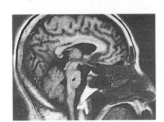

Chapter 7

KAZUO MINEMATSU

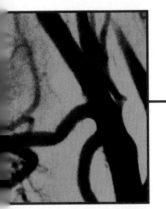

Cardioembolic Stroke

AN EMBOLISM IS A SUDDEN BLOCKAGE of an artery or vein by an obstruction that is carried into place by flowing blood (Figs. 7.1, 7.2). Although brain embolism was described clinically and pathologically over 150 years ago, cardioembolic stroke, a brain embolism of cardiac or transcardiac origin, has been considered as a common cause of ischemic stroke for only a couple of decades. The increased recognition is probably related to an enhanced awareness of potential cardiac source of emboli and improved technology to document cardiac abnormalities associated with embolization. In the *Classification of Cerebrovascular Diseases III,* reported in 1990 by the Ad Hoc Committee of the National Institute of Neurological Disorders and Stroke, cardioembolic stroke is described as one of three major clinical categories of brain infarction. Brain embolism caused by thrombus or microthrombus from a diseased arterial wall is also an important mechanism of transient ischemic attack (TIA) or brain infarction in patients with atherothrombotic arterial lesions. It should be separated from cardioembolic stroke, however, because of differences in etiologic mechanisms, clinical features, diagnostic tests, and preventive measures.

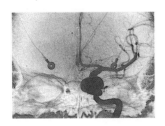

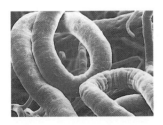

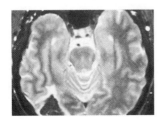

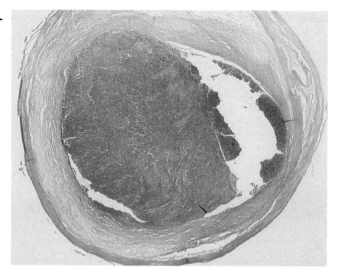

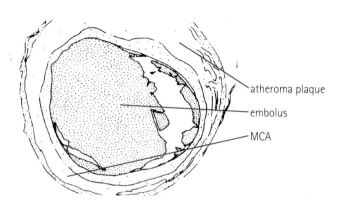

atheroma plaque

embolus

MCA

FIGURE 7.1 → This pathologic specimen shows a large embolus occluding the main trunk of the middle cerebral artery (MCA) with a minimal underlying atheroma.

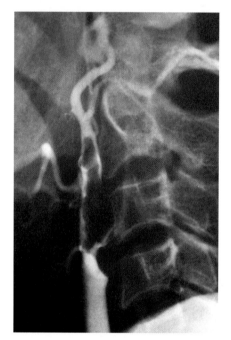

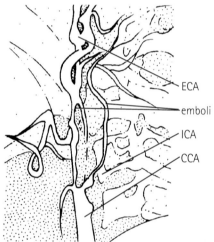

ECA

emboli

ICA

CCA

FIGURE 7.2 → Multiple occlusions of the internal and external carotid arteries (ICA, ECA) just distal to the common carotid bifurcation from cardiac emboli can be seen on this carotid angiogram. (CCA=common carotid artery)

FIGURE 7.3 → PREDISPOSING FACTORS FOR EMBOLIZATION FROM THE HEART

INTRACARDIAC THROMBUS FORMATION
Intracardiac blood stasis
Endothelial disruption
Systemic coagulopathy

INTRAVENEOUS THROMBUS FORMATION (BLOOD STASIS, ENDOTHELIAL DISRUPTION, AND COAGULOPATHY)
Intracardiac shunt (paradoxical embolism)

VALVULAR VEGETATION

INTRACARDIAC TUMOR

Of the 450,000 new strokes in the United States each year, approximately 85% are ischemic in origin. Cardioembolic stroke represents roughly 15% to 20% of ischemic strokes in recent clinical surveys, whereas autopsy studies indicate that 20% to 30% of ischemic strokes are of cardiac origin. The discrepancy may be explained by the higher mortality of cardioembolic stroke in comparison with other ischemic strokes. Younger patients with ischemic stroke and TIA are more susceptible to cardioembolic stroke than are older stroke patients; 23% to 36% of them are presumed to suffer from emboli of either a cardiac or transcardiac origin.

PATHOPHYSIOLOGY

INTRACARDIAC THROMBUS FORMATION
Intracardiac thrombus formation is unlikely under normal cardiac conditions, but certain abnormalities predispose to its development (Fig. 7.3). Intracardiac blood stasis—which may accompany atrial fibrillation (AF), acute myocardial infarction, ventricular aneurysm, and cardiomyopathy—is a predisposing factor, as are endothelial disruption and systemic coagulopathy. Endothelial disruption is particularly important in acute myocardial infarction or with a prosthetic cardiac valve. Systemic coagulopathy is a major influence in nonbacterial thrombotic endocarditis. Valvular vegetations associated with infective

endocarditis and intracardiac tumors, such as atrial myxoma, may dislodge into the blood stream, leading to arterial occlusion. Increasing evidence suggests that paradoxical embolism, an arterial embolism of venous origin that traverses an intracardiac shunt, occurs more frequently than previously considered. This mechanism appears to be particularly important in younger patients.

SITES OF OCCLUSION
Emboli in arteries travel primarily within the central current of blood flow and not peripherally. If an arterial branch is at a right angle to or is much smaller than the parent artery, only the peripheral layer of intraluminal flow enters the branch. This tendency explains the predominance of embolism to the middle cerebral artery (MCA) as compared to the anterior cerebral artery (ACA). Embolic occlusion is frequently documented just prior to sites of arterial branching, such as the tip of the internal carotid artery (ICA), the trifurcation of the MCA, and the top of the basilar artery (BA). Because the diameter of branches at these sites is considerably smaller than that of the parent artery, further passage of the clot may be prevented. Foci of atheroma at curves in an artery are another site where embolic material may arrest. In other cases, emboli stop at distal intracranial arterial branches (Fig. 7.4). The predominant sites of arterial occlusion with emboli can be con-

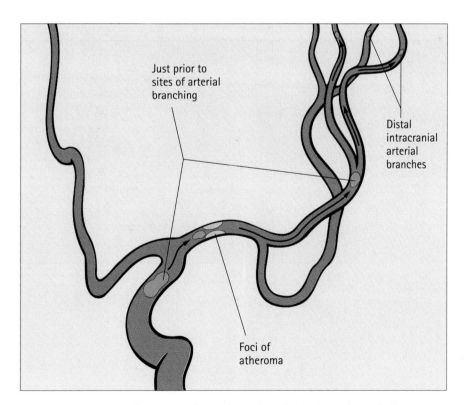

FIGURE 7.4 → Predominant sites of arterial occlusion by emboli.

trasted to the typical location of atheroma, which usually occur at proximal portions of the ICA, the trunk of the MCA, and the proximal BA (Fig. 7.5). Occlusion by emboli may take place at several distal arterial branches or even in multiple vascular territories, usually caused by a number of embolic fragments or repeated embolization. Consequently, a series of brain infarcts involving the cortex or cerebellum in several vascular territories is highly suggestive of cardioembolic stroke. Although the deep perforating arteries are particularly vulnerable to hypertensive arteriopathy, cardioembolic events may involve the origins of the perforating arteries, resulting in a subcortical infarct (Figs. 7.6, 7.7). A recent report found that 17 out of 100 patients with a subcortical infarct had a cardiac source of embolus.

VANISHING OCCLUSION

Embolic fragments occluding brain vessels may be dissolved and fragmented by intrinsic thrombolytic mechanisms, migrate to distal branches, and finally disappear within hours or days. These "vanishing occlusions" or "reopening of an occluded artery" are uncommon with other causes of ischemic stroke, but are frequently observed (up to 95%) in patients with cardioembolic stroke (Fig. 7.8).

HEMORRHAGIC TRANSFORMATION

Petechial hemorrhages or hematomas may occur within an infarction (Fig. 7.9). This pathologic change, hemorrhagic infarct, or hemorrhagic transformation, is characteristic of cardioembolic stroke and was once believed to be diagnostic. The frequency of hemorrhagic transformation in cardioembolic stroke has been reported as 51% to 78% in autopsy studies, and 2% to 50% on CT studies. Distal migration of embolic fragments with reperfusion of infarcted tissue is a hypothetical mechanism of hemorrhagic transformation. The reperfusion may result in leakage of blood across the vascular endothelium damaged by ischemia, producing varying degrees of hemorrhagic infarction (Fig. 7.10). However, a recent autopsy study demonstrated that hemorrhagic transformation can occur in areas distal to persistent embolic arterial occlusion. Leptomeningeal collaterals are the only possible route of reperfusion to the necrotic area in this circumstance. Hemorrhagic transformation appears to occur less frequently in atherothrombotic brain infarction (2–21% in autopsy series). Although hemorrhagic infarction per se is not specific for cardioembolic stroke, hemorrhagic infarctions with cardioembolic stroke occur more frequently, are more dense, and involve larger areas deep within the infarct than those caused by other mechanisms. Subcortical hemorrhagic infarcts seem to be highly indicative of cardioembolic stroke. Larger areas of infarction and older age appear to be associated with a higher incidence of hemorrhagic transformation. Massive hemorrhagic transformation causing a globular parenchymal hemorrhage that resembles primary

FIGURE 7.5 → SITES OF ARTERIAL OCCLUSION

	CARDIOEMBOLIC	ATHEROTHROMBOTIC*
Extracranial (proximal) carotid artery	6 (5%)	30 (32%)
Intracranial (distal) carotid artery	28 (26%)	9 (9%)
Middle cerebral artery, trunk	26 (25%)	45 (47%)
Middle cerebral artery, branch	46 (43%)	11 (12%)
Total	106	95

*The incidence of intracranial atherothrombotic arterial lesions is higher in Japan than in the North America and Europe.

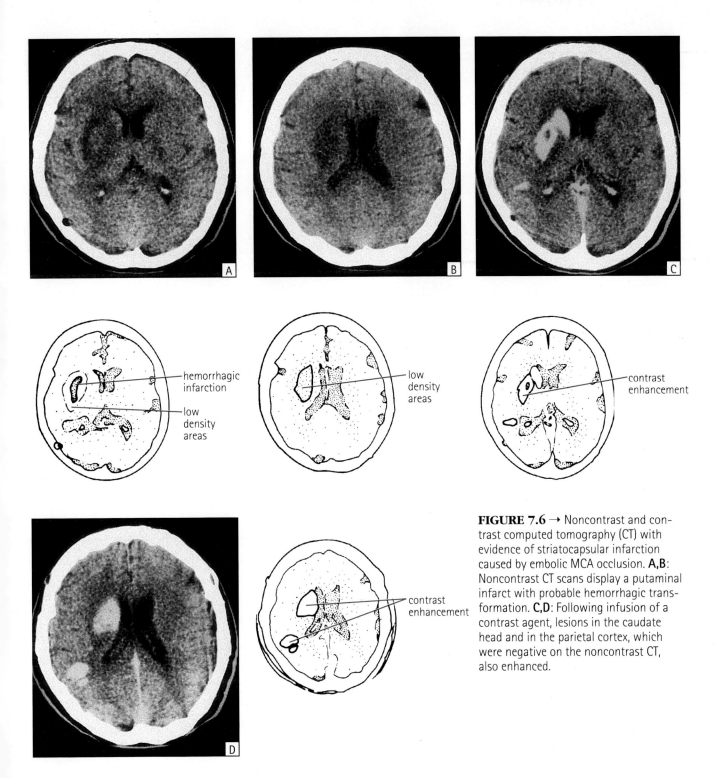

FIGURE 7.6 → Noncontrast and contrast computed tomography (CT) with evidence of striatocapsular infarction caused by embolic MCA occlusion. **A,B**: Noncontrast CT scans display a putaminal infarct with probable hemorrhagic transformation. **C,D**: Following infusion of a contrast agent, lesions in the caudate head and in the parietal cortex, which were negative on the noncontrast CT, also enhanced.

hemorrhagic infarction

low density areas

low density areas

contrast enhancement

contrast enhancement

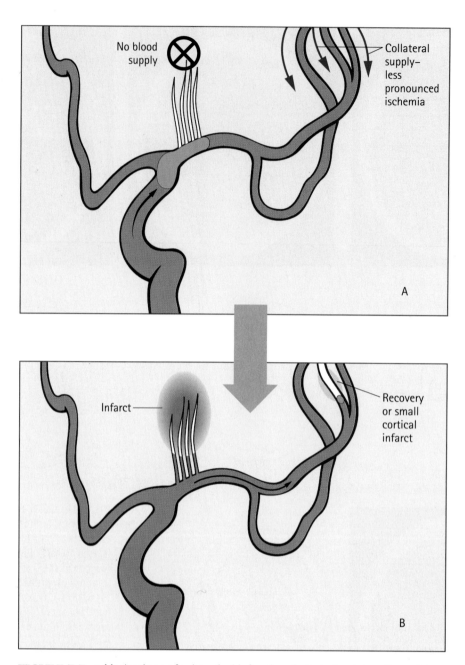

FIGURE 7.7 → Mechanisms of subcortical infarction. **A**, Embolic obstruction of the lateral striate arteries. **B**, Embolic migrations leading to recovery in cortical, but not subcortical, regions.

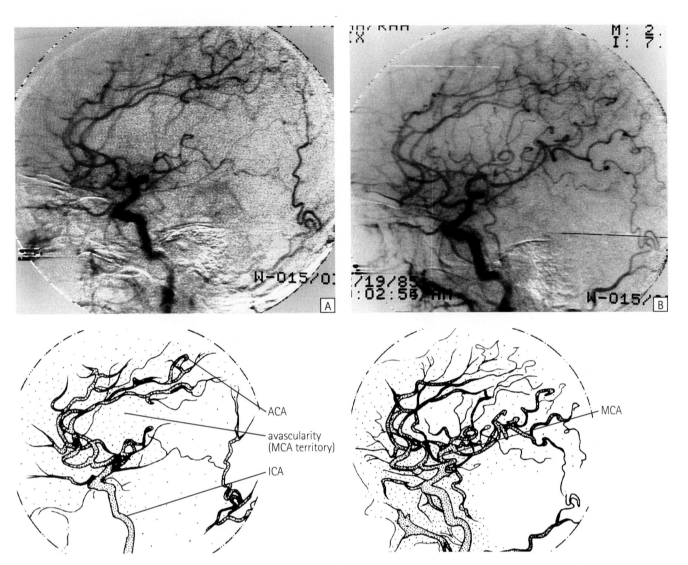

ACA

avascularity
(MCA territory)

ICA

MCA

FIGURE 7.8 → Angiographic evidence of vanishing occlusion. **A**, Initial angiogram on the day of stroke onset demonstrates multiple MCA occlusions. **B**, Follow-up angiogram 3 months later reveals normal arteries, indicating complete reopening of previously occluded arteries.

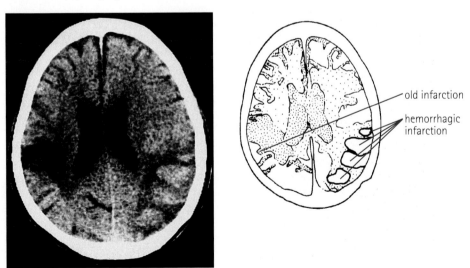

old infarction

hemorrhagic
infarction

FIGURE 7.9 → CT appearance of a hemorrhagic infarct in a patient with cardioembolic stroke. Contralateral hypodensity corresponds to a previous episode of cardioembolic stroke.

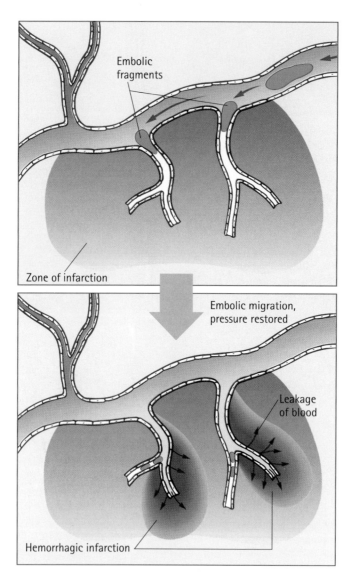

Embolic fragments

Zone of infarction

Embolic migration, pressure restored

Leakage of blood

Hemorrhagic infarction

FIGURE 7.10 → A hypothetical mechanism of hemorrhagic transformation.

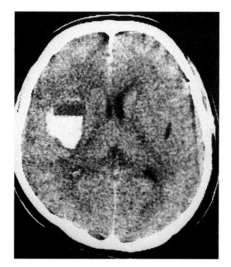

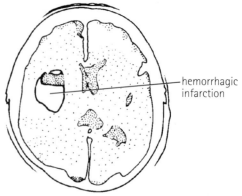

hemorrhagic infarction

FIGURE 7.11 → Massive hemorrhagic transformation, observed in a patient treated with anticoagulants.

intracerebral hematoma is observed in approximately 10% of hemorrhagic infarctions, and is more likely to occur in patients treated with anticoagulants (Fig. 7.11).

CARDIAC EVALUATION

There are no absolutely valid criteria to conclusively establish the diagnosis of cardioembolic stroke. The diagnosis is made by confirming the presence of several suggestive features. The presence of a potential cardiac or transcardiac source of emboli is a prerequisite for diagnosis. The common cardiac sources of emboli are outlined in Figure 7.12, and will be discussed in subsequent sections. Identifying these sources depends on how carefully patients are evalu-

ated (Fig. 7.13). A standard chest x-ray and electrocardiogram (ECG) in addition to a routine physical examination should be performed to detect cardiac abnormalities. Prolonged ECG monitoring, up to 48 hours, is recommended to uncover episodic cardiac arrythmias such as paroxysmal atrial fibrillation (AF) and the sick sinus syndrome (SSS) in selected patients, especially those under age 50. Transthoracic echocardiography may detect clinically silent cardiac diseases. These examinations do not often find unsuspected arrythmias (0–4%) or organic cardiac diseases (0–6%) when performed in consecutive patients with acute ischemic stroke or TIA. Therefore, definitive recommendations concerning the use of echocar-

FIGURE 7.12 → POTENTIAL CARDIAC SOURCES OF EMBOLISM

COMMON SOURCES
- Nonvalvular atrial fibrillation (NVAF)
- Sick sinus syndrome (SSS)
- Acute myocardial infarction
- Left ventricular aneurysm
- Nonischemic cardiomyopathy
- Rheumatic heart disease
- Prosthetic cardiac valves
- Mitral valve prolapse (MVP)
- Infective endocarditis
- Cardiac diseases with intracardiac shunt (paradoxical embolism), patent foramen ovale, atrial septal defect, etc.

LESS COMMON SOURCES
- Nonbacterial endocarditis (NBTE)
- Myxomas
- Mitral annuls calcification
- Calcific aortic stenosis
- Atrial septal defect

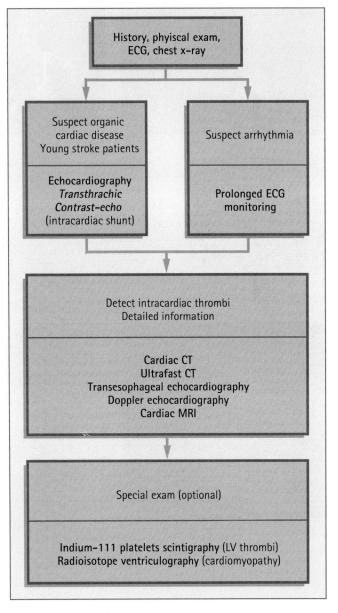

FIGURE 7.13 → Algorithm for cardiac evaluations of patients with presumed cardioembolic stroke.

diography and prolonged ECG monitoring cannot be made. Routine echocardiographic examination is recommended for ischemic stroke patients younger than 50 years because they are susceptible to cardioembolic stroke. Transthoracic echocardiography is relatively insensitive to detecting small intraventricular and atrial thrombi. Transesophageal echocardiography and ultrafast CT have recently been reported to be more sensitive in detecting potential cardiac sources and intracardiac thrombi (Fig. 7.14). Especially when the trans-

esophageal approach is taken, contrast echocardiography using saline, glucose, or a gelatinous solution containing air microbubbles injected intravenously can detect a patent foramen ovale—a potential cause of paradoxical embolism in young stroke patients who lack an obvious stroke mechanism. Patients with a potential cardiac source of brain embolism sometimes (13–48%) have concomitant cerebrovascular arterial lesions that could also be responsible for the brain ischemia. Six to 25% of patients with a suspected car-

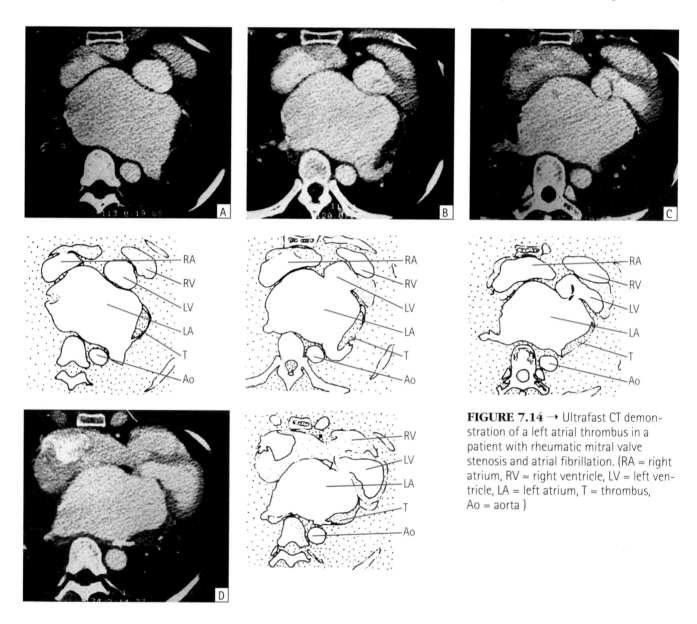

FIGURE 7.14 → Ultrafast CT demonstration of a left atrial thrombus in a patient with rheumatic mitral valve stenosis and atrial fibrillation. (RA = right atrium, RV = right ventricle, LV = left ventricle, LA = left atrium, T = thrombus, Ao = aorta)

dioembolic stroke have no obvious cardiac source despite an extensive search.

NEUROLOGIC EVALUATION

Individual neurologic features of the stroke do not usually identify the stroke mechanism.

Most of the clinical features that were considered relatively specific for cardioembolic stroke are also commonly observed in patients with other types of ischemic stroke, and therefore are not pathognomonic for cardioembolic stroke. The only clinical features correlating with the presence of a cardiac source of emboli are the abrupt onset of neurologic deficits, diminished level of consciousness at stroke onset, and a history of systemic embolism. Abrupt onset of the maximal neurologic deficit is frequently listed on diagnostic criteria for cardioembolic stroke. Although clinical symptoms and signs develop suddenly in the majority of patients, approximately 5% to 20% of patients develop symptoms gradually or intermittently at onset. The "nonsudden" onset is probably attributable to repeated embolization at short intervals or to changes in the cerebral circulatory status following distal migration of embolic materials. Approximately 40% of patients with other causes for ischemic stroke may also present with the sudden onset of deficits. Although a diminished level of consciousness at onset and a history of systemic embolization are significantly more frequent in patients with a high risk for cardioembolic stroke, these historical features are not often encountered (29% and 5%, respectively). Activity at onset, seizure at onset, headache, vomiting, or the presence of an isolated deficit, which were previously considered specific for embolic stroke, have been reported as infrequent and have no diagnostic value for conclusively establishing the presence of cardioembolic stroke.

Atherothrombotic and lacunar infarction may be preceded by TIAs, but they occur less frequently prior to cardioembolic stroke (11–30%). In a clinical study, 23% of 250 carotid TIA patients had a potential cardiac source of emboli. Multiple ipsilateral TIAs are more likely to precede atherothrombotic brain infarction, but a history of TIAs in multiple vascular territories suggests cardioembolic rather than atherothrombotic stroke.

More than 70% of cardioembolic strokes occur in the MCA territory. The posterior branches of the MCA are more frequently involved by embolic occlusion than the anterior branches. This observation explains why isolated Wernicke's aphasia and an acute confusional state, which correspond to cortical damage in the left and right posterior MCA territories, predominate in cardioembolic stroke. Global aphasia without hemiparesis, caused by two separate infarct foci involving both the Broca and Wernicke areas, appears to be specific for cardioembolic stroke. Rapid recovery from a major hemispheric syndrome at onset, "spectacular shrinking deficit," has recently been reported to occur in some patients with cardioembolic stroke. A rapidly migrating embolus, which initially lodges in the ICA or the trunk of the MCA, is the mechanism for this phenomenon. Occlusion at the top of the BA is more common with cardioembolic than atherothrombotic brain infarction. Combinations of characteristic oculomotor, visual, and neuropsychologic deficits, called "top of the basilar" syndrome by Caplan, indicate cardioembolic stroke. Isolated PCA syndromes are most often cardioembolic.

BRAIN IMAGING AND ANGIOGRAPHY

Imaging studies of the brain with computed tomography (CT) and magnetic resonance imaging (MRI) often provide suggestive evidence of a cardioembolic stroke, such as infarction in other vascular territories, visualization of embolic material in the brain vessels, and hemorrhagic infarction. The early CT finding of a hyperdense portion of the MCA in patients with acute supratentorial infarction, which is called "hyperdense MCA sign," often indicates an embolic occlusion (Fig. 7.15). In approximately 20% of cardioembolic strokes, CT taken within 2 to 4 days after stroke onset shows hyperdensity within a hypodense infarct area, evidence of hemorrhagic transformation. Cerebral angiography may demonstrate intraluminal defects representing embolic fragments within a couple of days after stroke onset (see Fig. 7.2). More than 70% of embolic occlusions can be displayed within the first

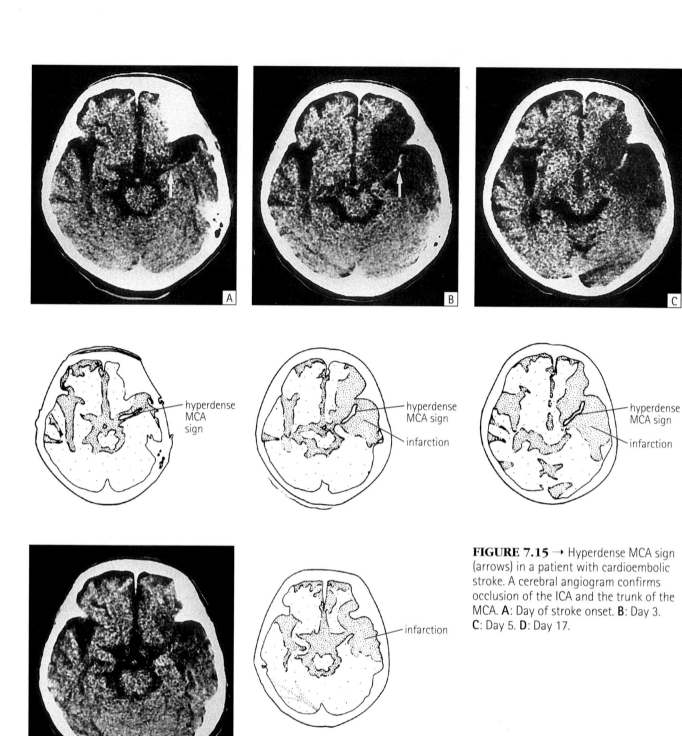

FIGURE 7.15 → Hyperdense MCA sign (arrows) in a patient with cardioembolic stroke. A cerebral angiogram confirms occlusion of the ICA and the trunk of the MCA. **A**: Day of stroke onset. **B**: Day 3. **C**: Day 5. **D**: Day 17.

2 days, whereas angiograms after the second day show an occlusion in less than 30% of patients. These vanishing occlusions can be documented by repeat angiography (up to 95%), and strongly suggest embolism (see Fig. 7.8). A normal angiogram, without evidence of arterial pathology, may offer some indirect support for a cardioembolic stroke if patients have cortical or cerebellar infarcts, a potential cardiac source, or both. Distal branch occlusion without ipsilateral, proximal, atherosclerotic lesions also suggests a cardioembolic mechanism. Cerebral angiography may be valuable in establishing the cause of stroke as cardioembolic, but it is invasive and cannot be routinely recommended. Magnetic resonance angiography can display vascular pathology noninvasively, and may soon become the procedure of choice for demonstrating embolic arterial occlusion.

DIAGNOSTIC CRITERIA

A large number of diagnostic criteria for cardioembolic stroke have been suggested in the literature (Fig. 7.16). A potential cardiac source of emboli and the abrupt onset of maximal deficit are included in almost all criteria. Multiple brain infarcts, hemorrhagic infarcts, van-

ishing occlusion, branch occlusion, and systemic embolism are also frequently suggested. It should be emphasized that there is no absolute gold standard for diagnosing cardioembolic stroke. The history, physical examination, and the results of appropriate laboratory evaluation should lead the clinician to an educated best approximation of diagnosis.

CARDIAC SOURCES

NONVALVULAR ATRIAL FIBRILLATION

Nonvalvular (nonrheumatic) atrial fibrillation (NVAF) is the most common cardiac disorder responsible for cardioembolic stroke, accounting for approximately 45% of cardioembolic stroke patients in recent clinical studies. NVAF affects 3% of the population over 65 years of age. The Framingham study reported that NVAF patients have a fivefold increased risk of cerebral infarction and that more than two thirds of their strokes are due to cardiac embolism. The annual stroke incidence in NVAF patients is 5% (2.8–8.8%). Approximately one third of all patients with NVAF will experience a stroke if preventive measures are not employed. NVAF is one of the most important risks

---

FIGURE 7.16 → DIAGNOSTIC CRITERIA FOR CARDIOEMBOLIC STROKE

A. PRIMARY
   Potential cardiac or transcardiac source of emboli

B. SECONDARY
   Abrupt onset of maximal neurological deficit
   Evidence of embolism to other organs
   Evidence suggesting embolic infarcts with a brain imaging study (CT, MRI)
   • Multiple cortical or cerebellar infarcts in multiple vascular territories
   • Hemorrhagic infarcts
   Angiographic evidence suggesting embolic occlusion
   • Vanishing occlusion
   • Distal branch occlusion
   • Intraluminal filling defect presenting embolic fragments

C. SUPPLEMENTARY
   A history of TIAs in multiple vascular territories
   Specific stroke syndromes
      • Global aphasia without hemiparesis, spectacular shrinking deficit, top of the basilar syndrome, and isolated posterior cerebral artery syndrome
   Absence of atherosclerotic vascular disease by angiography

DIAGNOSIS OF CARDIOEMBOLIC STROKE, MOST LIKELY:
A + more than 2 items of B
A + single item of B + more than 2 items of C

DIAGNOSIS OF CARDIOEMBOLIC STROKE, POSSIBLE:
A + single item of B

for stroke in the elderly because it is associated with more than one third of their strokes. The cardiovascular conditions that most often coexist with NVAF are hypertension and ischemic heart disease. Some NVAF-patient subgroups, which may have increased stroke risk, are older patients, those with congestive heart failure, coronary heart disease, a history of prior stroke (and silent stroke on CT), or intracardiac thrombus. In contrast, idiopathic AF (lone AF), which is defined as AF in predominantly young men without clinical, ECG, or chest x-ray evidence of other heart disease, is associated with a very low risk of stroke (0.5%/y in patients under age 60 at diagnosis). Although intracardiac thrombus formation predisposes patients with NVAF to cardioembolic stroke, transthoracic echocardiography (TTE) can detect left atrial thrombi in only 30% of patients when examined after stroke. Transesophageal echocardiography (TEE) can detect thrombi more accurately (sensitivity 89%) than TTE (56%).

SICK SINUS SYNDROME

Another important arrythmia that causes embolic stroke, SSS increases the risk from 8% to 10% per year. SSS patients with the greatest risk for embolization have brady-tachyarrhythmias. It should be noted that SSS is commonly associated with AF. Although a ven-

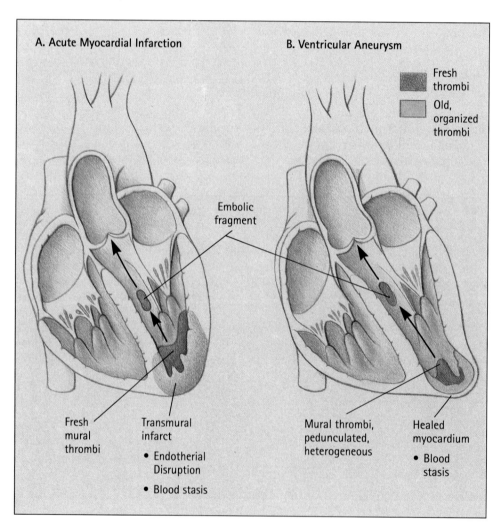

FIGURE 7.17 → Intracardiac thrombus formation and embolization in acute myocardial infarction (**A**) and ventricular aneurysm (**B**) .

tricular demand cardiac pacemaker can prevent bradycardias that result in Stokes-Adams attack, it may cause an increase in embolization for SSS patients. Sequential cardiac pacing may be more appropriate, as it may reduce stroke incidence.

ACUTE MYOCARDIAL INFARCTION AND VENTRICULAR ANEURYSM

Acute myocardial infarction causes approximately 15% of all cardioembolic strokes, next in frequency to NVAF. One to 6% of patients with acute myocardial infarction experience clinically evident systemic embolism. Mural thombi are detected in 10% to 17% of patients with transmural myocardial infarction, and are more frequent in anterior wall infarction (30–56%) than in inferior wall infarction (0–4%). Strokes complicate about 6% of cases in the former, but only 1% in the latter. Mural thrombi usually develop within 7 days following an acute myocardial infarction. Embolic stroke is most likely to occur within the initial 4 weeks. Although chronic myocardial infarction is less likely to cause embolization, patients with ventricular aneurysm have a potential for embolic stroke of app-roximately 13% over their lifetimes (0.35%/patient/y), and account for 10% of all cardioembolic stroke (Fig. 7.17). Mural thrombi within an aneurysm do not always predict the potential for future embolization. Pedunculated, mobile, or heterogeneous thrombi are more apt to embolize than flat homogeneous thrombi and may warrant anticoagulation.

NONISCHEMIC CARDIOMYOPATHY

Brain embolism is not rare in patients with nonischemic cardiomyopathy (idiopathic, peripartum, alcoholic, with cardiac amyloidosis, Chagas disease, or endocardial fibroelastosis). An echocardiographic study revealed a 36% incidence of left ventricular thrombus, usually accompanied by globally impaired ventricular contractility. Embolism has been reported in 18% of patients with dilated cardiomyopathy who do not receive anticoagulants, or up to 12% per year. Brain embolism can be the presenting feature of cardiomyopathy. Despite the lack of prospective studies, the general consensus is that long-term anticoagulation is indicated even if left ventricular thrombi are not demonstrated, especially if AF is present.

RHEUMATIC HEART DISEASE

Rheumatic heart disease, particularly mitral valvular disease with AF, was the most important cause of cardioembolic stroke several decades ago, and is still a major factor in countries where the disease is prevalent. An epidemiologic survey revealed that rheumatic heart disease associated with AF has a 17-fold risk increase of brain infarction as compared with a normal age-matched control population. About 20% of unanticoagulated patients with mitral stenosis experience embolism over their lifetimes, with 60% to 75% having a brain embolism.

PROSTHETIC CARDIAC VALVE

Since the advent of cardiac valve replacement as an important approach for treating several valvular diseases, including rheumatic heart disease, prosthetic cardiac valves have become one of the common causes of embolic stroke. Patients with a mechanical valve in the mitral position have the greatest risk of emboli and need long-term anticoagulation. Anticoagulation is recommended for the first few months for patients with bioprosthetic valves, especially if they have concommitant AF.

MITRAL VALVE PROLAPSE

Mitral valve prolapse (MVP), a myxomatous degeneration of the valve leaflet, leads to a redundancy and prolapse of the valve during systole, and was recently recognized as a potential embolic source for young stroke patients (Fig. 7.18). Although this abnormality occurs in 5% to 10% of the population, predominantly women (F:M ratio, 7.6%:2.5%), it is found in up to 40% of stroke patients under 45 years of age. The true incidence of embolic events in the MVP population is much lower, probably only 1/6000/y. Emboli from MVP are generally transient, reflecting the small size of the thrombi arising from this valvular degeneration.

PATENT FORAMEN OVALE AND PARADOXICAL EMBOLISM

Paradoxical embolism can be diagnosed if patients have venous thrombosis or pulmonary embolism, arterial embolism without a cardiac embolic source, and a right-to-left cardiac shunt (Fig. 7.19). The incidence of paradoxical embolism has probably been underestimated because of clinically silent venous thrombosis or pulmonary embolism, and because detecting a right-to-left cardiac shunt is difficult. Since color Doppler or contrast transesophageal echocardiography began to be used for detecting intracardiac shunt, physiologic shunting via a patent foramen ovale (PFO) has been recognized more often in normal people (10–18%). PFO is detected in 40% to 58% of young stroke or TIA patients, versus 10% of age-matched controls (Fig. 7.20). This anomaly must be searched for in young stroke patients without an

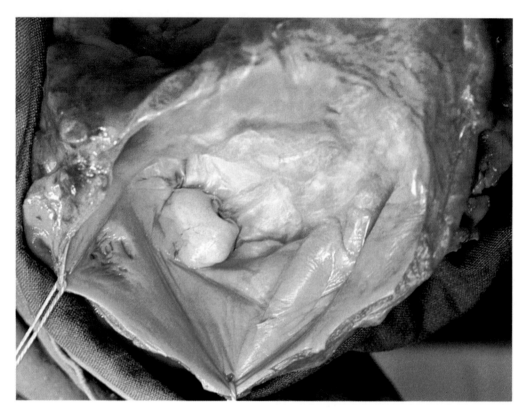

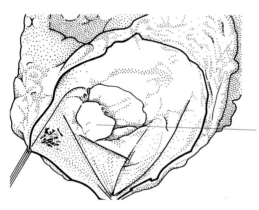

FIGURE 7.18 → A prolapsed mitral valve observed from the left atrium. (From Perkin GD, 1986)

prolapsed mitral valve

apparent cause of stroke. Contrast echocardiography, particularly with the transesophageal approach, should be used whenever possible.

INFECTIVE ENDOCARDITIS

Approximately 20% (13–33%) of patients with infective endocarditis experience an embolic stroke (Fig. 7.21). A study reported that 74% of ischemic strokes had occured by the time of presentation and an additional 13% occurred less than 48 hours after diagnosis of infective endocarditis. Intracerebral or subarachnoid hemorrhage may also occur in patients with infective endocarditis, secondary to hemorrhagic transformation of embolic infarct or rupture of mycotic aneurysms. Serial blood cultures are essential for diagnosis and treatment. Emboli frequently

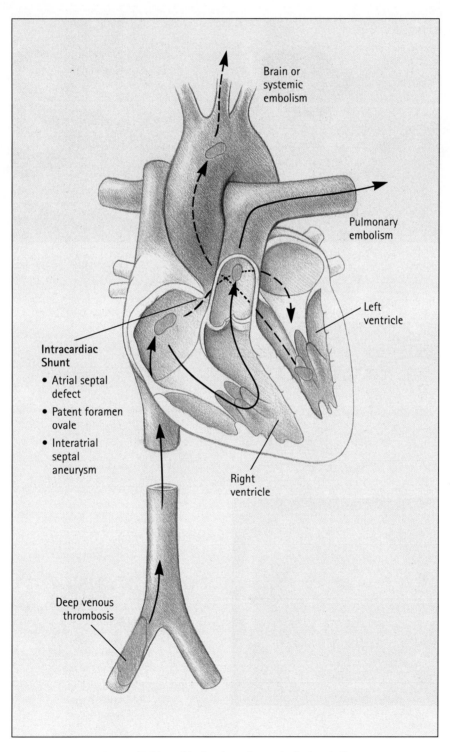

FIGURE 7.19 → Mechanism of paradoxical embolism.

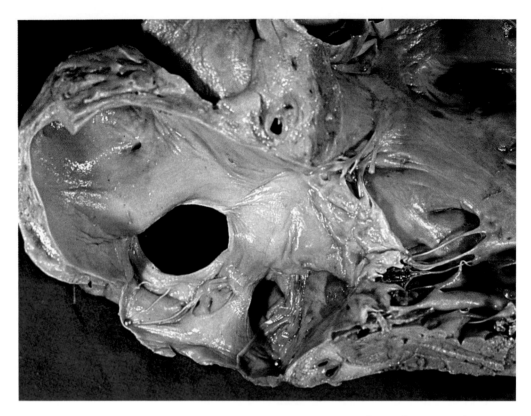

FIGURE 7.20 → Patent foramen ovale observed from the right atrium. (From Perkin GD, 1986)

right atrium

tricuspid valve

foramen ovale

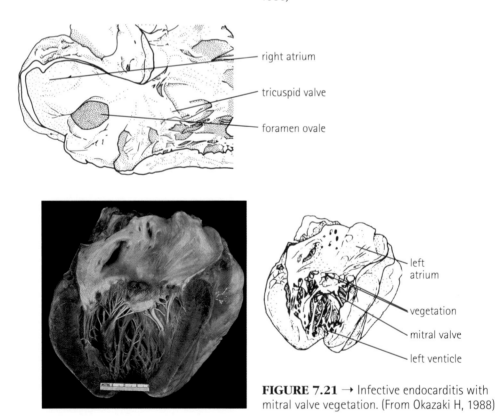

left atrium

vegetation

mitral valve

left venticle

FIGURE 7.21 → Infective endocarditis with mitral valve vegetation. (From Okazaki H, 1988)

accompany fungal and Staphylococcal infections. Echocardiography can identify vegetations as small as 2 mm and may establish the diagnosis. Vegetations detected by echocardiography are associated with an increasing risk of embolic stroke. Aortic valve vegetations have a higher incidence of embolization than other valves (44% vs. 5%). Antibiotic therapy is definitely recommended, but emergency broad-spectrum antibiotic therapy should be delayed until samples for blood culture have been obtained. Valve replacement may be indicated in patients with severe congestive heart failure, uncontrolled sepsis, and persistent embolization. Anticoagulant therapy should be avoided early in the course of native valve endocarditis because evidence suggests an unacceptably high incidence of hemorrhagic central nervous complications.

NONBACTERIAL THROMBOTIC ENDOCARDITIS
Nonbacterial thrombotic endocarditis (NBTE) should always be suspected when ischemic stroke occurs in patients with malignancy or a chronic wasting illness. The incidence of embolic stroke in patients with NBTE has been reported to be approximately 30%. The clinical onset may be "stuttering" due to frequent small emboli preceding the major embolic event. Initial minor episodes may be misdiagnosed as an epileptic seizure. The embolism may antedate the recognition of the background illness. Cardiac murmurs are unusual and the lesion (valve vegetations) may escape detection with 2-dimensional echo-cardiography. Recent studies indicate that transesophageal echocardiography can accurately detect vegetations (sensitivity 98%, specificity 100%).

MYXOMAS
Myxomas are the only cardiac tumors that regularly embolize. Embolic complications, resulting in ischemic extremities, loss of peripheral pulses, or permanent motor or sensory neurologic deficits are the presenting symptoms of atrial myxoma in 32% to 36% of patients. Emboli are most often composed of a tumor fragment. Atrial myxomas are usually detected by echocardiography (Fig. 7.22) and/or cardiac CT. Although cerebral and/or systemic emboli often recur before surgery, surgical therapy is usually curative.

MISCELLANEOUS
Recent clinical investigations have demonstrated several potential cardiac sources of emboli that were not previously recognized as origins of embolic stroke, including mitral annulus calcification, calcific aortic stenosis, atrial septal aneurysm, and idiopathic hypertrophic subaortic stenosis. Their contribution to overall incidence of cardioembolic strokes is very low.

OUTCOME
Emboli from cardiac sources often cause severe neurologic deficits or death. Many clinical studies have demonstrated that the average infarct size is larger in cardioembolic stroke than in infarct associated with other causes (Fig. 7.23). Intact consciousness or som-

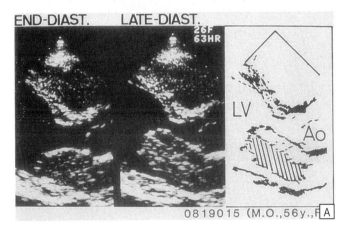
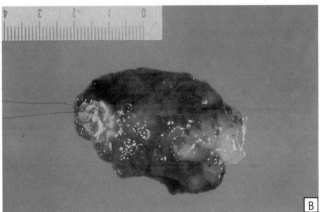

FIGURE 7.22 → **A**, An atrial myxoma is well visualized on echocardiography. **B**, The myxoma after surgical removal. (From Alpert JS, 1993, in press)

nolence within days after stroke onset may be followed by rapid deterioration caused by brain edema and/or hemorrhagic transformation. Mortality and morbidity are common. This disastrous outcome is typical in patients with occlusion of large brain vessels such as the ICA and the main trunk of the MCA. Patients with occlusion of a distal intracranial artery, however, usually present with minor cortical symptoms such as homonymous hemianopia, apraxia, agnosia, and minor aphasia syndromes with no or slight consciousness disturbance (Fig. 7.24). Approximately 10% to 14% of patients with an initial major hemispheric syndrome recover suddenly within hours after stroke onset, leaving minor or no neurologic manifestations. The mechanism has been assumed to be an embolus, initially lodged in a large artery of the carotid system, which migrates to the distal branches. Similar improvement may occur in patients with cardioembolic occlusion of the vertebrobasilar system. Migrating embolus within minutes or hours after the onset causes no residual deficits. TIA of cardioembolic origin may be common. The outcome of patients with cardioembolic stroke is correlated with the initial site of arterial occlusion and timing of distal migration of the embolus.

RECURRENCE AND PREVENTION

Risk of recurrence of cardioembolic stroke varies with the time after the stroke onset, associated cardiac diseases, as well as hematologic and hemodynamic conditions. Approximately 10% (2–22%) of patients with cardioembolic stroke will experience a second

---

FIGURE 7.23 → DISTRIBUTION OF CT INFARCT SIZE IN CONSECUTIVE PATIENTS WITH CARDIOEMBOLIC STROKE

INFARCT SIZE	INFARCT INDEX*	# CASES (%)
No infarct**	0	24 (7)
Small (<3 cm in diameter)	< 5%	21 (6)
Medium (<single lobe)	<25%	164 (45)
Large (<entire MCA area)	<50%	101 (28)
Extensive (≥entire MCA area)	≥50%	52 (14)
Total		362

*Infarct Index: The ratio of the maximum hypodense area to the entire ipsilateral hemisphere area on CT
**Including cardioembolic TIA patients

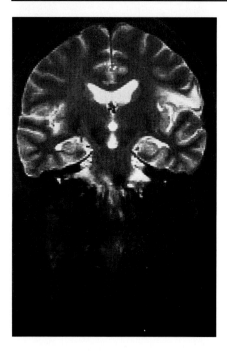

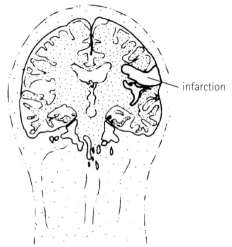

infarction

FIGURE 7.24 → A T2-weighted MRI demonstrates a small hyperintensity area in the left parietal cortex. The patient presented with an isolated conduction aphasia.

embolic stroke within two weeks, although recent studies suggest a lower risk (4%). Little difference in early recurrence rate is found between NVAF and other cardiac sources. A hypercoagulable state and/or dehydration in the early post-stroke period reportedly promotes intracardiac thrombus formation, resulting in recurrent embolism. Immediate anticoagulation has been recommended to prevent recurrent embolism within 2 weeks after stroke onset. Early recurrent embolism may be reduced by approximately one third with this measure, without a significant increase in symptomatic hemorrhagic complications, if patients with considerable risk of hemorrhagic complications are avoided (Fig. 7.25).

Cardioembolic stroke patients generally have a significant risk of recurrence for long periods after the initial stroke. Recurrent embolism occurs in 30% to 75% of patients with rheumatic heart disease, if preventive measures are not taken. Long-term chronic anticoagulation has been recommended for patients with cardioembolic stroke caused by rheumatic heart disease, NVAF, and other cardiac diseases if patients have no contraindications and can be monitored carefully. In patients with anterior myocardial infarct, recurrent embolism is rare after several months; long-term anticoagulation should be maintained only in those with ventricular wall motion abnormalities.

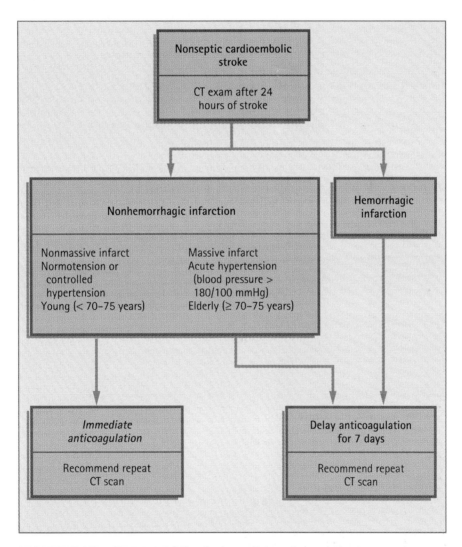

FIGURE 7.25 → Recommendation for immediate anticoagulation to prevent recurrent cardioembolic stroke during the initial 2 weeks. (Modified from the recommendation by the Cerebral Embolism Study Group, 1989)

REFERENCES

Alpert JS, Hurst JW. *Diagnostic Atlas of the Heart*. New York: Raven Press. 1993 (In press).

Bladin PF, Berkovic SF. Striatocapsular infarction: large infarcts in the lenticulostriate arterial territory. *Neurology*. 1984; 34:1423–1430.

Bozzao L, Fantozzi LM, Bastianello S, et al. Ischemic supratentorial stroke; angiographic findings in patients examined in the very early phase. *J Neurol*. 1989; 236:340–342.

The Boston Area Anticoagulation Trial for Atrial Fibrillation Investigators. The effect of low-dose warfarin on the risk of stroke in patients with nonrheumatic atrial fibrillation. *N Engl J Med*. 1990; 323:1505–1511.

Caplan LR. "Top of the basilar" syndrome. *Neurology*. 1980; 30:72–79.

Cerebral Embolism Study Group. Immediate anticoagulation of embolic stroke: brain hemorrhage and management options. *Stroke*. 1984; 15:779–789.

Cerebral Embolism Task Force. Cardiogenic brain embolism. *Arch Neurol*. 1986; 43:71–84.

Cerebral Embolism Task Force. Cardiogenic brain embolism: the second report of the Cerebral Embolism Task Force. *Arch Neurol*. 1989; 46:727–743.

Kittner SJ, Sharkness CM, Price TR, et al. Infarcts with a cardiac source of embolism in the NINCDS Stroke Data Bank: historical features. *Neurology*. 1990; 40:281–284.

Lechat P, Mas JL, Lascault G, et al. Prevalence of patent foramen ovale in patients with stroke. *N Engl J Med*. 1988; 318:1148–1152.

Minematsu K, Yamaguchi T, Omae T. 'Spectacular shrinking deficit': rapid recovery from a major hemispheric syndrome by migration of an embolus. *Neurology*. 1992; 42:157–162.

Okada Y, Yamaguchi T, Minematsu K, et al. Hemorrhagic transformation in cerebral embolism. *Stroke*. 1989; 20:598–603.

Okazaki H, Scherthauer BW. *Atlas of Neuropathology*. New York: Gower Medical Publishing. 1986.

Perkin GD, Rose FC, Blackwood W, Shawdon HH. *Atlas of Clinical Neurology*. London: Gower Publishing. 1986.

Ringelstein EB, Koschorke S, Holling A, et al. Computed tomographic patterns of proven embolic brain infarctions. *Ann Neurol*. 1989; 26:759–765.

Vandenberg B, Biller J. Cardiac evaluation of the patients with stroke. *Cerebrovasc Dis*. 1991; 1(suppl 1):73–82.

Wolf PA, Dawber TR, Thomas HE Jr, Kannel WB. Epidemiologic assessment of chronic atrial fibrillation and risk of stroke: the Framingham Study. *Neurology*. 1978; 28:973–977.

Yamaguchi T, Minematsu K, Choki J, Ikeda M. Clinical and neuroradiological analysis of thrombotic and embolic cerebral infarction. *Jpn Circ J*. 1984; 48:50–58.

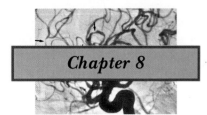

Chapter 8

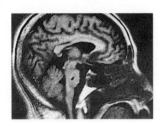

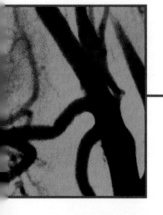

KAZUO MINEMATSU

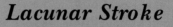

Lacunar Stroke

IN MOST PATIENTS with ischemic stroke due to cardioembolic or atherothrombotic occlusion of large cerebral arteries, both the infarct and arterial abnormalities can be easily demonstrated with computed tomography (CT), magnetic resonance imaging (MRI), cerebral angiography, ultrasound studies, and gross inspection of the vessels at surgery or necropsy. The complex features of stroke pathophysiology, symptomatology, outcome, and recurrence demand that patients be carefully monitored and treated. Another subgroup of ischemic stroke, lacunar stroke, is caused by small-vessel diseases. Lacunar stroke represents a small infarction in a unique location, resulting in relatively simple neurologic symptoms and an excellent outcome (Fig. 8.1). CT studies often miss such small infarcts. Cerebral angiography routinely fails to document abnormalities of the small vessels. Although the clinical diagnosis is not completely reliable, physicians should always try to differentiate lacunar strokes from the other categories of ischemic strokes. Lacunes, which are very common, do not require extensive diagnostic testing or aggressive therapeutic interventions such as anticoagulation or vascular surgery.

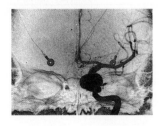

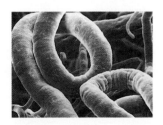

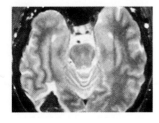

DEFINITION

The term "lacune" (French for a small fluid-filled cavity) applies to a brain infarct, ranging from 0.2 mm^3 to as large as 15 mm^3 in volume, that remains after macrophages carry off infarcted tissue (Fig. 8.2). The extensive clinicopathologic observations by Miller Fisher and his colleagues established ischemic stroke with a lacune as an independent stroke entity. They described four clinical subtypes according to the neurologic symptoms, calling them lacunar syndromes.

The term lacunar stroke (or infarction) is currently used for several different conditions, ranging from a small ischemic stroke to a small infarct in the territory of a single penetrator due to in situ small-vessel disease (Fig. 8.3). This semantic confusion is probably attributable to: 1) the capability of CT and MRI to display some, but not all, small deep infarcts; and 2) the inability of angiography to demonstrate involvement of one or more penetrators in addition to the presence or absence of in situ disease. In this chapter, the term 'lacunar stroke' will be used for stroke caused by a small (<15 mm in diameter) infarct, restricted to the territory of a penetrating branch, that is probably caused by small-vessel disease.

INCIDENCE

Lacunar stroke accounts for approximately 15% (10–26%) of symptomatic ischemic stroke patients in the United States. A recent epidemiologic survey revealed that the age- and sex-adjusted average annual incidence rate of lacunar stroke in the United States is 13.4/100,000 persons, or 12% of all first cerebral

---

FIGURE 8.1 → CLINICAL CATEGORIES OF BRAIN INFARCTION

CATEGORY	ETIOLOGY	INVOLVED ARTERY	LOCATION OF INFARCT
Atherothrombotic	Atherosclerosis	Extracranial or major intracranial	Cortical, watershed or deep (large)
Cardioembolic	Cardiac sources of emboli	Extracranial or major intracranial	Cortical, or deep (large)
Lacunar	In situ pathology of a small artery	Penetrators	Deep and small (<15mm in diameter)

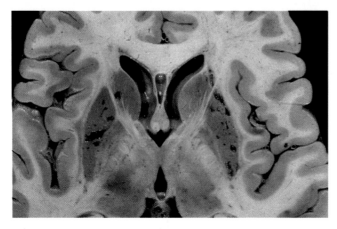

FIGURE 8.3 → DEFINITIONS OF LACUNAR STROKE

DEFINITION
1. Small void in the brain
2. Small infarct in the territory of a single penetrator
3. Small (by size) ischemic stroke
4. Stroke caused by a small infarct in the territory of a single penetrator likely to be due to small-vessel disease
5. Same as "4"; + lacunar syndrome
6. Lacunar syndrome with no visible lesion on CT or MRI imaging

---

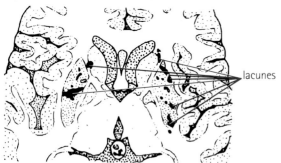

lacunes

FIGURE 8.2 → A pathologic specimen of the brain with multiple small bilateral old lacunes in the basal ganglia. (From Okazaki H, 1988)

infarcts. In an autopsy-based study, lacunes were documented in 169 (6%) of 2859 consecutive brains; as many as 81% of the patients with lacunes had been asymptomatic.

PATHOLOGY

LOCATION OF LACUNES AND THE PENETRATOR

Almost all lacunes occur in the territories of the lenticulostriate and thalamoperforant arteries, the paramedian branches of the basilar artery (BA) and the branches of the anterior choroidal artery (AChA) (Fig. 8.4). Lacunes are rarely found in the cortical gray matter, the white matter of the cerebral hemispheres, visual radiations, corpus callosum, medulla, or spinal cord, despite the presence of small intracortical vessels similar to those found in regions where lacunes are frequent. All the vessels related to lacunes (i.e., the "penetrators") share: 1) a similar small size, 2) a tendency to arise directly from much larger arter-

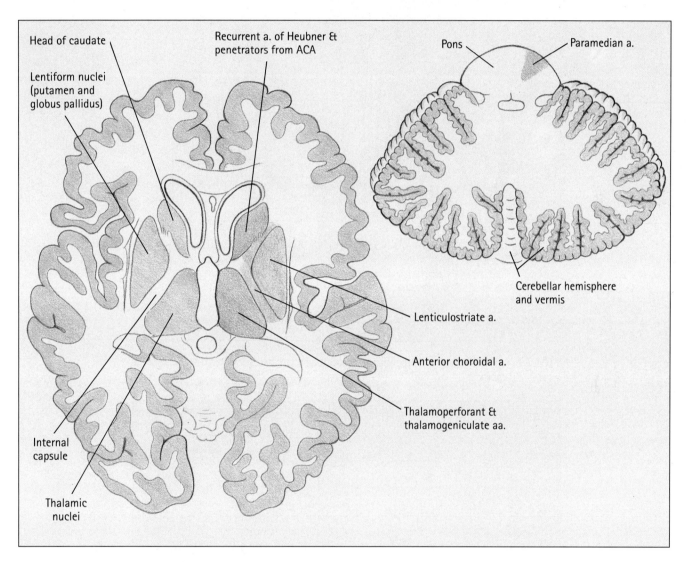

FIGURE 8.4 → Vascular territories of the penetrator as they relate to lacunes.

ies, and 3) an unbranching end-artery anatomy (Fig. 8.5). The size of these penetrators varies depending on their sites. These variations in size may cause the predominant pathologic features of small-vessel disease to differ (Fig. 8.6). Occlusions at the origin of a penetrator may yield a swath of infarction larger than 15 mm³, called superlacunes.

ARTERIAL PATHOLOGY OF LACUNES

There are four major vascular processes associated with lacunes: 1) *lipohyalinosis,* 2) atherosclerosis *(microatheroma),* 3) *presumed microembolism,* and 4) atherosclerotic plaque in the wall of the parent artery *(mural plaque)* blocking the orifice of a penetrator (Fig. 8.7). When cardioembolism, large-artery

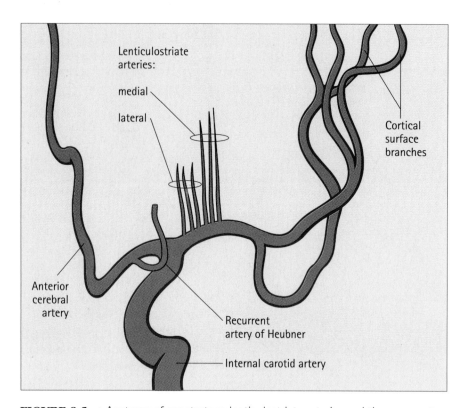

FIGURE 8.5 → Anatomy of penetrators: lenticulostriate arteries and the recurrent artery of Heubner.

FIGURE 8.6 → SIZE OF THE PENETRATOR AT VARIOUS SITES		
PENETRATORS	DIAMETER	PREDOMINANT PATHOLOGY
Lenticulostriate arteries		
• the medial group	100–200 μ	Lipohyalinosis
• the lateral group	200–400 μ	Microatheroma
Thalamoperforant arteries	100–400 μ	Lipohyalynosis or microatheroma
Paramedian branches of the basilar artery	40–500 μ	Lipohyalinosis, microatheroma, or mural plaque

atherosclerosis, or any other etiology is more likely on clinical grounds, the term "lacune" should be avoided.

Lipohyalinosis affects the smaller penetrating arteries, resulting in smaller lacunes, most of which are asymptomatic (Fig. 8.8). This pathologic change occurs in a setting of chronic, nonmalignant hypertension. Microatheroma, miniature focus of a typical atherosclerotic plaque found in the penetrators of advanced hypertensives, is another common cause of lacunes, and may be responsible for many of the larger, symptomatic lacunes. Microembolism cases have a normal small-vessel pathology, but a luminal thrombus. Mural plaque may incidentally affect a penetrator at its origin, producing the largest lacunes, particularly in the BA territory. Although this mechanism is not a true in situ small-vessel disease, it causes infarcts that

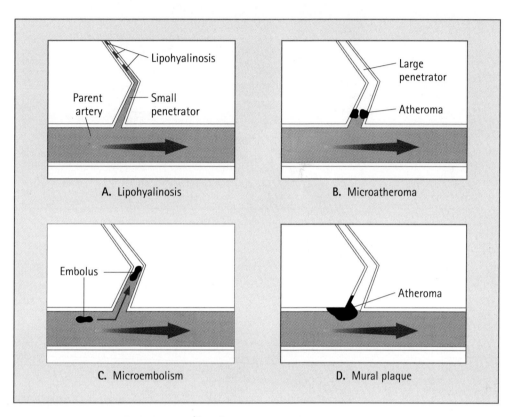

FIGURE 8.7 → Arterial pathologies that produce lacunes.

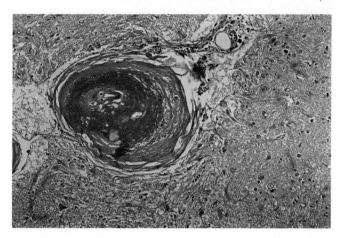

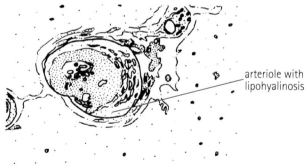

FIGURE 8.8 → Cross-sectional histopathologic demonstration of an arteriole with lipohyalinosis. Hematoxylin and eosin. (From Okazaki H, 1988)

cannnot be reliably separated from true lacunes. On rare occasions, arteritis due to chronic meningitis, such as Heubner's arteritis secondary to neurosyphilis, may involve a penetrator during its short subarachnoid course, resulting in a lacune.

CLINICAL FEATURES

Lacunar stroke at any lesion location appears to have relatively common clinical features, which may aid in diagnosis (Fig. 8.9).

FIGURE 8.9 → CLINICAL FEATURES COMMON TO ALL LACUNAR STROKES	
RISK FACTORS	Hypertension (65–80% of cases), diabetes mellitus
PRIOR TIAS	20% (less common than in atherothrombotic stroke)
MODE OF ONSET	Relatively slow (sudden onset in 40%)
DISTURBANCE OF CONSCIOUSNESS	None
PRESENTING SYMPTOMS	Highly focal (lacunar syndrome)
NEUROPSYCHOLOGICAL DEFICITS	Rare or none
PROGNOSIS	Excellent in most cases

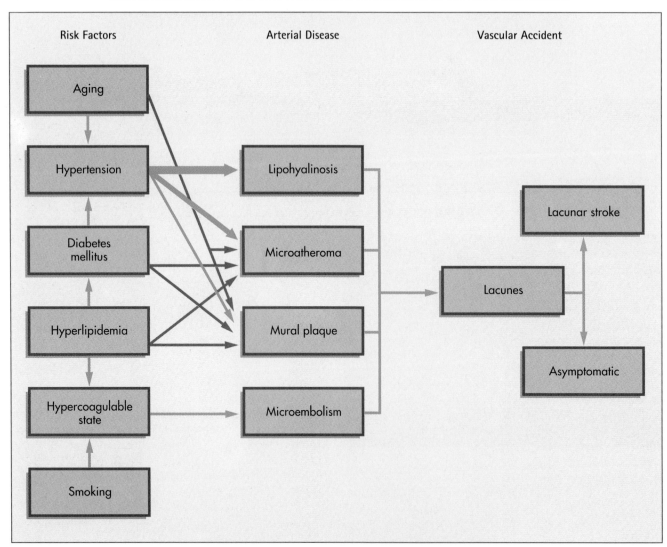

FIGURE 8.10 → Relationship of risk factors to lacunes.

HYPERTENSION AND OTHER RISK FACTORS

Pathologic and epidemiologic studies have demonstrated that hypertension has a close relationship to in situ small-vessel diseases and is the most important risk factor for lacunar stroke. Microatheroma and lipohyalinosis are closely linked to the presence of high blood pressure. Pathologically, the presence of atherosclerosis in cerebral arteries that are smaller than 1 mm almost always suggests a history of hypertension. In 167 autopsy patients with symptomatic or asymptomatic lacunes, hypertension was documented in 64%, diabetes in 34%, smoking in 46%, and no known risk factors in 18%. The Framingham Study proved hypertension to be the most common and potent precursor of "atherothrombotic brain infarction," which perhaps included lacunar stroke. A recent epidemiologic study found an 81% prevalence of hypertension in lacunar stroke, significantly higher than for nonlacunar stroke. In Fig. 8.10, relationships of risk factors with lacunes and lacunar stroke are demonstrated.

TIA AND LACUNAR STROKE

Transient ischemic attacks (TIAs) are observed in approximately 20% of patients before lacunar stroke. As compared with TIA associated with atherothrombotic stroke, TIA in lacunar stroke occurs less commonly, is more likely to recur, is usually longer in duration, and is more likely to have a shorter latency between the TIA and stroke. TIA is not correlated with the type of subsequent lacunar stroke, its severity, or prognosis.

SYMPTOMATOLOGY OF LACUNAR STROKE

A relatively slow or stuttering mode of onset is observed in many lacunar stroke cases. As many as 30% of lacunar strokes develop over a period of up to 36 hours. The initial deficit intensifies or occasionally spreads into limbs not affected initially. A sudden onset occurs, however, in 40% of cases. Presenting symptoms are almost always highly focal. A few nonfocal symptoms have been reported, including headache, lightheadedness, hiccough, asterixis, or mood lability. Consciousness is not disturbed. Higher cortical function deficits have been reported in only a few patients (see the following section). Patients with lacunar stroke usually present with one or more focal neurologic deficits, which have been classified into several neurologic syndromes called the lacunar syndromes. The prognosis is generally excellent.

Recently, several studies have suggested that higher cortical function deficits such as aphasia, apraxia, and agnosia may result from lacunar strokes. Small caudate lacunes are often incidentally found with CT or MRI, or at necropsy, without any clinical history of stroke. Presenting manifestations in several patients with caudate lacunes have been reported to be mild and transient hemiparesis, dysarthria, abulia, agitation and hyperactivity, contralateral neglect (right caudate), or language abnormalities (left caudate). Infarctions in the AChA territory have been reported to usually result from small-vessel disease, and to consistently be accompanied by hemiparesis. Dysarthria and hemisensory loss are less common; hemianopia is rare. Although an AChA territorial infarction on the right side can produce a neglect syndrome and one on the left side can cause a mild language disorder, there is no evidence that an AChA infarct caused by small-vessel disease produces these deficits. Small infarctions in the anterior thalamus, or territory of the tuberothalamic branches, can present with dysphasia or neglect, but small-vessel disease does not always account for these cases. In 530 consecutive patients with ischemic strokes, three patients who presented with amnestic aphasia were observed to have a small, left anterior, thalamic infarct. The etiology of these thalamic infarcts, however, was not lacunar but cardioembolic (Fig. 8.11). Consequently, higher cortical function disturbances caused by definite lacunes have not reliably been documented.

PSEUDOBULBAR SYNDROME AND LACUNAR STATE

The accumulation of lacunes in the white matter of the brain and basal ganglia, with or without multiple episodes of lacunar stroke, may occur during extended hypertension (Fig. 8.12). These multiple lacunes may produce the pseudobulbar syndrome, which is characterized by spasmodic laughing and crying (emotional incontinence), primitive reflexes, dysarthria, and swallowing problems with an enhanced gag reflex. Multiple lacunes scattered over the brain may cause the lacunar state, a pseudobulbar syndrome with a short-stepped gait, generalized akinesia, fixed facial expression, and urinary incontinence. This syndrome may be associated with a mental deterioration that can range from minimal to overt vascular dementia.

LACUNAR SYNDROMES

The essential clinical features of lacunar stroke are attributable to their small size and unique locations. These characteristics produce distinctive syndromes, which are not mimicked by larger lesions in the same locations or by small lesions in other locations that were caused by other stroke mechanisms. Since Miller Fisher and his colleagues reported the four classical lacunar syndromes based on clinicopathologic correlations, including pure motor hemiparesis (PMH),

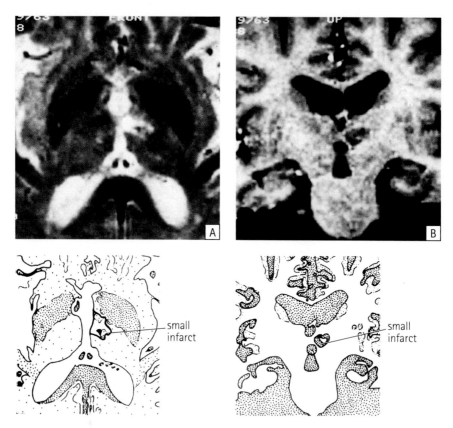

FIGURE 8.11 → Small, anterior thalamic infarct caused by cardioembolic stroke. The patient presented with amnestic aphasia. **A:** T2-weighted axial slice. **B:** T1-weighted coronal slice. A tiny T2-WI hypointense and T1-WI hyperintense area observed in the core of the lesion represent hemorrhage within an infarct (hemorrhagic transformation).

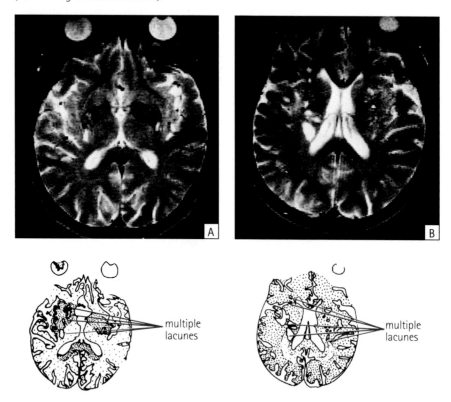

FIGURE 8.12 → **A,B:** Multiple lacunar infarcts as demonstrated by MRI.

pure sensory stroke (PSS), ataxic hemiparesis (AH), and dysarthria–clumsy hand syndrome (Fig. 8.13), many new syndromes have been proposed mainly based on clinico-CT and MRI correlations (Fig. 8.14).

PURE MOTOR HEMIPARESIS

Pure motor hemiparesis (PMH) is most easily diagnosed when the stroke equally affects motor function of the face, arm, and leg contralateral to the lesion, sparing sensation, vision, language, and behavior.

There are many variations in the degree of deficit among the face, arm, and leg. In a few cases, the face is essentially spared and in the other cases, weakness of the arm may exceed that of the leg. Sensory complaints by patients with PMH are not rare (numbness, heaviness, and loss of feeling), but patients may be describing weakness.

The lesions responsible for PMH are typically in the corona radiata, internal capsule, pons, and medullary pyramid. Lacunes are most frequently

---

FIGURE 8.13 → CLASSICAL LACUNAR SYNDROMES

SYNDROMES	MANIFESTATIONS	LESION SITES
Pure motor hemiparesis*	Hemiparesis	Posterior limb of the internal capsule, basis pontis
Pure sensory stroke	Hemisensory deficits	Thalamus (VPN)
Ataxic hemiparesis**	Hemiparesis + ipsilateral ataxia	Posterior limb of the internal capsule or corona radiata, basis pontis
Dysarthria–clumsy hand syndrome	Dysarthria + clumsiness of a hand	Dorsal-pontine base, internal capsule or corona radiata?

Original terms are *pure motor hemiplegia, and **homolateral ataxia and crural paresis.

FIGURE 8.14 → OTHER LACUNAR SYNDROMES

PURE MOTOR HEMIPARESIS, PLUS
- Modified PMH with "motor aphasia"
- PMH sparing face
- PMH with horizontal gaze palsy
- PMH with crossed third nerve palsy (Weber syndrome)
- PMH with crossed sixth nerve palsy
- PMH with confusion
- Locked-in syndrome (bilateral PMH)

VARIATIONS OF THALAMIC LACUNAR STROKE
- Sensorimotor stroke (thalamocapsular)
- Mesencephalothalamic syndrome
- Thalamic dementia

BRAIN STEM LACUNAR STROKE
- Cerebellar ataxia with crossed third nerve palsy (Claude syndrome)
- Lower basilar branch syndrome
- Lateral medullary syndrome
- Lateral pontomedullary syndrome

MISCELLANEOUS
- Hemichorea-hemiballism
- Pure dysarthria
- Acute dystonia of thalamic origin
- Weakness of one leg with ease of falling
- Loss of memory (?)

Modified from Miller Fisher, 1982.

located in and around the internal capsule (66% in one series) (Fig. 8.15). Capsular lesions responsible for PMH are classified into the following three distinct categories, corresponding to lesion location and the responsible artery: 1) capsulo-putamino-caudate infarcts (type 1), in the territory of the larger, lateral lenticulostriate arteries; 2) capsulo-pallidal infarcts (type 2), in the territory of the smaller, medial lenticulostriate branches; and 3) anterior capsulo-caudate infarcts (type 3), in the territory of the anterior cerebral artery (ACA) including the recurrent artery of Heubner. A typical, profound hemiparesis is observed only in type 1, but partial, incomplete syndromes may occur in all subtypes.

The major anatomic focus of capsular hemiparesis is the hind portion of the capsule's posterior limb. This location corresponds to the approximate capsular position for the motor fibers found by whole brain anatomic dissection. In a CT study, all 36 cases involving the internal capsule had a hemiparesis that affected the face, arm, and leg similarly. In 21 cases involving the corona radiata, or at extreme ends of

the capsule, an incomplete syndrome that commonly spared the face was seen. A lacune with pure facial weakness was located at the genu. Another with pure leg weakness was found at the extreme posterior end of the capsule. In patients with capsular PMH, lesion volume and severity of the hemiparesis are correlated, except for the few cases where the infarct involves the lowest portion of the internal capsule.

PURE SENSORY STROKE

Pure sensory stroke (PSS) usually arises from a thalamic lacune. The patient's complaints are described as striking spontaneous sensations: stretched, hot, sunburned, "stuck with pins," larger, smaller, heavier. The disturbance in sensation typically extends over the entire side of the body. Axial structure may be involved, even splitting the two sides of the nose, tongue, etc. This midline split, with its characteristic distribution of deficits, is diagnostic for thalamic sensory disturbances. However, individual patients may have sensory deficits of a parietal type in the face, the arms, the legs, the oral cavity, as well as the peribuccal area and forearm.

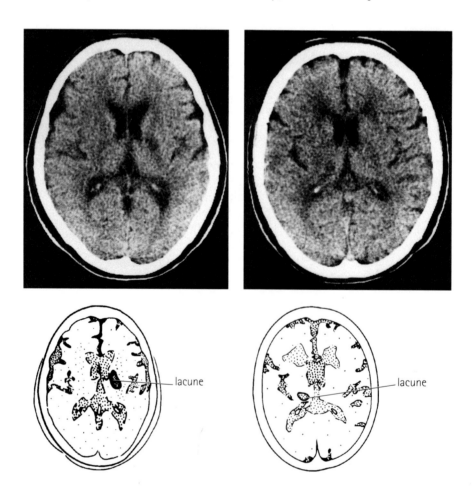

FIGURE 8.15 → Computed tomography (CT) study in a patient presenting with pure motor hemiparesis. Hypodensity was located at the posterior limb of the internal capsule.

FIGURE 8.16 → CT study in a patient presenting with sensorimotor stroke. Hypodensity was documented at the thalamocapsular region.

The most common location of PSS lacunes is the ventral posterior nuclei of the thalamus. In contrast to PMH lacunes, thalamic lacunes with PSS are sometimes too small to be displayed by CT, and are frequently caused by lipohyalinosis. In one autopsy case, the lesion lay completely outside the thalamus, involving the corona radiata of the internal capsule's posterior limb. PSS due to a pontine lacune was documented with MRI.

SENSORIMOTOR STROKE

Sensorimotor stroke is a combined syndrome, in which both the motor and sensory deficits occur contralaterally to the ischemic lesion. Although this subgroup was reported as next in frequency (20%) to PMH (57%) in CT studies, only a few autopsy cases have been documented. Pathologically verified locations of the lesion for this syndrome are the posteroventrolateral nucleus of the thalamus, posterior limb of the internal capsule, and pons (Fig. 8.16). The genu/posterior limb of the internal capsule or the corona radiata are the lesion sites found on a CT study.

ATAXIC HEMIPARESIS AND DYSARTHRIA–CLUMSY HAND SYNDROME

Ataxic hemiparesis is defined as hemiparesis with ipsilateral ataxia. Dysarthria–clumsy hand syndrome is classified as severe dysarthria and dysphagia combined with a slight weakness and clumsiness of the hand. In the former, paresis is more commonly crural. Facial weakness could be present in the latter. These two syndromes are sometimes discussed as varieties of basilar branch occlusion syndromes. Ataxic hemiparesis is the result of infarction of the basis pontis at the junction of the upper one third and inferior two thirds (Fig. 8.17). Dysarthria–clumsy hand syndrome has a similar lesion location to ataxic hemiparesis, or a lacune at the genu of the internal capsule. Dysarthria–clumsy hand syndrome is probably best regarded as a variant of ataxic hemiparesis.

HEMICHOREA-HEMIBALLISMUS

This relatively rare syndrome, which usually occurs suddenly, consists of distal choreiform movements, proximal ballistic movements, or both. In one case

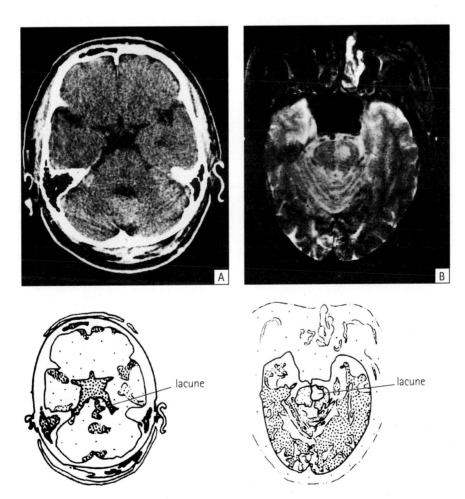

FIGURE 8.17 → **A,B;** CT and T2-weighted MRI studies in a patient presenting with ataxic hemiparesis. Infarcted lesion was demonstrated at the basis pontis.

with distal choreiform movements of the arm and leg as well as rare ballistic movements, CT documented a putaminal infarct of a size consistent with a lacune. The subthalamic nucleus, striatum, and thalamus are considered to be the lesion locations responsible for this syndrome. The lesion must spare the adjacent internal capsule, because motor strength is normal. The specificity of this syndrome for lacunar stroke is not great. In a recent study, almost half (10 of 21) of patients with hemichorea-hemiballism had some other, nonstroke cause.

VARIETIES OF BASILAR BRANCH OCCLUSION SYNDROMES

In the brain stem, small lacunar-size infarcts are caused not only by true small-vessel diseases but also by a mural plaque of the BA that occludes a single penetrating artery. A striking number of syndromes have been described arising from small infarcts of various brain stem parts. They include not only some classical lacunar syndromes but also specific vascular syndromes previously not listed as lacunar syndromes (Fig. 8.18).

LACUNAR STROKE VERSUS LACUNAR SYNDROME

It may be expected that nonlacunar brain pathology can produce the lacunar syndromes. Lacunar syndromes following hemorrhagic stroke were documented in 11% of clinically diagnosed lacunar syndrome patients (Fig. 8.19). Sensorimotor stroke and ataxic hemiparesis were the most frequent syndromes. Cortical infarcts, brain abscesses, brain tumors and other pathologies have reportedly produced lacunar syndromes. Recently, the sensitivity and specificity of the lacunar syndromes for the diagnosis of lacunar stroke were tested; 95% sensitivity and 93% specificity were reported when in 103 lacunar and 144 cortical infarctions were analyzed. This result suggests that the lacunar syndrome is highly diagnostic of lacunar stroke, if other nonischemic mechanisms are excluded with CT or MRI.

In a recent CT study of 337 consecutive lacunar stroke patients, PHM constituted 57% of all lacunar strokes, followed in frequency by sensorimotor stroke (20%), ataxic hemiparesis (10%), PSS (7%) and dysarthria–clumsy hand syndrome (7%). These figures are almost comparable to those in the author's study, in which 141 consecutive lacunar stroke patients (99 male, 42 female, mean age of 65 years) diagnosed with CT and MRI were analyzed (Fig. 8.20). The most frequent lesion sites in this series were the lenticulostriate arterial territory with pure motor hemiparesis, the thalamoperforant arterial territory with sensorimotor and pure sensory stroke, and the BA-paramedian arterial territory with ataxic hemiparesis. Patients with sensorimotor stroke frequently had a lesion in the lenticulostriate territory. In 22 (20%) of 131 patients with a classic lacunar syndrome, particularly in sensorimotor stroke patients, the imaging studies did not display a lacune, or demonstrated multiple lacunes at two or more sites that were potentially responsible for the syndrome.

Only 20 patients with larger or symptomatic lacunar stroke have been reported with detailed clinical information and a vascular pathologic examina-

---

FIGURE 8.18 → VARIETIES OF BASILAR BRANCH OCCLUSION SYNDROMES

- Dysarthria–clumsy hand syndrome
- Homolateral ataxia and crural paresis
- Pure dysarthria with no focal signs
- Pure hemiparesis sparing the face
- Oculomotor paresis with cerebellar ataxia
- Abducens palsy with pure motor hemiparesis
- Contralateral paralysis of lateral gaze
- Internuclear ophthalmoplegia and pure hemiparesis
- Dysarthria with cerebellar ataxia and internuclear ophthalmoplegia
- Pure sensory stroke and its variants

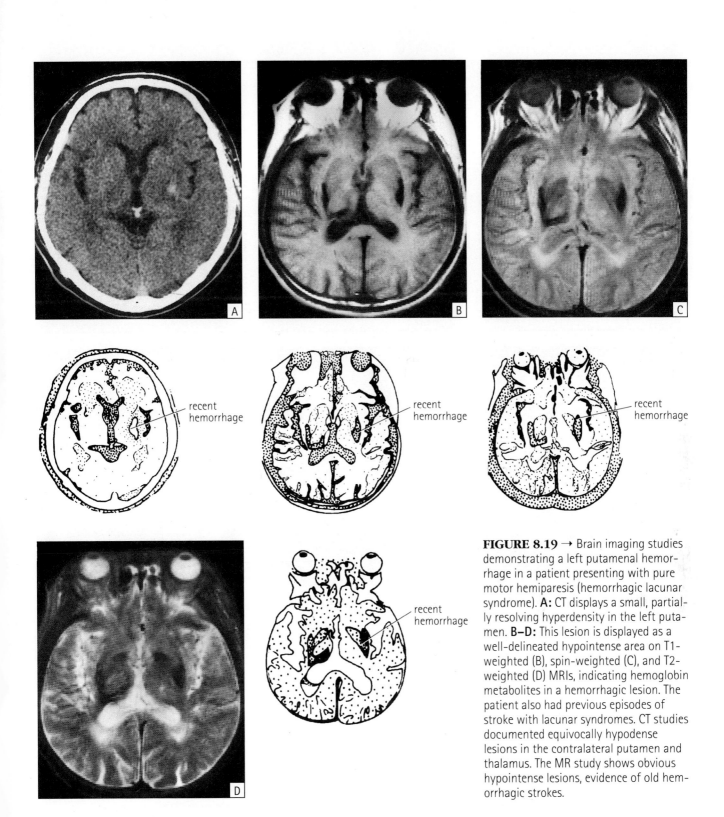

FIGURE 8.19 → Brain imaging studies demonstrating a left putamenal hemorrhage in a patient presenting with pure motor hemiparesis (hemorrhagic lacunar syndrome). **A:** CT displays a small, partially resolving hyperdensity in the left putamen. **B–D:** This lesion is displayed as a well-delineated hypointense area on T1-weighted (B), spin-weighted (C), and T2-weighted (D) MRIs, indicating hemoglobin metabolites in a hemorrhagic lesion. The patient also had previous episodes of stroke with lacunar syndromes. CT studies documented equivocally hypodense lesions in the contralateral putamen and thalamus. The MR study shows obvious hypointense lesions, evidence of old hemorrhagic strokes.

	LENTICULOSTRIATE ARTERY	THALAMOPERFORANT ARTERY	BA-PARAMEDIAN ARTERY	UNDETERMINED	TOTAL (%)
PMH	69	0	4	7	80 (57)
SMS	6	11	0	11	28 (20)
PSS	0	6	0	2	8 (6)
AH	2	0	9	2	13 (9)
D-CHS	2	0	0	0	2 (1)
Misc.	3	1	5	1	10 (7)
Total (%)	82 (58)	18 (13)	18 (13)	23 (16)	141

PMH: pure motor hemiparesis, SMS: sensorimotor stroke, PSS: pure sensory stroke, AH: ataxic hemiparesis, D-CHS: dysarthria–clumsy hand syndrome, Misc: miscellaneous

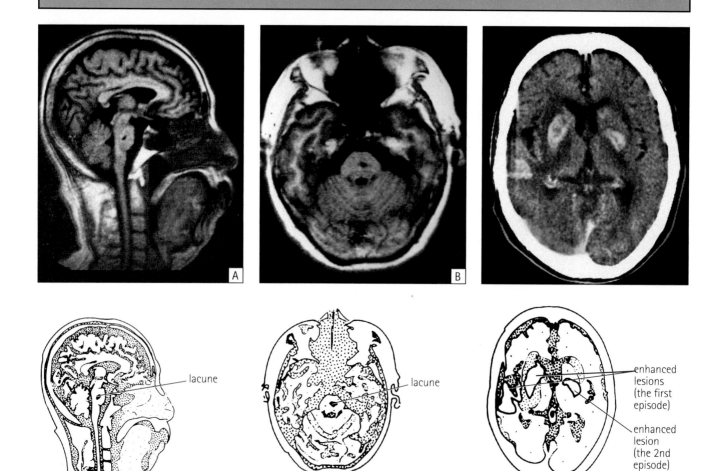

FIGURE 8.21 → MRI demonstration of a lacune in the basis pontis. T1-weighted images in saggital (**A**) and axial views (**B**).

FIGURE 8.22 → A contrast CT study demonstrates deep cerebral infarcts in cardioembolic stroke. Patients experienced two episodes over several days, initially deep and cortical infarcts in the right side, and subsequently a deep infarct in the left basal ganglia.

tion. Microatheroma was the predominant arterial pathology, particularly in cases with pure motor hemiparesis. Lipohyalynosis was observed in patients with thalamic, pure sensory stroke, and thalamocapsular sensorimotor stroke.

DIAGNOSIS

The clinical diagnosis of lacunar stroke should be made principally by the signs and symptoms that occur during the early stage of stroke. Also helpful, but not always possible, are brain imaging studies that demonstrate a deep infarct smaller than 15 mm (or 20 mm) in diameter. The majority of patients have hypertension; absence of hypertension may suggest another etiology for the stroke. Absence of symptoms such as consiousness disturbance, higher cortical function deficits, and headache may distinguish lacunar stroke from other strokes. Typical lacunar syndromes are highly indicative of lacunar stroke but are not the gold standard for the diagnosis.

LABORATORY STUDIES

Because they are small, individual lacunes do not damage the brain enough to disturb the electroencephalogram (EEG). Somatosensory evoked potentials have been reported as routinely abnormal in sensorimotor stroke and ataxic hemiparesis, but consistently normal in pure motor hemiparesis and pure sensory stroke.

Computed Tomography

Although lacunar strokes were clinically diagnosed before the advent of CT, this imaging technique has greatly improved the speed and accuracy of diagnosis. If a small, deep, hypodensity is displayed in a penetrator territory that corresponds to the presenting lacunar syndrome, the diagnosis of lacunar stroke can reliably be made. CT studies greatly help to exclude other pathologies that may cause lacunar syndromes. Small lacunes, however, are frequently missed by CT studies. Even larger lacunes are often missed in the brain stem, partly because CT artifacts are common in the infratentorial structures. In a report with CT examinations, only 33% of patients with clinically evident lacunar stroke had a positive CT scan within the first week of stroke, significantly less than the 67% of those with nonlacunar minor stroke. Therefore, a negative CT study does not exclude, and may actually support, the diagnosis of lacunar stroke. A CT study sometimes overestimates the size of lacunes by as much as 100%, resulting in difficulty in differentiating lacunes from nonlacunar small deep infarcts. The larger the lacune observed on CT, the more disease involving the parent major cerebral artery should be suspected. In a CT study, 33% of patients with small deep infarcts on CT had a possible carotid or cardiac source of embolism.

Magnetic Resonance Imaging

Recent studies revealed that MRI detection of responsible lacunes is definitely superior to CT (74% vs. 15%). The clinico-MRI correlation was 98% when scanning was carried out within 13 days of symptom onset in 100 consecutive cases of lacunar stroke. Lacunes at a brain stem location can reliably be displayed only with MRI (Fig. 8.21). However, MRI may fail to show the small infarct of pure sensory stroke, the infarct of pure motor stroke in the lowermost pons, or smaller lacunes in the range of 3 to 4 mm. MRI is often sensitive enough to display asymptomatic lacunes or other small cavities in the brain such as *état criblé*. Therefore, a small lesion demonstrated with MRI does not always indicate a lacunar stroke.

Cerebral Angiography and Other Noninvasive Tests

Cerebral angiography is not routinely recommended for diagnosing lacunar stroke because it rarely demonstrates small-vessel abnormalities. In a recent study, severe carotid or MCA disease on the ipsilateral side was documented in only 3.3% of lacunar stroke with angiography, significantly less than the 79% of nonlacunar, minor stroke. If other stroke mechanisms are suspected, patients with presumed lacunar stroke should initially be evaluated with other noninvasive tests, including duplex carotid sonography, transcranial doppler sonography, and MR angiography. The prevalence of significant ipsilateral extracranial carotid stenosis, determined by carotid duplex sonography, was reported to be 13% in lacunar stroke, significantly less than the 41% prevalence in nonlacunar hemispheric stroke.

DIFFERENTIAL DIAGNOSIS OF LACUNAR STROKE

When a patient presents with a minor stroke deficit, there is the danger of interpreting it as a lacunar process when in fact it is the prodrome or the early phase of a major carotid or basilar stroke. Deep brain infarcts caused by major arterial occlusive diseases should be routinely excluded, because the prognosis and therapeutic measures are different from those of lacunar stroke. An atherothrombotic or cardioembolic occlusion of the parent large artery can produce a deep infarct alone on CT or MRI if 1) the duration of the parent artery's occlusion by migrating emboli is too short to cause cortical damage, but sufficient to produce an infarct in the deeper structures (Fig. 8.22); 2) the blood supply via collaterals is developed enough to spare the cortical regions distal to the occlusion from infarcts; or 3) the cortical infarcts are missed by imaging studies. These nonlacunar deep brain infarcts can often be differentiated from lacunar stroke because of their larger size, associated angiographic findings, absence of hypertension, presence of potential cardiac source for emboli, or clinical manifestations. Nonlacunar deep infarcts should be suspected if 1) deep infarcts exist with a border-zone distribution; 2) the lacune is larger than 20 to 30 mm in diameter (Fig. 8.23); 3) multiple small infarcts are distributed within the terminal zone; and 4) a clinical picture suggests the possibility of cardioembolic stroke (e.g., an accompanying old cortical infarct, potential cardiac sources, a younger stroke patient, or sudden onset).

Lacunar syndromes may be caused by nonlacunar mechanisms. Timely imaging studies are necessary to exclude these mechanisms. In particular, small brain hemorrhage occurs at almost the same sites as lacunes and may rapidly resolve from hyperdensity to normo- or hypodensity on CT. A CT study performed days or weeks after stroke onset may not only miss the hyperdensity—direct evidence of hemor-

rhage—but can cause an erroneous diagnosis of lacunar stroke, due to a small, deep hypodensity. T2-weighted MRI can display distinct evidence of metabolites from hemorrhage for a long time, allowing the differential diagnosis of a hemorrhagic lacunar syndrome (see Fig. 8.19).

OUTCOME AND RECURRENCE

Lacunar strokes show improvement in a large percentage of cases within days or months, usually more rapidly than in larger cerebral infarctions with a similar initial motor deficit. An incomplete, partial hemiparesis syndrome has the best prognosis. In a study of presumed lacunar pure motor stroke patients 3 weeks after stroke onset, 63% had no or minor residua, 26% had moderate residua, and 11% experienced severe hemiparesis. Patient survival is significantly better after a lacunar rather than a nonlacunar infarct. In an analysis of 1122

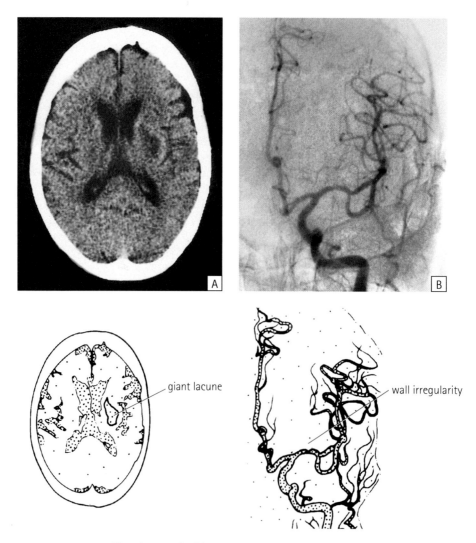

giant lacune

wall irregularity

FIGURE 8.23 → Giant lacune. **A:** CT demonstrates a large hypodensity in the left basal ganglia. **B:** Carotid angiogram shows wall irregularity, suggesting an atheromatous lesion in the main trunk of the left MCA, where the lenticulostriate arteries branch off.

consecutive stroke patients admitted to the National Cardiovascular Center (Osaka, Japan), approximately 85% of lacunar stroke patients survived for 5 years after stroke onset, a significantly better survival rate than in other ischemic strokes and brain hemorrhage.

Recently, stroke was reported to recur annually in 7.3% to 11.8% of patients with lacunar stroke. In our study, the cumulative recurrence rate during the initial 5 years after stroke was approximately 30% (annual rate 6%) in 312 patients with lacunar stroke, less frequent than in cardioembolic (40%) and atherothrombotic stroke patients (46%). However, multiple recurrences of lacunar stroke are not rare and may cause a pseudobulbar syndrome and lacunar state, resulting in profound functional and social disabilities.

PREVENTION AND TREATMENT

Controlling hypertension has been the primary prevention for lacunar stroke. Several pathologic, epidemiologic, and clinical surveys have provided evidence that treating hypertension probably does reduce the incidence of lacunar stroke. The role of antihypertensives remains controversial in patients with established lacunar stroke, but hypertension should still be treated, particularly if patients are younger or have moderate to severe hypertension. Antihypertensive therapy should be delayed until clinical manifestations stabilize (the first two or three weeks after stroke onset), because reduction in blood pressure during the early and unstable stage may further diminish blood flow, resulting in clinical deterioration.

No special treatment during the acute stage has been shown to improve the lacunar stroke's clinical course. Patients should be kept in bed and given appropriate hydration during the first few days to avoid orthostatic hypotension and dehydration, which may result in deterioration. This is particularly important when major cerebral arterial disease has not been completely excluded. Anticoagulant therapy is not recommended because it may cause brain hemorrhage through the arterial wall affected by lipohyalinosis. Antiplatelet therapy with aspirin or ticlopidine has been shown to significantly reduce recurrence of ischemic stroke, and is therefore recommended for lacunar stroke patients whose blood pressure is controlled in the normotensive to mildly hypertensive range.

REFERENCES

Bladin PF, Berkovic SF. Striate capsular infarction: large infarcts in the lenticulostriate arterial territory. *Neurology*. 1984; 34:1423–1430.

Boiten J, Lodder J. Lacunar infarcts. Pathogenesis and validity of the clinical syndromes. *Stroke*. 1991; 22: 1374-1378.

Bruno A, Graff-Radford NR, Biller J, Adams HP. Anterior choroidal artery territory infarction: a small vessel disease. *Stroke*. 1989; 20:616-619.

Caplan LR, Schmahmann JD, Kase CS, et al. Caudate infarcts. *Arch Neurol*. 1990; 47:133-143.

Chamorro A, Sacco RL, Mohr JP, et al. Clinical-computed tomographic correlations of lacunar infarction in the stroke data bank. *Stroke*. 1991; 22:175-181.

Fisher CM. Lacunar stroke and infarcts: a review. *Neurology*. 1982; 32:871-876.

Fisher CM. Lacunar infarcts: a review. *Cerebrovasc Dis*. 1991; 1:311-320.

Ghika JA, Bogousslavsky J, Regli F. Deep perforators from the carotid system. Template of the vascular territories. *Arch Neurol*. 1990; 47:1097-1100.

Hier DB, Foulkes MA, Swiontoniowski M, et al. Stroke recurrence within 2 years after ischemic infarction. *Stroke*. 1991; 22:155-161.

Hommel M, Besson G, LeBas JF, et al. Prospective study of lacunar infarction using magnetic resonance imaging. *Stroke*. 1990; 21:546-554.

Mohr JP, Caplan LR, Melski JW, et al. The Harvard Cooperative Stroke Registry: a prospective registry. *Neurology*. 1978; 28:754-762.

Mohr JP. Lacunes. *Stroke*. 1982; 13:3-11.

Mori E, Tabuchi M, Yamadori A. Lacunar syndrome due to intracerebral hemorrhage. *Stroke*. 1985; 16:454-459.

Norrving B, Cronquist S. Clinical and radiologic features of the lacunar versus nonlacunar minor stroke. *Stroke*. 1989; 20:59-64.

Pullicino P, Nelson RF, Kendall BE, Marshall J. Small deep infarcts diagnosed on computed tomography. *Neurology*. 1980; 30:1090-1096.

Rothrock JF, Lynden PD, Hesselink JR, et al. Brain magnetic resonance imaging in the evaluation of lacunar stroke. *Stroke*. 1987; 18:781-786.

Sacco SE, Whisnant JP, Broderick JP, et al. Epidemiological characteristics of lacunar infarcts in a population. *Stroke*. 1991; 22:1236-1241.

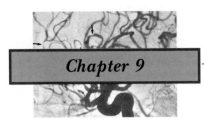

Chapter 9

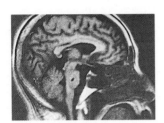

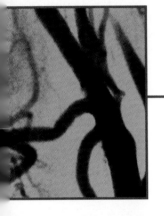

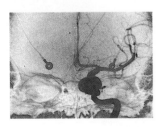

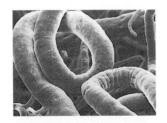

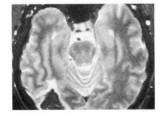

MARK J. GORMAN

NABIH M. RAMADAN

STEVEN R. LEVINE

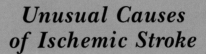

Unusual Causes of Ischemic Stroke

WHEN A PATIENT PRESENTS with an acute neurologic deficit, a detailed history followed by a complete physical and neurologic examination usually leads to an anatomic localization and a probable cause (differential diagnosis). Confirmatory diagnostic studies commonly employed in the first 48 hours include cranial computed tomography (CT) or magnetic resonance imaging (MRI) to rule out hemorrhage, neoplasm, or infectious lesions. When the presumed cause of the acute deficit is cerebral ischemia, a minimal investigation may include carotid artery ultrasound, electrocardiography and, if indicated, echocardiography. Blood tests such as complete blood count with differential, platelets, prothrombin time, and partial thromboplastin time are also performed. This initial work-up helps to determine the common causes of ischemic stroke, such as atherosclerosis or cardioembolism. Despite a comprehensive initial evaluation, however, the physician is often left without a firm etiologic diagnosis and may abandon further investigations in favor of maintaining low health-care costs.

Unusual causes of stroke may be hereditary; a thorough diagnostic search is important, not only to determine appropriate therapy, but also because the correct diagnosis of a hereditary condition can affect the patient's family. A thoughtful and detailed reevaluation of the patient's history and physical examination are important first steps. Occasionally, clues can be found in the family or employment histories. Knowledge of a supposedly innocuous infection, or a dilated ophthalmologic examination, may also yield pertinent facts. These clues are generally subtle and must be specifically inquired about or they may be overlooked. Unusual causes of ischemic stroke can be divided into five major categories: 1) cardiac, 2) arteriopathic, 3) hematologic, 4) toxic, and 5) miscellaneous.

CARDIOEMBOLIC STROKE

Cardiac sources for cerebral embolism are second in frequency to carotid artery tree atherosclerosis and at times can be quite difficult to ascertain on routine testing. A simple anatomic organization is shown in Figure 9.1. Cardioembolic stroke has no single clinical presentation. Although questions about cardiac symptomatology should be asked, stroke is commonly the presenting complaint of underlying heart pathology.

VALVE-RELATED CAUSES

Infective endocarditis, occasionally caused by rare organisms, is a well documented cause of ischemic stroke and is covered in Chapter 7 (Fig. 9.2).

In *nonbacterial thrombotic endocarditis* (NBTE or marantic), platelet-fibrin complexed material is deposited on the surface of the valve without causing specific valvular damage. NBTE occurs in response to a variety of systemic diseases (Fig. 9.3) and may account for up to 27% of strokes in patients with known cancer. The vegetations are usually small (≤3 mm) but can range to over 1 cm in size. Generally, the stroke is heralded by a prodrome of transient neurologic deficits and often presents as an encephalopathy. Pathologically, platelet-fibrin embolic material may be found occluding the cerebral artery that supplies the infarcted area. Hemorrhagic transformation may occur. In cases of NBTE associated with cancer, a high concurrence with lower extremity thrombophlebitis has been found; a prothrombotic state may underlie both conditions. NBTE must be suspected in a patient with ischemic stroke in the setting of lupus or cancer, especially since a heart murmur is often absent and the physical examination may be unremarkable except when evidence of systemic emboli is present.

FIGURE 9.1 → UNUSUAL CARDIAC CAUSES OF ISCHEMIC STROKE

VALVE RELATED
- Infective endocarditis (rare organisms)
- Nonbacterial thrombotic endocarditis (marantic)
- Libman-Sacks endocarditis
- Calcific aortic stenosis

AORTIC-ROOT RELATED
- Marfan's syndrome
- Aortic dissection
- Syphilitic, tuberculous aortitis
- Ulcerated plaques of aortic arch

CHAMBER RELATED
- Nonischemic cardiomyopathies
- Patent foramen ovale
- Atrial septal defects
- Idiopathic hypertrophic subaortic stenosis
- Cardiac tumors (atrial myxoma, metastatic melanoma, rhabdomyosarcoma, etc.)

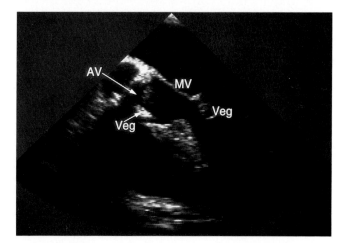

FIGURE 9.2 → Aortic valve (AV) and mitral valve (MV) vegetations in a case of endocarditis shown on transesophageal echocardiography (TEE).

FIGURE 9.3 → CAUSES OF NBTE

- Systemic lupus erythematosus (SLE)
- Pregnancy/puerperium
- Mucin-producing carcinoma
- AIDS
- Antiphospholipid antibody syndrome

Calcific aortic stenosis (CAS) is an age-related degeneration of the valve. It may cause systemic as well as cerebral embolism. The diagnosis is made when a patient has evidence of embolic infarct and calcific material is found lodged in the artery appropriate to the lesion (usually exhibited on CT scan). Echocardiography must confirm the CAS, which can also be visualized on catheterization (Fig. 9.4). Therapy is currently empiric. Because CAS is a fairly common lesion in the elderly, its recent recognition as a cause for embolic stroke should lead to a more accurate estimate of its true prevalence and attributable risk for stroke.

CHAMBER-RELATED CAUSES

Nonischemic cardiomyopathies (Fig. 9.5), often related to alcohol, postinfectious or familial conditions, or to the postpartum period, can cause stroke if a thrombus forms in a quiescent area of a dilated ventricle or atrium.

Patent foramen ovale (PFO) has recently been given importance in the etiology of "cryptogenic" stroke. In the study by Lechat et al., the prevalence of PFO in patients without an identifiable cause for their stroke was 49% as compared to 10% for a control group. It was previously believed that constantly elevated pulmonary or right ventricular pressure was a necessary prerequisite to right-to-left shunt in patients with interatrial wall defects and subsequent strokes. However, it is now thought that a momentary reversal of the normal interatrial pressure gradient occurs early in ventricular systole and is sustained for a more significant amount of time during maneuvers that increase venous pressure (cough, straining for bowel movement, positional changes, etc.). In one study, saline contrast echocardiography identified spontaneous right-to-left shunting in about 70% of patients with PFO, while the other 30% were identified during cough or Valsalva maneuver. Likewise, atrial septal defects can cause an embolic stroke (Fig. 9.6).

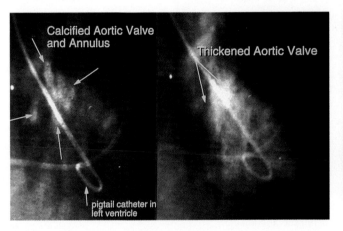

FIGURE 9.4 → Cardiac catheterization ventriculogram showing aortic valve calcification (calcific aortic stenosis).

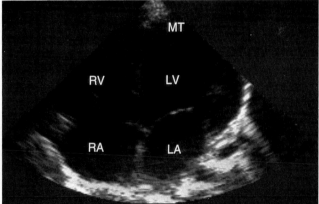

FIGURE 9.5 → Transthoracic echocardiography (TTE) showing dilated cardiomyopathy of right ventricle (RV); left ventricle (LV); right atrium (RA); and left atrium (LA). Note apical/mural thrombus (MT).

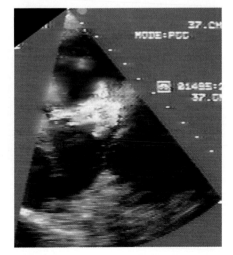

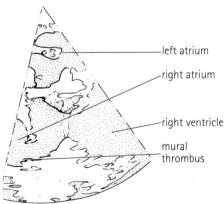

FIGURE 9.6 → TEE showing an atrial septal defect with a right-to-left shunt. Yellow-orange color indicates blood flow from right atrium to left atrium. Thrombus is seen in the right atrium.

Idiopathic hypertrophic subaortic stenosis (IHSS) has been linked to stroke. Between 2.6% and 22% of patients with IHSS have had a stroke. An ischemic cerebral event is sometimes the presenting symptom. Concomitant left atrial enlargement, mitral annular calcification, atrial fibrillation, hypertension, and increased atrioventricular conduction delay add to the risk of stroke. Interestingly, echocardiography has not yet revealed intracardiac thrombus in patients with IHSS and stroke.

Atrial septal aneurysm, sinus of Valsalva aneurysm, and other structural chamber abnormalities occur rarely and carry a risk of thromboembolism. They may be difficult to visualize on transthoracic echocardiography (TTE) (Fig. 9.7).

Atrial myxoma, the most common cardiac tumor, can lead to ischemic stroke in up to 45% of cases. Arising in either atrium, myxoma is a high risk for ischemic stroke (> 6% per year). Right-sided myxoma has also been documented to cause stroke when a patent foramen ovale or ASD exists (Fig. 9.8). Neurologic symptoms are the presenting complaint in about 30% of cases. Emboli generally consist of myxomatous material but can also be thrombotic if an adherent clot breaks loose. Myxomatous embolization has been implicated in causing cerebral aneurysms, which may rupture, leading to a primary presentation of subarachnoid hemorrhage (SAH). Large myxomas are easily visualized on TTE or transesophageal echocardiography (TEE), but small ones may require gated cardiac MRI or catheterization for diagnosis. Other rare tumors of the heart (e.g., rhabdomyosar-coma) may also cause stroke.

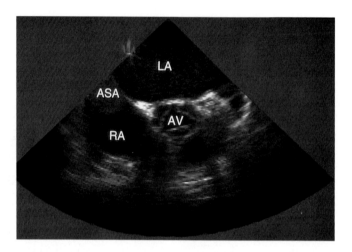

FIGURE 9.7 → TEE view of atrial septal aneurysm (ASA) at the level of the aortic valve (AV) as well as the right and left atriums, with spontaneous contrast within the aneurysm.

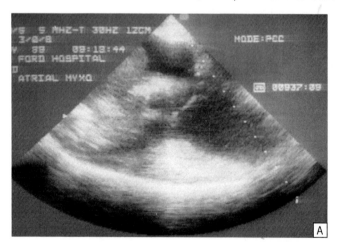

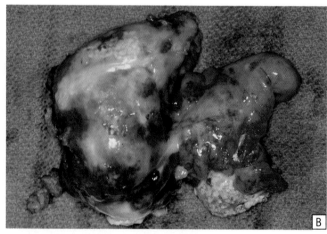

FIGURE 9.8 → TEE **(A)** and gross pathologic specimen **(B)** of a large myxoma in the right atrium.

AORTIC ROOT DISEASES

Aortic root diseases known to cause stroke include Marfan's syndrome (Fig. 9.9), aortic dissection (Fig. 9.10), syphilitic and tuberculous aortitis, and ulcerated plaques of the aortic arch.

Ulcerated plaques of the aortic arch have until recently been thought of as rare causes of embolic stroke. However, a recent autopsy series identified ulcerated aortic plaques proximal to the origin of the common carotids in 61% of stroke patients who had no known cause for their strokes, as opposed to only 22% in stroke patients who had an identifiable cause. The underlying mechanism of the ulcerations is atherosclerosis, but no correlation was found between the presence of aortic plaques and the degree of stenosis in the extracranial internal carotid artery (ICA). Ulcerated plaques of the aortic arch are difficult to diagnose in vivo, although they occasionally may be spotted on TEE. More accurate in vivo diagnosis awaits further technical advances.

ARTEROPATHIC CAUSES OF STROKE

In situ thrombosis, artery-to-artery embolism, and distal field ischemia (watershed infarct) represent the main known mechanisms of infarction in atherosclerotic disease. The mechanisms of cerebral ischemia in nonatherosclerotic arteropathies are similar; vasospasm is an additional postulated mechanism. Often, systemic or historic features are suspicious for a process other than atherosclerosis. Figure 9.11 lists the less frequently seen arteropathies.

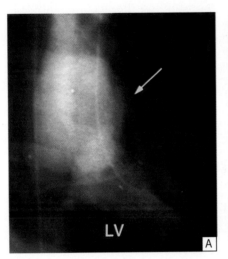 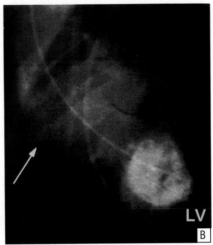

FIGURE 9.9 → **A,** Left ventriculogram, right anterior oblique view. **B,** Left anterior oblique view. Note dilated aortic root and sinus of Valsalva (arrows) consistent with Marfan's syndrome.

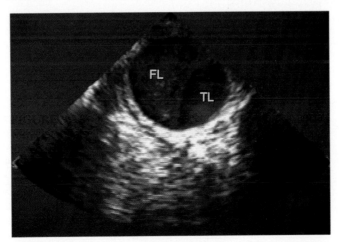

FIGURE 9.10 → TEE showing dissection of the thoracic aorta with clot in false lumen (FL) and Doppler color flow in true lumen (TL).

VASCULOPATHIES

Infective

Bacterial meningitides sometimes involve the meningeal vessels directly, producing an acute vasculitis. Involvement can also be indirect, causing extrinsic compression of the vessels. Either situation can precipitate an ischemic event. In bacterial infections, polymorphonuclear leukocytes (PMNs) usually infiltrate the vessels, whereas in other types of infection, the infiltrate is predominantly lymphocytic. If the infection itself does not cause stroke, the stenosis that results from scarring may produce a progressive vascular insufficiency syndrome. In fact, leptospiral infection has been implicated in moyamoya syndrome. Neurotuberculosis characteristically forms a thick exudate at the base of the brain, often encasing the vessels of the circle of Willis, and in this manner can cause stroke. The abbreviated list in Figure 9.11 illustrates the wide range of organisms known to cause stroke in the setting of meningitis.

Noninfective

Stroke related to the *multiple cholesterol emboli syndrome* occurs when cholesterol crystals embolize to cerebral vessels from an ulcerated plaque of the proximal aorta, carotid arteries or, less commonly, intracranial vessels. Spontaneous plaque disruption, warfarin therapy, and invasive procedures such as angiography or open heart surgery can lead to this condition. When the cholesterol clefts disrupt the vascular intima, they may cause a hypersensitivity vasculopathy with inflammatory changes on vessel biopsy, an elevated erythrocyte sedimentation rate (ESR),

peripheral eosinophilia, and multiple organ system involvement. Diagnosis is made by skin, renal, or cerebral biopsy. Treatment is directed toward lowering cholesterol levels and removing the offending lesion. The role of steroids is controversial; warfarin may exacerbate clinical symptomatology.

Isolated angiitis of the central nervous system (IAC), a necrotizing angiitis affecting mainly small- to medium-sized vessels, is almost completely restricted to the central nervous system (CNS). It usually appears in the middle-aged and elderly. Clinically characterized by its lack of systemic signs, it often begins with headache, confusion, lethargy, and memory loss, reflecting its diffuse multivessel involvement. Stroke, seizure, or myelopathy caused by larger-vessel angiitis, may be presenting signs or may become prominent later in the course of the illness, representing the accumulation of small defects over time. Evidence of increased intracranial pressure and cranial nerve abnormalities are common. The etiology of IAC is unknown (some cases have been linked to Hodgkin's disease, sarcoidosis, or herpes zoster) and temporary spontaneous improvement of symptoms often makes the diagnosis difficult. Hematologic and serologic studies are normal; cerebral spinal fluid (CSF) shows a nonspecific mild to moderate elevation in pressure, protein, or white blood cell count (predominantly lymphocytes) in over 75% of patients. The diagnosis is made when an angiogram shows features typical of vasculitis; however, completely normal angiographic studies (< 10%) and nonspecific arterial changes are often found. In such instances, biopsy of both leptomeninges and parenchyma may be required. A vas-

---

FIGURE 9.11 → UNUSUAL ARTERIOPATHIES

INFECTIVE VASCULOPATHIES
  BACTERIAL
  • Spirochetes (syphilis, leptospirosis, Lyme disease)
  • Mycobacterium tuberculosis

  FUNGAL
  • Mucormycosis
  • Aspergillosis

  VIRAL
  • Herpes zoster
  • Cytomegalovirus

  HELMINTHS
  • Cysticercosis

  RICKETTSIAL
  • Rocky mountain spotted fever

NONINFECTIVE VASCULOPATHIES
  • Multiple cholesterol emboli syndrome
  • Isolated angiitis of the CNS
  • Giant cell arteritis
      Takayasu's disease
      Temporal arteritis
  • Systemic necrotizing vasculitis
      Polyarteritis nodosa
      Allergic angiitis and granulomatosis (Churg-Strauss syndrome)
      Overlap syndrome
  • Systemic lupus erythematosus
  • Hypersensitivity vasculitis
  • Wegener's granulomatosis
  • Scleroderma
  • Sarcoidosis
  • Inflammatory bowel disease

NONSPECIFIC ANGIOPATHIES
  • Fibromuscular dysplasia
  • Nontraumatic spontaneous dissection
  • Moyamoya
  • Oral contraceptive–related
  • Vanishing cerebral vasculopathy of pregnancy
  • Homocystinuria
  • Mitochondrial angiopathy
  • Postirradiation arteriopathy
  • Malignant atrophic papulosis (Kohlmeier-Degos disease)
  • Alpha-glucosidase deficiency
  • Sneddon's syndrome
  • Malignant endotheliomatosis

cular inflammatory infiltrate with occasional granuloma formation and surrounding areas of parenchymal hemorrhage or infarction are typical findings. The prognosis of patients with IAC is generally poor, but cortico-steroids, often in combination with immunosuppressive agents, may induce remission.

Polyarteritis nodosa (PAN) is a systemic necrotizing vasculitis that has prominent neurologic symptoms. Systemic nonspecific symptomatology is prominent early in its course, with a predilection for nephritis and subsequent hypertension. Neurologic problems occur in approximately 75% of patients; peripheral neuropathy, headache, and retinopathy are the most common complaints. Either hemorrhagic or ischemic stroke occurs in 14% of cases, generally late in the course, representing significant vascular scarring. Stroke is often a contributing cause of mortality. Abnormal laboratory studies include elevated erythrocyte sedimentation rate, anemia, leukocytosis, proteinuria, circulating immune complexes, and the presence of hepatitis B surface antigen (30% of cases). Biopsy of involved tissue reveals necrotizing vasculitis of small- and medium-sized muscular arteries. Treatment with corticosteroids and immunosuppressive agents has lowered the mortality rate to about 20%.

Allergic angiitis and granulomatosis (AAG) is closely related to PAN but has an allergic component and more prominent lung involvement. It is clinically similar to PAN, except for the presence of asthma. The vessel wall infiltrates contain many eosinophils and tend to involve capillaries and venules as well as the arteries. Granulomas are often found in the vessel wall.

Overlap syndrome has clinical and pathologic features of both PAN and AAG. Stroke may occur in either AAG or PAN overlap syndrome.

Temporal arteritis (Fig. 9.12) is a disease of the elderly (>60 years) that affects mostly whites. Headache, generally centered on one or both temples, is often an initial complaint but systemic symptoms of a nonspecific nature (malaise, low-grade fever, night sweats, muscular aches, weight loss) are much more prominent early in the disease's course. Jaw claudication in addition to superficial temporal artery swelling and tenderness may be present. Most patients have anemia and a elevated ESR, often over 80. Unilateral permanent visual loss, which occurs in almost 50% of cases, is probably due to ischemic optic neuropathy. Cerebral infarction is less common, occurring in about 10%, but may present in any arterial territory. The diagnosis is made when a long-segment temporal artery biopsy reveals a patchy granulomatous arteritis with minimal necrosis and characteristic multinucleated giant cells. Long-term corticosteroid treatment prevents the ocular and cerebral complications of the disease.

Takayasu's arteritis (Fig. 9.13) predominantly affects Asian females in their third and fourth decades.

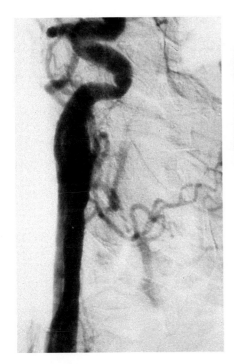
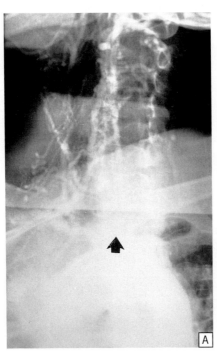
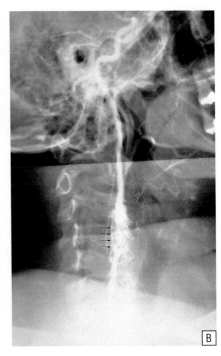

FIGURE 9.12 → Selective carotid arteriogram showing dissection in an autopsy-proven case of temporal/giant-cell arteritis. True lumen (darker area) superimposed on false lumen (lighter area).

FIGURE 9.13 → **A,** Arch aortogram showing complete obliteration of both subclavian arteries (arrowhead). **B,** Muscular collaterals (small arrows) reconstitute the carotid arteries distally.

It is a giant-cell arteritis, as is temporal arteritis, but with a predilection for the aorta and its major branches. Early systemic symptoms are of a nonspecific nature (malaise, fevers, muscular aches, weakness) and are followed by hypertension and vascular occlusive events (myocardial infarction, claudication of extremity, transient ischemic attack [TIA], or stroke). Cataracts are often present. Neurologic symptoms relate to the territory of the occluded artery. Subclavian steal may occur secondary to subclavian artery occlusion. Pathologically, Takayasu's disease is characterized by thickening of the aorta, often with obliteration of one or more of the vessels arising from the arch. Administration of corticosteroids is the currently accepted treatment.

Stroke in lupus can be ischemic or hemorrhagic and is often related to Libman-Sacks endocarditis, thrombocytopenic purpura, fibrin-platelet occlusive disease associated with antiphospholipid antibodies and, possibly, a noninflammatory vasculopathy. Stroke due to true cerebral vasculitis has rarely been documented.

The *hypersensitivity vasculitides* have in common a PMN invasion of small vessels, especially postcapillary venules. They are usually associated with a known predisposing event and often involve the skin, causing rash and urticaria. Henoch-Schönlein purpura is the prototype syndrome, but the group also includes drug-induced allergic vasculitis, serum sickness, postinfectious vasculitis, and some cases of mixed cryoglobulinemia. To our knowledge, stroke has only rarely been shown in this group of diseases.

Wegener's granulomatosis is a systemic vasculitis with necrotizing granulomatous invasion of small arteries and veins. Typically involving both upper and lower respiratory tracts and sometimes causing glomerulonephritis, it has rarely been implicated in ischemic stroke. The most common neurologic complications of Wegener's granulomatosis are peripheral and cranial neuropathies. Ophthalmologic involvement via direct granulomatous invasion from contiguous nasal sinuses is present in 30% of cases.

Sarcoidosis is a granulomatous disease of unknown etiology that frequently affects the CNS. Although patients are often found to have granulomatous invasion of small blood vessels and small infarcts at autopsy, it is a very rare sarcoid patient who has symptomatic cerebral infarction (CI). Angiography is usually normal; diagnosis may be made based on accompanying systemic and laboratory findings of sarcoidosis. Because of the rarity of stroke in sarcoidosis, the usefulness of prednisone in this circumstance is unknown.

Scleroderma (Fig. 9.14) has only been related to stroke in a few case reports. Limited evidence implicates a vasculopathy, either inflammatory or noninflammatory, cardiac embolism, or hypercoagulability.

Inflammatory bowel disease (IBD) (Fig. 9.15) is listed here mainly because of its well known association with the other systemic vasculitides. IBD also may cause

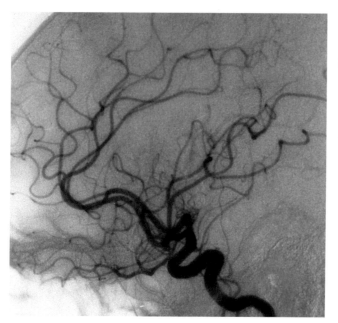

FIGURE 9.14 → Selective carotid arteriogram reveals complete MCA occlusion in a patient with scleroderma and stroke.

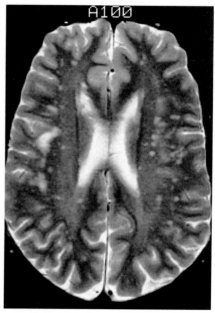

FIGURE 9.15 → Multifocal, bilateral white-matter ischemic changes seen on T2-weighted MRI (TR2500, TE90) from a patient with Crohn's disease.

a separate vasculitis, resulting in skin necrosis that resolves with bowel resection. It has also been postulated to cause stroke from a variety of hematologic mechanisms, including increased factor VIII levels, thrombocytosis, hyperfibrinogenemia, decreased antithrombin III levels, high plasminogen activator inhibitor levels, and impaired release of tissue plasminogen activator. Despite all of its associated coagulation abnormalities, stroke is a very rare consequence of IBD.

NONSPECIFIC ANGIOPATHIES

Fibromuscular dysplasia (FMD) is a nonatherosclerotic disease of medium-sized arteries that predominantly affects women in their sixth or seventh decade. Usually asymptomatic, it can present as thrombo-embolic stroke related to spontaneous dissection, aneurysm formation, or carotid artery fistulas. Pathologically, segmental fibromuscular hypertrophy leading to luminal compromise alternates with areas of medial thinning and loss of the elastic membrane, producing dilation. This alternating pattern of stenosis with dilation is responsible for the characteristic "string of beads" configuration on angiography (Fig. 9.16), although it can also present with a focal or multifocal tubular stenotic appearance. The etiology and natural history of FMD are unknown. Originally described in the renal arteries as a cause of hypertension, it can affect any medium-sized artery; in the cervicocephalic circulation, multi-vessel involvement is the rule. Therapy is controversial and should be individualized.

Spontaneous cervicocephalic arterial dissection (SD) occurs mainly in women in their fourth or fifth decade. SD is defined as an arterial dissection that occurs without trauma, although most authors implicate minor trauma as a possible causative factor (Fig. 9.17). The etiology appears to vary, having been linked with FMD (in up to 15% of cases) and cystic medial necrosis, but most have no clear specific defect. A high incidence of hypertension (nearly 50%) provides one clue. A debatable association with oral contraceptive use, together with a much higher incidence in women, indicates a possible hormonal influence.

Clinically, SD ranges from asymptomatic to a severe unilateral headache (the most common symptom) to symptoms of transient or permanent cerebral ischemia. Lateral medullary syndrome is the most common symptom complex seen with vertebral dissection. Middle cerebral artery (MCA) territory infarct and Horner's syndrome are frequently seen with ICA dissection. SD was found to occur in about 0.5% of patients with ischemia who underwent cerebral angiography. Pathologically, the dissection can be found: 1) immediately subintimal, in which case the accumulation of blood in the false lumen constricts the true lumen, causing ischemic symptoms downstream; or 2) in the media or subadventitia, producing aneurysmal dilation, which may rupture and lead to SAH when the dissection extends into the intradural segment of the involved vessel.

Patients with SD appear to fall into two categories: those with underlying arteriopathy, who usu-

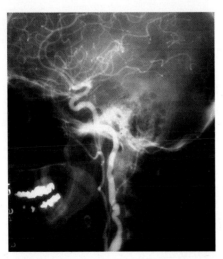
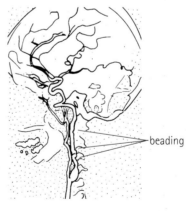

FIGURE 9.16 → Selective carotid arteriogram with characteristic beading in the proximal ICA in fibromuscular dysplasia.

ally present with multiple dissections, and those with otherwise normal arteries, who present with a single dissection. Surgical repair should be contemplated for those with accessible ruptured dissecting aneurysms. Antiplatelet or anticoagulation therapy is generally recommended for patients with extracranial dissections and ischemic symptoms. Patients with SD tend to do well and the arterial lesions are generally resolved on repeat angiography months later.

Moyamoya disease is an angiographically defined syndrome of unproven etiology that consists of recurrent TIA and/or stroke (Fig. 9.18). It usually affects young women, with about 40% presenting after their second decade. The characteristic angiographic picture consists of stenosis or occlusion of the supraclinoid ICA and/or proximal anterior cerebral artery (ACA) and MCA, along with an abnormal vascular network seen in the arterial phase near the occlusion (Fig. 9.19). This vascular network has been likened to a puff of smoke, which in Japanese is "moyamoya." It is believed to represent tiny local collateral vessel dilation compensating for the occlusion until larger transdural anastamoses can be established to supply the area formerly fed by the occluded vessel. Neuropathology reveals laminated fibrosis of the intima and multiplication of the elastica without an inflammatory reaction. Involvement of the vasculature is generally bilateral and clinical recurrence of ischemia is characteristic. Intracranial hemorrhage is a common presentation of moyamoya disease in Japan.

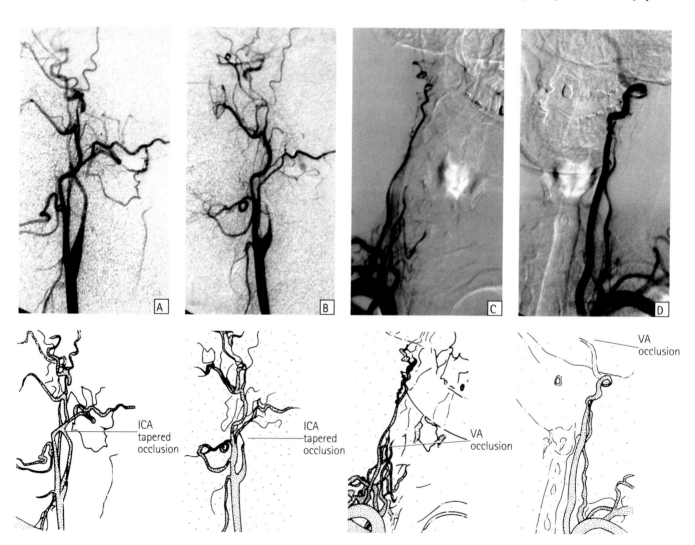

FIGURE 9.17 → Cerebral arteriogram consistent with 4-vessel dissection. Note bilateral ICA tapered occlusion (**A,B**) and occlusion of both vertebral arteries (**C,D**).

The use of *oral contraceptives* (OC) has been associated with an increased risk of vascular complications of all types, as well as ischemic and hemorrhagic stroke and SAH. The risk of stroke with the older, higher-dose OC has been estimated at 5 to 26 times higher than matched nonusers. The risk related to the newer, low-dose pill, however, has not been established. The increased risk has been correlated with high estrogen and progestogen pill dosage, older age, and smoking. Proposed mechanisms have included increased embolic tendency (but without a clear-cut embolic source), arterial intimal hyperplasia leading to focal narrowing, increased thrombotic tendency, and induction of hypertension with its attendant risks. Typically, these patients have a low mortality rate and tend to do well.

One of the etiologic mechanisms of ischemic cerebrovascular disease in pregnancy may be a variation of the OC-related angiopathy. It is postulated to be secondary to reproductive hormone-related intimal hyperplasia that resolves after the peripartum period has passed. Likewise, FMD, SD, and possibly moya-moya all have several features in common: 1) they have a significant predilection for women; 2) they are often seen during pregnancy, the puerperium, or OC use; and 3) although they are apparently distinct entities, they have at least some similar pathologic features. No specific etiology has been worked out for any of them, but a hormonal contribution seems probable.

Homocystinuria represents a group of hetero-

FIGURE 9.18 → POSSIBLE CAUSES OF MOYAMOYA SYNDROME

Leptospiral arteritis	Tuberculous meningitis
Oral contraceptives and cigarette smoking	Vasospasm following SAH
Sickle-cell anemia	Sneddon's syndrome
Atherosclerotic cerebrovascular disease	Pseudoxanthoma elasticum
Neurofibromatosis	Tuberous sclerosis
Trisomy 21	Retinitis pigmentosa
Mitochondrial encephalopathy	Fanconi's anemia
Postirradiation cerebrovascular disease	Type I glycogenosis
Head trauma	Fibromuscular dysplasia

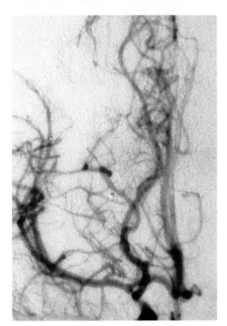

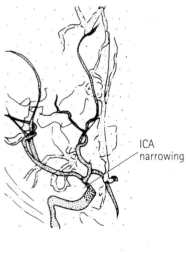

ICA narrowing

FIGURE 9.19 → Moyamoya disease: note severe narrowing of the supraclinoid ICA with collateral reconstitution distally.

geneous (mainly inherited; occasionally acquired) abnormalities of the cysteine synthetic pathway that results in low levels of cysteine and excessive levels of homocysteine. The most common cause of the disease is cysteine-β-synthetase deficiency. Prevalence of homozygosity is between 1 in 80,000 and 1 in 200,000 in whites, but climbs to as high as 1 in 70 for heterozygosity. While homozygotes usually have certain physical attributes that facilitate the diagnosis (ectopia lentis, mental retardation, skeletal deformities similar to Marfan's syndrome, and often microcephaly), heterozygotes are phenotypically normal.

The main cause of morbidity and mortality (most homozygotes die by their third decade of life) is multiple vascular occlusions leading to stroke, peripheral ischemia, and—more rarely—myocardial infarction. Heterozygotes have an increased incidence of peripheral and cerebral arterial occlusions. Superior sagittal sinus thrombosis has also been reported in association with homocystinuria. The high levels of homocysteine appear to cause intimal damage, followed by a vasculopathy that is neuropathologically characterized by intermittent fibrous plaques leading to luminal narrowing. An increased tendency to thrombosis, in addition to the vasculopathy, may play a role, but has not been well characterized to date. The diagnosis of heterozygosity, which should be pursued in young stroke victims without other apparent cause, is made by a methionine loading test. Diagnosis may be confirmed by measuring cystathionine-β-synthetase levels in cultured skin fibroblasts, but doing so does not eliminate other possible variants. Treatment is threefold: 1) dietary restriction of methionine, 2) Vitamin B$_6$ in those responsive to it, 3) aspirin or other platelet antagonist to help prevent vascular occlusion.

A subgroup of the inherited mitochondrial disorders known as *MELAS* (mitochondrial myopathy, encephalopathy, lactic acidosis, and strokelike episodes) presents a unique stroke syndrome. Those affected are usually young. The characteristic deficits (recurrent episodes of alternating hemiparesis, hemianopsia and/or cortical blindness) are mainly transient, but over time these patients become retarded and encephalopathic. The lesions on CT scan, which probably represent infarctions (although not in classic pial arterial distributions), can resolve with clearing of the symptoms. Neuropathologically, multiple necrotic areas, which involve mainly cortical and, to a lesser degree, subcortical and brainstem regions, correspond to those pial arterioles and small arteries from 50 to 250 µm in diameter that are affected by the mitochondrial angiopathy. Arteriolar occlusion has not been confirmed; the immediate cause of damage has been postulated to arise from impaired autoregulation in the areas supplied by these vessels. Patients usually die by the age of thirty.

People who have had head or neck irradiation may develop stenotic and/or ulcerative lesions in the parts of the vessels included in the field of irradiation. Seen anywhere from 4 to 36 years later, *postirradiation arteriopathy* usually presents as TIA or cerebral infarction in the appropriate territory. Pathology reveals periarterial fibrosis, thickening, and hypertrophy of the intima as well as general signs of calcific atherosclerosis. Postirradiation arteriopathy is thought to represent a form of accelerated atherosclerosis. Surgical repair by endarterectomy or patch is curative, but is technically demanding.

Also known as Kohlmeier-Degos disease, *malignant atrophic papulosis* is a systemic vasculopathy of unknown etiology. Occurring at any age, it is characterized by a pathognomonic skin rash consisting of scaly papules up to about 1 inch in diameter on the trunk and proximal extremities. It is followed within a few months by gastrointestinal (GI) and neurologic symptoms. The GI complications are most often related to viscous perforation and are usually the immediate cause of mortality. Neurologic findings relate almost exclusively to infarction, although symptoms like headache and memory loss are less specific. The pathology has shown fibrous intimal proliferation with obliteration of the lumen or thrombosis. No specific etiology or hereditary pattern has been confirmed, nor has a successful treatment been found. The prognosis is poor, especially for those with GI or neurologic complications.

Alpha-glucosidase deficiency is a rare, inherited cause of stroke due to basilar artery (BA) aneurysm formation. A vacuolar arteriopathy from the deposition of glycogen in the tunica media and intima has been postulated to result in the aneurysmal dilation and has been documented to cause SAH and CI.

Sneddon's syndrome is an unusual dermatocerebral syndrome of livedo reticularis and ischemic stroke of unknown cause. Patients tend to be young, have antiphospholipid antibodies (up to 25% of cases), and the vessel pathology is one of noninflammatory vasculopathy. The diagnosis is confirmed by biopsy of the purple-blue, mottled skin lesions found in the affected areas.

Malignant endotheliomatosis is an extremely rare malignancy of the cerebral vessel endothelial cell. As the cells proliferate and grow, they may obstruct blood flow and lead to ischemic stroke. This condition is diagnosed by leptomeningeal and cerebral par-enchymal biopsy and should be considered in patients with subacute stroke syndromes that have no apparent cause.

HEMATOLOGIC CAUSES OF STROKE

Many types of *blood dyscrasias* have been linked to ischemic stroke. Often tested for, they are actually rare, accounting for less than 5% of strokes in general and approximately 5% to 15% of strokes in young people. Abnormalities of the blood can lead to enhanced intravascular thrombosis under a variety of circumstances. The delicate balance between prothrombotic and antithrombotic tendencies involves many interwoven systems and the clinical separation of these states is sometimes difficult. Laboratory tests can help to pinpoint the specific abnormality. Many of the known hematologic causes are listed in Figure 9.20

HYPERCOAGULABLE STATES

Maintaining hemostasis in vivo is accomplished by a balance between the clotting system, naturally occurring anticoagulants, and the fibrinolytic system. An interplay between clotting factors II (prothrombin), VII, IX, and X, the anticoagulants protein C (PC), protein S (PS), and antithrombin III (AT III), in addition to the fibrinolytic components, plasminogen, its activator and its inhibitor, determines the degree of circulating anticoagulation/coagulation activity.

Hereditary AT III deficiency is believed to occur in up to 1 out of 2000 persons. Heterozygotes have antigen or activity levels 40% to 60% of normal (homozygosity is thought to be incompatible with life). Several types or subclasses are known, some with decreased antigen levels, others with normal antigen levels but decreased activity. Thrombosis can occur at any age but most frequently is seen between 15 and 30 years of age.

Acquired AT III deficiency is found in nephrotic syndrome, severe liver disease, disseminated intravascular coagulation, and in patients taking oral contraceptives and L-asparaginase chemotherapy. *AT III deficiency,* usually the qualitative dysfunction, has been linked in a few cases to stroke, mainly in patients who have had prior venous thrombosis.

PC deficiency can also be inherited (probably autosomal dominant with variable penetrance) or acquired. Hereditary PC deficiency has been identified in many families, both in reduced concentrations (quantitative), as well as in normal concentrations with reduced activity (qualitative). Acquired PC deficiency has been documented in disseminated intravascular coagulation, acute leukemia, and marked liver dysfunction. PC deficiency may be subclinical but can be made manifest with coumarin anticoagulants. Under these circumstances, because of its short half-life (about six hours), its already diminished concentration drops below a critical level when compared to the other vitamin K-dependent proteins with longer half-lives (e.g., factors IX and X). Thus, diffuse coagulation in capillaries with ensuing tissue necrosis may occur,

---

FIGURE 9.20 → CATEGORIES OF UNUSUAL HEMATOLOGIC CAUSES OF ISCHEMIC STROKE

FACTORS THAT TIP THE BALANCE
OF THE FIBRIN-GENERATING SYSTEM
TOWARD HYPERCOAGULABILITY
Absent or Poorly Active Factors That
Limit the Coagulation Cascade
- Antithrombin III deficiency
- Protein C deficiency
- Protein S deficiency

Increased Levels of Coagulation Factors
That Promote the Coagulation Cascade
- Factor V elevation
- Factor VIII elevation

Absent or Poorly Active Factors of the
Fibrinolytic Pathway
- Plasminogen deficiency
- Plasminogen activator deficiency
- Factor XII/prekallikrein deficiency

Dysfibrinogenemias

FACTORS THAT INCREASE THE
TENDENCY OF CELLS TO AGGREGATE
Abnormalities of cellular elements
predisposing to thrombosis
- Hemoglobinopathies
  (Hb SS, Hb SA, Hb SC)
- Platelet hyperaggregability
  syndromes

Overproduction of abnormal or normal
plasma proteins (hyperviscosity syndromes)
- Paraproteinemias
  Waldenström's macroglobulinemia
  Multiple myeloma
  Lymphoma
- Cryoglobulinemia
- Heavy chain diseases

Overproduction of cellular elements
- Polycythemia rubra vera
- Relative polycythemia
- Erythrocytosis
- Leukemia
- Essential thrombocythemia

IMMUNE-MEDIATED
PROTHROMBOTIC STATES
- Thrombotic thrombocytopenic
  purpura
- Antiphospholipid antibody syndrome

---

usually limited to the skin. PC deficiency has rarely been associated with arterial thrombosis but has been clearly linked with stroke on several occasions.

PS deficiency, which is also believed to be transmitted by an autosomal gene, has a controversial association with stroke in heterozygotes with low free levels. A recent report of a family with stroke and PS deficiency has provided a stronger link. A more recent case-control study has shown that acquired PS deficiency does not increase the risk of ischemic stroke.

Thrombosis in the deficiency syndromes of PC, PS, and AT III occurs predominantly in the venous system and is usually associated with a predisposing event such as surgery, pregnancy, delivery, infection, or trauma. The explanation given for this observation is that thrombomodulin, which binds thrombin and redirects its function to activate PC, is attached to the endothelial cell surface; free thrombin generated during the constant movement of blood does not come into contact with enough thrombomodulin to adequately activate the PC system nor enough heparan-bound AT III to neutralize it, making the patient vulnerable to venous thrombosis. This is probably a contributing factor in deep venous thrombosis in all immobilized patients and would tend to occur more frequently with a deficiency of one of the above named factors.

Relative elevations of factors V and VIII have been postulated to contribute to a prothrombotic state. Although a clear causal relationship to stroke has not been established, levels of greater than 2½ times normal were highly correlated to stroke. Recently, a case linking familial factor V deficiency with stroke in a young man has been reported.

Plasminogen disorders are also just being recognized for their role in stroke and we are aware of only a single case report of two patients with cerebellar infarction in association with isolated abnormalities of plasminogen. Both of the cases occurred in young men without a history of venous thrombosis and both were apparently successfully treated with antiplatelet agents. In separate reports, factor XII deficiency has been implicated in stroke.

Elevated levels of plasminogen activator inhibitor and defective release of tissue plasminogen activator are found with greatly increased frequency in patients with quiescent inflammatory bowel disease (IBD), suggesting a possible role in the occurrence of cerebral infarction in these patients. Circulating immune complexes have also been associated with active IBD and may contribute to the thrombotic tendency.

Pregnancy and the puerperium have been linked to stroke via a variety of hypercoagulable mechanisms. Factors VII, VIII, IX, X, and fibrinogen are elevated during pregnancy. Reports of both enhanced and decreased fibrinolysis during pregnancy may indi-cate systemic alterations that contribute to thrombosis; platelets seem to become more likely to aggregate as the patient approaches term.

Dysfibrinogenemias have been associated with mainly venous, but also arterial, thromboses. As yet, there is no report of ischemic stroke in patients with dysfibrinogenemia in the absence of other concomitant stroke risk factors.

HEMOGLOBINOPATHIES

The most devastating of the hemoglobinopathies, *sickle-cell disease* (SCD), has a high rate of morbidity and mortality from stroke (approximately 5.5–17%). TIAs are frequently present initially, followed by cerebral infarction, most commonly in the border zone between the vascular territories of the MCA and ACA (Fig. 9.21).

An associated large intracranial vessel fibrous intimal hyperplasia with occasional accompanying thrombosis, hypothesized to result from years of high-velocity, flow-induced damage to the endothelium, is the underlying pathologic alteration. Endothelial damage has been found mainly in the supraclinoid ICA, proximal MCA, ACA, and to a lesser extent posterior cerebral artery (PCA). It is coupled with a high-volume, maximally dilated arteriolar system believed to represent physiologic compensation for the lower hematocrit and the lower oxygen-carrying/delivery capacities of hemoglobin (Hb) SS and the sickled red blood cells (RBCs). Cerebral infarction probably arises by one of several mechanisms: 1) progressive stenotic occlusion in combination with an already compromised vasodilatory reserve, which can lead to downstream border zone infarctions when even mild episodes of hypotension occur; 2) emboli arising from the intimal lesions, which may travel to smaller arteries, causing cessation of flow and small focal infarcts; 3) progressive stenotic occlusion with superimposed thrombosis at the point of large-vessel damage, leading to large infarctions appropriate to the territory. All of these mechanisms may interact in the setting of intravascular sickling and small vessel occlusion to produce a mixed large- and small-vessel infarction.

Typically, ischemic stroke affects SCD sufferers in their first or second decade. These people often recover well, probably due to the enhanced neuronal plasticity in young people. However, recurrent strokes with the resultant additive effect of several small deficits are always feared. A predisposition to cerebral infarction can generally be reliably predicted by noninvasive transcranial Doppler (TCD), which identifies progression of high-velocity flow in intracranial vessels. Long-term exchange transfusion in these patients appears to prevent progression of vasculopathy and reduces the risk of recurrent infarction. Isolated case reports of Hb SC- and Hb SA-related ischemic strokes have been published.

HYPERVISCOSITY SYNDROMES

The viscosity of blood is the result of an interaction between blood cells and plasma proteins. This interaction, mediated by cell-protein-cell bridges, causes the cells to have an increased affinity for one another. The resulting tendency of RBCs to aggregate diminishes blood flow, which is especially important in naturally slow-flowing channels such as capillaries, poststenotic arterioles, and veins. Manifesting frequently as rouleaux formation, it can ultimately lead to thrombosis. The degree of this interaction, and thus the degree of blood viscosity, depends mainly on the size, density, and charge of the plasma proteins, but also on the number of blood cells.

Plasma proteins that have the correct shape, charge, and adequate molecular weight to precipitate a hyperviscosity syndrome include fibrinogen and immunoglobulins. Diseases specifically known to cause stroke by hyperviscosity attributable to plasma proteins include multiple myeloma (Fig. 9.22), Waldenström's (IgM) macroglobulinemia, heavy chain disease, and malignant lymphomas. Lymphomas may additionally cause strokes by perivascular infiltrations of malignant cells or abnormal proliferation of endothelial cells, resulting in obstruction. Disseminated intravascular coagulation (DIC) may also play a role in stroke, both in lymphoma and generally. However, almost every reported case of focal lesions in the setting of DIC is complicated by many factors and it is difficult to attribute focal cerebral infarction solely to this widespread process. Cryoglobulinemia has been asso-

ciated with cerebral thrombosis in at least one case, but generally manifests peripherally with symptoms of Raynaud's phenomenon and visual disturbances in cold weather.

A hyperviscosity syndrome can occur because of the shape and resiliency of the RBC (sclerocythemic hyperviscosity; e.g., SCD and other hemoglobinopathies) and also because of increase in the sheer number of RBCs (polycythemic hyperviscosity). Polycythemia rubra vera (PRV), a myeloproliferative disorder involving increased production of all cell lines in the bone marrow, results in an accumulation of RBCs, white blood cells, and platelets in the blood. The risk for thrombosis correlates mainly with the elevated hematocrit. Stroke is clearly associated with PRV, and probably complicates the other myeloproliferative disorders (leukemias, erythrocytosis, and essential thrombocythemia) by similar mechanisms (Fig. 9.23). Stroke has also been reported in secondary polycythemias, but this is a very rare occurrence.

IMMUNE-MEDIATED PROTHROMBOTIC STATES

Thrombotic thrombocytopenic purpura (TTP) is an uncommon disease of unknown etiology that primarily affects young women (20–50 years of age). Characterized by hemolytic anemia, thrombocytopenia, fever, as well as neurologic and renal dysfunction, nearly half of those affected die in the first attack. Neurologic symptoms occur in the majority of patients with TTP and include stupor, coma, seizures, and stroke. Usually a monophasic illness, a relapsing type of TTP has been described that may also be associated with stroke. The mechanism of ischemic stroke in TTP is hypothesized to be an abnormal platelet/vessel-wall

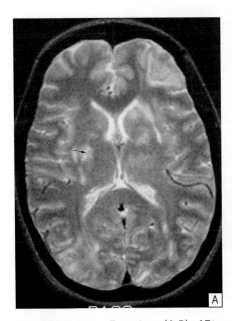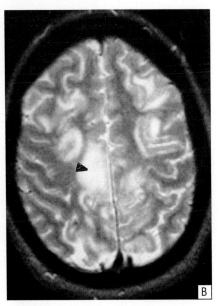

FIGURE 9.21 → Two views (**A,B**) of T2-weighted (TR2800, TE90) MRI scan of a patient with sickle-cell anemia. The multiple increased signal intensity is consistent with small (arrow) and large (arrowhead) cerebral infarcts.

interaction or an immune-mediated platelet hyperaggregability and consumptive process. Small vessels become plugged with platelet-fibrin aggregates, leading to ischemia, although large-vessel occlusion has also been reported. Platelet secretory products may also be involved in the injury process (Fig. 9.24).

Ischemic stroke can be associated with antibodies that bind phospholipids (aPL) (Fig. 9.25). The two most clinically relevant aPLs are the lupus anticoagulant and anticardiolipin antibody. Up to 10% of all first ischemic stroke patients and up to 45% of all ischemic stroke patients under age 50 harbor aPLs. They can be associated with left-sided cardiac valvular lesions, especially mitral thickening and regurgitation (which may represent Libman-Sacks endocardi-

tis), a false-positive VDRL, a positive ANA (usually low titer, homogeneous pattern), and thrombocytopenia. Women may have a higher risk of recurrent thromboembolic events, including myocardial infarction, pulmonary embolus, as well as deep vein and peripheral vascular thrombosis. Patients with aPL syndrome tend to be younger. Women are more commonly involved than in typical atherothrombotic stroke. Treatment is empiric, and patients with cardiac sources of stroke may benefit from warfarin.

DRUG-RELATED STROKE

Opiates, especially the intravenous use of heroin and pentazocine/tripelennamine (Talwin), have been linked to cerebral infarction and hemorrhage. In the

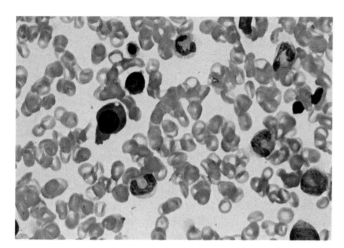

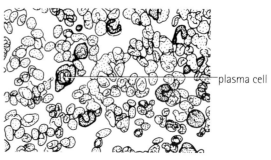

plasma cell

FIGURE 9.22 → Bone marrow biopsy (x 200) from a patient who presented with recent cerebral ischemia and was found to have smoldering multiple myeloma. An increased number of plasma cells can be seen.

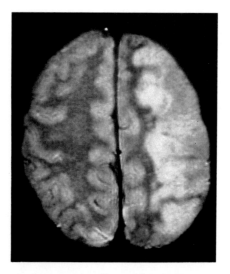

FIGURE 9.23 → T2-weighted MRI (TR2800, TE90) showing large area of hyperintensity consistent with right hemispheric infarction in a patient with thrombocytosis.

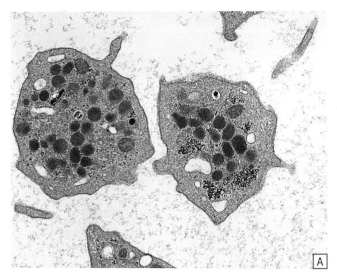
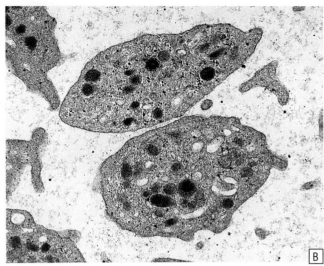

FIGURE 9.24 → Electron microscopic views (x 27,000). **A,** Platelet from a normal person shows numerous α-granules, dense bodies and mitochondria. **B,** Platelets from a patient with acute ischemic stroke show a depletion of the α-granules.

dense body

α-granule

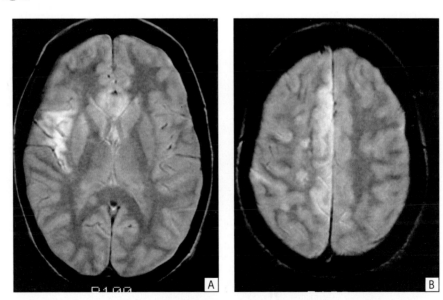

FIGURE 9.25 → T2-weighted (**A:** TR2800, **B:** TE90) cranial MRI shows increased signal intensity in multiple arterial territories. Patient has history of fetal loss and elevated antiphospholipid antibody titers.

past, Talwin injection and its impurities (talc, starch, pieces of crushed tablets) have led to embolization of these foreign materials, resulting in stroke. Heroin has also been related to a hypersensitivity-type small-vessel vasculitis leading to stroke.

Sympathomimetics, particularly methamphetamine, have been associated with intracerebral hemorrhage, SAH, and CI. Many of the CI cases seem to be related to a necrotizing angiitis of arterioles and small muscular arteries, although segmental constrictions and occlusions of penetrators have also been reported, indicating possible varied effects on the vasculature. There is a renewed concern with amphetamines since the recent appearance of "ice"—a smokable form of methamphetamine that can deliver very high doses. At present, we are unaware of any documented reports of stroke with this form of the drug.

Cocaine, both in the conventional hydrochloride form and in the smokable "crack" alkaloidal form, has been associated with SAH, as well as with ischemic and hemorrhagic infarctions. It is probably the most common illicit drug associated with stroke. Surprisingly, it has not been associated with vasculitis. Postulated mechanisms include one or a combination of the following: acute hypertension, cerebral vasoconstriction, or increased platelet aggregation. On angiography, vasospasm, intraluminal clot, as well as large- and medium-sized vessel occlusion have been seen (Fig. 9.26).

MISCELLANEOUS

TUBEROUS SCLEROSIS

Tuberous sclerosis is an autosomally inherited syndrome clinically characterized by epilepsy, mental retardation, and angiofibromata of the skin known as adenoma sebaceum. Although the particular gene defect is unknown, it appears to be related to hyperplasia of ectoderm- and mesoderm-derived cells. This syndrome usually presents in childhood with infantile seizures and progressive mental deficiency, although its clinical expression varies widely. The skin manifestations of adenoma sebaceum typically arise later on, in the last half of the first decade. Strokes can occur by hemorrhage into affected cerebral areas or by cardioembolism arising from cardiac rhabdomyomas. More than half of these patients die before adulthood.

FABRY'S DISEASE

Fabry's disease, an X-linked lysosomal enzyme(α-galactosidase) deficiency that produces accumulation of ceramide trihexoside (CTH), predominantly affects hemizygote males and, to a lesser extent, heterozygote females. The lipid tends to deposit systemically in the glomerulus, skin, cornea, and diffusely throughout the vasculature. Accordingly, the systemic clinical manifestations, which usually begin in the second decade, include 1) proteinuria, hypertension, and progressive renal failure; 2) characteristic angio-

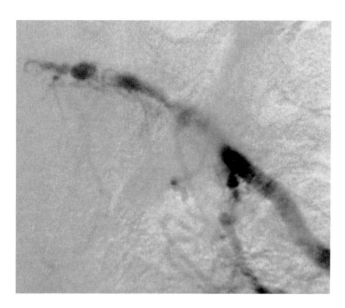

FIGURE 9.26 → Basilar artery narrowing and distal occlusion in a chronic cocaine user.

keratomas of the skin; 3) corneal opacifications; 4) myocardial infarction; and 5) stroke relating to vascular occlusion. CTH also forms deposits in the CNS, mainly in areas of the brain where the blood-brain barrier is more permeable, such as 1) the supraoptic and paraventricular nuclei of the hypothalamus, 2) the hippocampus, 3) parahippocampal gyrus, 4) inferior temporal cortex, 5) median eminence, 6) dorsal root ganglia of the spinal cord, as well as 7) certain brainstem nuclei that are involved mainly in the autonomic system, including the intermediolateral cell column of the spinal cord.

Patients with Fabry's disease quickly manifest CNS dysfunction, usually beginning with painful paresthesias relating to fever or exercise (which may be secondary to lipid deposition in the peripheral nerves). The mechanisms of cerebral vessel occlusion that arise later in Fabry's disease include 1) occlusion from lipid deposition in the vessel walls; 2) cardioembolism from valvular lesions secondary to lipid deposition, mitral valve prolapse, or 3) cardiomyopathy secondary to accelerated hypertension from renal disease. Angiography in presumed vasculogenic stroke has revealed marked dilation of the cerebral arteries similar to observations of tortuous and dilated retinal and scleral vessels. Patients often die in their 40s or 50s from myocardial infarction, stroke, or renal failure.

MIGRAINE-RELATED STROKE

Migraine headaches are probably a risk factor for stroke. The relationship of migraine to stroke can be separated into four distinct categories: 1) *coexisting stroke and migraine*—a stroke that arises in a migraineur, occurring remote in time from a typical migraine attack; 2) *stroke with clinical features of migraine*—a stroke that presents as a typical migraine, either in a patient with an established history of migraine (symptomatic migraine) or as a first-time occurrence (migraine mimic); 3) *migraine-induced stroke*—a stroke that occurs during a typical migraine attack and appears to be an extension of the aura into a permanent deficit. These may occur in the presence or absence of stroke risk factors, but other causes of stroke must be excluded. 4) The *"uncertain"* category is for migraine-related strokes not falling clearly into the other types. The etiology of migraine-induced stroke is uncertain.

Acknowledgments
Lori Douthat, Laura Brenton and Dr. Steve Smith, Department of Cardiology; Dr. Jean Riddle, Department of Rheumatology; Drs. Ken Kapphahn and Gretchen Tietjen, Department of Neurology, Henry Ford Hospital, Detroit.

REFERENCES

Adams RD, Vander Eecken HM. Vascular diseases of the brain. *Ann Rev Med.* 1952; 213–252.

Amarenco P, Duyckaerts C, Tzourio C, et al. The prevalence of ulcerated plaques in the aortic arch in patients with stroke. *N Engl J Med.* 1992; 326:221–225.

Amico L, Caplan LR, Thomas C. Cerebrovascular complications of mucinous cancers. *Neurology.* 1989; 39:522–526.

Biller J, Adams HP Jr. Non-infectious granulomatous angiitis of the central nervous system. In: Toole JF (ed). *Handbook of Clinical Neurology,* Vol. 55 (11): Vascular Diseases, Part III, 1989; 387–400.

Bleck TP. Takayasu's disease. In: Toole JF (ed). *Handbook of Clinical Neurology,* Vol. 55 (11): Vascular Diseases, Part III, 1989; 335–340.

Brown MM, Swash M. Polyarteritis nodosa and other systemic vasculitides. In: Toole JF (ed). *Handbook of Clinical Neurology,* Vol. II (55): Vascular Diseases, Part III, 1989; 353–368.

Cerebral Embolism Task Force. Cardiogenic brain embolism. *Arch Neurol.* 1989; 46:727–743.

Conlan MG, Haire WD, Burnett DA. Prothrombotic abnormalities in inflammatory bowel disease. *Dig Dis Sci.* 1989; 34:1089–1093.

D'Angelo A, Landi G, Vigano'D'Angelo S, et al. Protein C in acute stroke. *Stroke.* 1988; 19:579–583.

Demers C, Ginsberg JS, Hirsh J, et al. Thrombosis in antithrombin-III-deficient persons. *Ann Intern Med.* 1992; 116:754–761.

Fisher CM, Adams RD. Observations on brain embolism with special reference to hemorrhagic infarction. In: Furlan AJ (ed). *The Heart and Stroke.* 1987; 17–36.

Furie B, Furie BC. Molecular and cellular biology of blood coagulation. *N Engl J Med.* 1992; 326:800–806.

Furlan AJ, Lucas FV, Craciun R, Wohl RC. Stroke in a young adult with familial plasminogen disorder. *Stroke.* 1991; 22:1598–1602.

Gomez-Aranda F, Dominguez JML, Fernandez VR, Garcia EM. Stroke and familial protein S deficiency (letter). *Stroke.* 1992; 23:299.

Hart RG, Kanter MC. Hematologic disorders and ischemic stroke: a selective review. *Stroke.* 1990; 21:1111–1121.

Kaku DA, Lowenstein DH. Emergence of recreational drug abuse as a major risk factor for stroke in young adults. *Ann Intern Med.* 1990; 113:821–827.

Kaye EM, Kolodny EH, Logigian EL, Ullman MD. Nervous system involvement in Fabry's disease: clinicopathological and biochemical correlation. *Ann Neurol.* 1988; 23:505–509.

Lechat P, Mas JL, Lascault G, Loron P, Theard M, Klimczac M, Drobinski G, Thomas D, Grosgogeat Y. Prevalence of patent foramen ovale in patients with stroke. *N Engl J Med.* 1988; 38:1148–52.

Levine J, Swanson PD. Nonatherosclerotic causes of stroke. *Ann Intern Med.* 1969; 70:807–816.

Levine SR, Welch KMA. Antiphospholipid antibodies. *Ann Neurol.* 1989; 26:386–389.

Levinson SA, Close MB, Ehrenfeld WK, Stoney RJ. Carotid artery occlusive disease following external cervical irradiation. *Arch Surg.* 1973; 107:395–397.

Longstreth WT Jr, Swanson PD. Oral contraceptives and stroke. *Stroke.* 1984; 15:747–750.

Makos MM, McComb RD, Hart MN, Bennett DR. Alpha-glucosidase deficiency and basilar artery aneurysm: report of a sibship. *Ann Neurol.* 1987; 22:629–633.

Mayer SA, Sacco RL, Hurlet-Jensen A, Shi T, Mohr JP. Free protein S deficiency in acute ischemic stroke: a case-control study. *Stroke.* 1993; 24:224–227.

Makori B, Sundt TM Jr, Houser OW, Piepgras DG. Spontaneous dissection of the cervical internal carotid artery. *Ann Neurol.* 1986; 19:126–138.

Moore PM. Diagnosis and management of isolated angiitis of the central nervous system. *Neurology.* 1989; 39:167–173.

Moore PM, Cupps TR. Neurological complications of vasculitis. *Ann Neurol.* 1983; 14:155–167.

Mumenthaler M. Cranial arteritis. In: Toole JF (ed). *Handbook of Clinical Neurology,* Vol 55 (11): Vascular Diseases, Part III, 1989; 341–351.

Ohene-Frempong K. Stroke in sickle cell disease: demographic, clinical, and therapeutic considerations. *Semin Hematol.* 1991; 28:213–219.

Ott E. Hyperviscosity syndromes. In: Toole JF (ed). *Handbook of Clinical Neurology,* Vol. 55 (11): Vascular Diseases, Part III, 1989; 483–492.

Roach ES. Malignant atrophic papulosis (Kohlmeier-Degos disease). In: Toole JF (ed). *Handbook of Clinical Neurology,* Vol 55 (11): Vascular Diseases, Part III, 1989; 275–281.

Ross Russell RW, Wade JPH. Haematological causes of cerebrovascular disease. In: Toole JF (ed). *Handbook of Clinical Neurology,* Vol 55 (11): Vascular Diseases, part III, 1989; 463–481.

Sakuta R, Nonaka I. Vascular involvement in mitochondrial myopathy. *Ann Neurol.* 1989; 25:594–601.

Sandok BA. Fibromuscular dysplasia of the cephalic arterial system. In: Toole JF (ed). *Handbook of Clinical Neurology,* Vol 55 (11): Vascular Diseases, part III, 1989; 283–292.

Schafer AI. The hypercoagulable states. *Ann Intern Med.* 1985; 102:814–828.

Stern BJ. Cerebrovascular disease and pregnancy. In: Goldstein PJ (ed). *Neurological Disorders of Pregnancy,* 1986; 19–40.

Vonsattel JPG, Hedley-Whyte ET. Homocystinuria. In: Toole JF (ed). *Handbook of Clinical Neurology,* Vol. 55 (11): Vascular Diseases, Part III, 1989; 325–334.

Welch KMA, Levine SR. Migraine-related stroke in the context of the international headache society classification of head pain. 1990; 47:458–462.

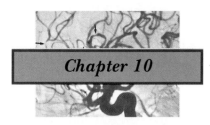

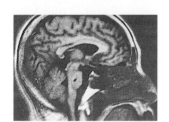

Chapter 10

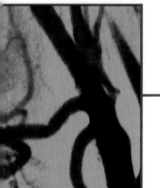

LAWRENCE M. BRASS

Stroke in Younger Patients

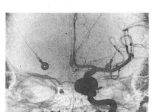

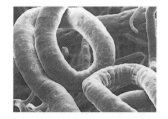

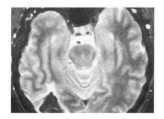

STROKE IN THE YOUNG usually refers to patients from the middle teen years to age 45 or 50. Stroke occurring in young adults is doubly dramatic. Not only does it strike previously healthy people, but the survivors face decades of disability. Physicians caring for young patients with stroke are confronted with special challenges. First, there are many nonvascular syndromes which can present as a stroke. Second, when the patient does have a stroke, there are many possible etiologies with a wide range of prognoses and therapeutic alternatives.

The goal of this chapter is to provide an overview of stroke in younger patients and to present various medical and surgical approaches. The details of many of the diseases are covered in greater detail elsewhere in this volume.

EPIDEMIOLOGY

The reported incidence of stroke in young adults is much lower than older adults (Fig. 10.1). Incidence estimates vary from 2.5 to 40 out of 100,000 and account for 4% to 10% of all strokes (i.e., 20,000–50,000 new strokes in young people each year in the U.S.). Over the age of 30, the incidence of stroke is slightly higher in men. Under the age of 30, some reports indicate a female preponderance. This difference has been attributed to the use of oral contraceptives by women. Over the past decade, low dose estrogen preparations have become standard and these differences may not persist. Even though the incidence of stroke is much less than usually reported for older age, stroke in the young is still a common cause of neurologic disease. For adults 18 to 44 years old, cerebrovascular disease is twice as prevalent as multiple sclerosis.

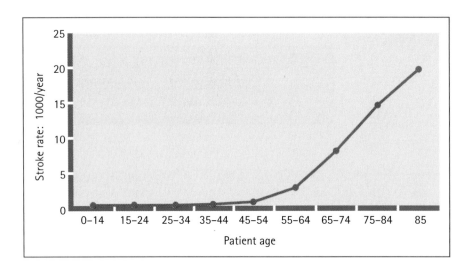

FIGURE 10.1 → Stroke rate by age group.

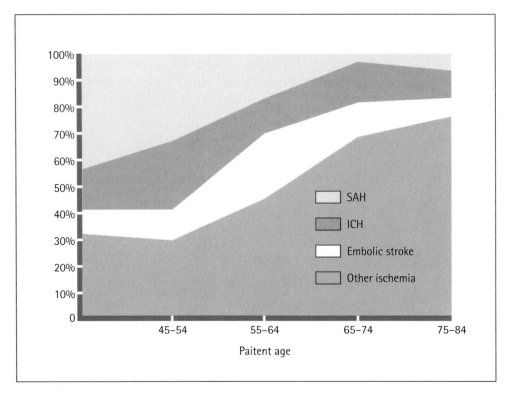

FIGURE 10.2 → Stroke type by age group.

TYPES OF STROKE IN THE YOUNG

In patients over the age of 60, 80% of strokes are ischemic. In younger patients, only half of strokes are due to ischemia (Fig. 10.2). As with older patients, the differentiation between hemorrhagic and ischemic stroke has important diagnostic and therapeutic implications and should be part of the initial evaluation of a stroke patient at any age.

Hemorrhage. Intracranial hemorrhage accounts for a larger portion of young strokes than strokes in older adults. This is due to the peak frequency of subarachnoid hemorrhage in younger adults and the relative rarity of atherosclerotic disease.

Subarachnoid Hemorrhage. About 25% of all subarachnoid hemorrhages (SAH) occur in patients under age 45. As with older adults, the most common cause is a ruptured saccular aneurysm. The diagnosis, evaluation, and treatment does not differ much for younger patients except, perhaps, to consider more strongly the diseases associated with intracranial aneurysms, including coarctation of the aorta, polycystic kidney disease, arteriovenous malformations (AVMs), Marfan's disease, and Ehlers-Danlos syndrome.

Younger patients with SAH often do not appear as ill as older adults. Warning (sentinel) bleeds may present as only a mild headache or change in a headache pattern. The outcome after SAH is probably better for younger patients because they are generally healthier. The diagnosis and management of younger patients with SAH does not differ significantly from older age groups and is covered in Chapter 12.

Intracerebral Hemorrhage. As with SAH, the causes and management of intracerebral hemorrhage (IH) are similar for young and old patients. The relative contribution of various sources, however, is different (Fig. 10.3). Trauma, drugs, and AVMs are more common in the younger groups. Hypertension plays a greater role in the older groups.

Ischemic Stroke. The lack of a satisfactory classification for ischemic stroke is even more of a problem for younger stroke patients. Etiology may be classified according to hemodynamics (e.g., large-vessel occlusion, small-vessel disease, or embolus) or pathophysiology (e.g., vasculopathy or coagulopathy). Problems arise because a single pathophysiologic process, such as coagulopathy, could be associated with more than one hemodynamic mechanism (e.g., embolus or thrombosis). An underlying disease process may also be associated with more than one pathophysiologic process. For example, antiphospholipid antibodies may have effects on both coagulation and the vascular endothelium.

CAUSES OF ISCHEMIC STROKE IN THE YOUNG

In patients past their sixth decade, atherosclerosis is the major underlying pathology. A greater variety of pathologies exist for younger patients. A systematic approach is essential for a thorough investigation. In careful studies of large numbers of young patients with stroke, including angiography, cardiac embolism appears to be the single most common cause of stroke, followed by thrombosis, arterial dissection, and atherosclerosis (Fig. 10.4). Major diseases associated with stroke in younger patients will be described.

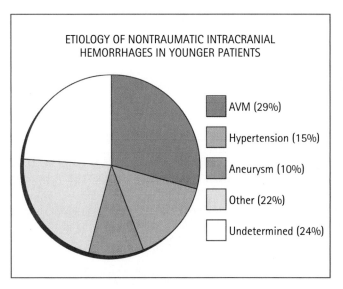

ETIOLOGY OF NONTRAUMATIC INTRACRANIAL HEMORRHAGES IN YOUNGER PATIENTS

- AVM (29%)
- Hypertension (15%)
- Aneurysm (10%)
- Other (22%)
- Undetermined (24%)

FIGURE 10.3 → Etiology of nontraumatic intracranial hemorrhages in younger patients.

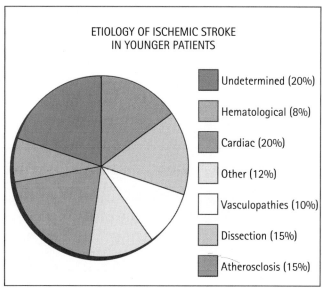

ETIOLOGY OF ISCHEMIC STROKE IN YOUNGER PATIENTS

- Undetermined (20%)
- Hematological (8%)
- Cardiac (20%)
- Other (12%)
- Vasculopathies (10%)
- Dissection (15%)
- Atherosclosis (15%)

FIGURE 10.4 → Etiology of ischemic strokes in younger patients.

VASCULOPATHY

Atherosclerosis. Although signs of atherosclerotic disease can be found by the late teens in most Americans, it usually remains asymptomatic until late middle age. Atherosclerosis is strongly age dependent. Atherosclerosis can cause stroke through a variety of mechanisms, the most common being large-vessel occlusive disease and sources for emboli.

Overall, only about 25% of ischemic stroke in the young is ascribed to atherosclerosis. Patients with atherosclerosis usually have classical risk factors such as hypertension, diabetes, a history of smoking, lipid abnormalities, or a family history of premature vascular disease. As with cardiovascular disease, younger patients with atherosclerosis associated with stroke may be more likely to have genetic traits associated with premature atherosclerosis.

Lipoproteins. The association between lipid abnormalities and stroke is not settled. The evidence is far less strong than for cardiac disease. Low levels of high-density lipoprotein cholesterol may be associated with an increased risk for stroke. It is widely believed, however, that lipid abnormalities probably play a role in younger patients with advanced atherosclerosis. Lipid abnormalities may also work synergistically with other vascular risk factors, especially in younger patients with accelerated atherosclerosis.

Elevation of lipoprotein Lp(a) is associated with an increased risk of stroke. Although its overall impact as a risk factor is unknown, it is believed to contribute to stroke risk by inhibiting the thrombolytic action of plasminogen. Other lipoprotein abnormalities possibly associated with stroke include type III hyperlipoproteinemia, type IV hyperlipoproteinemia, Tangier disease, and lipoprotein Lp(b).

Even in the absence of any definite association with stroke, attention to lipid abnormalities is important for reducing the risk of other manifestations of accelerated atherosclerotic vascular disease (e.g., early myocardial infarction and vascular death).

Dissection. Arterial dissection is a leading cause of stroke in the young and the most common nonatherosclerotic vasculopathy. This diagnosis should be considered in any young stroke patient, especially when vascular risk factors are absent.

Although classically associated with flexion or extension injuries to the neck, many cases of arterial dissection found in young patients are not associated with any clear history of neck injury. Even when there is a history of neck injury, it is often minor. A wide variety of activities has been associated with dissection (Figs. 10.5, 10.6).

In dissection, a tear in the vessel wall allows blood to accumulate in a "false lumen" within the medial layer of the arterial wall. As the false lumen fills with blood, it expands and can result in significant narrowing of the vessel lumen or lead to local thrombus formation with secondary embolization.

Classically, the patient may complain of head or neck pain. For the carotid artery, pain is often referred to the eye, temple, or forehead. There may also be an associated Horner's syndrome. With vertebral artery (VA) dissection, pain is often referred to the neck or the back of the head.

The most common location for a dissection is about 2 cm beyond the origin of the internal carotid artery (ICA). The diagnosis usually requires standard or MR angiography (Fig. 10.7). Ultrasound cannot reliably image much beyond the carotid bifurcation.

Some diseases appear to be associated with an increased tendency for arterial dissection and should be considered during the work-up of all patients with cervical dissection. These include: fibromuscular dysplasia, Marfan's syndrome, cystic medial degeneration, atherosclerosis, luetic arthritis, and Ehlers-Danlos syndrome.

Moyamoya is an arterial reaction to intracranial occlusive disease. Moyamoya (Japanese for a puff of smoke) refers to the angiographic finding of an arterial blush of fine vessels that resemble smoke

---

FIGURE 10.5 → ACTIVITIES ASSOCIATED WITH ARTERIAL DISSECTION

Coughing	Sports activities (tennis, skiing, basketball,	Neck flexing with child abuse
Brushing teeth	volleyball, polo, football, bowling, swim-	(scolding)
Nose blowing	ming, hockey)	Chewing
Chiropractic manipulation	Old whiplash injury	"Head banging" during dancing
Head-turning during a parade	Car sliding on ice	Strangulation
Straightening up after bending	Intraoral trauma (fall with object in mouth)	Childbirth
Trampoline exercises	Motor vehicle accident	"Downing" shots of liquor

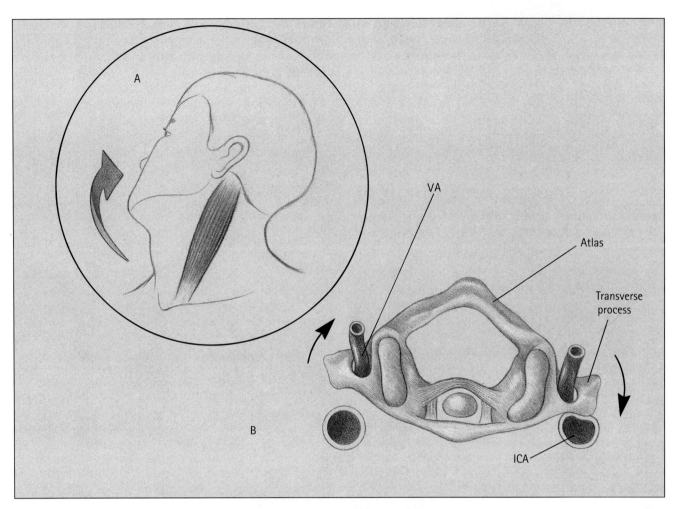

FIGURE 10.6 → The carotid arteries can be injured by neck rotation.
A, A hyperextended neck. **B,** The vertebral artery is impinged on the vertebral process.

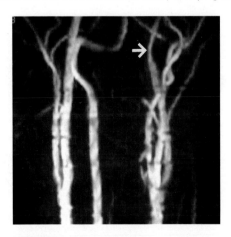

FIGURE 10.7 → An MRA is essential
for diagnosing arterial dissection (arrow).

at the base of the brain. These vessels are collaterals that form around an occlusion of large arteries at the brain's base. Arterial occlusion is the disease, not the formation of the collateral network. Any process associated with the occlusion of the proximal intracranial arteries (e.g., neurofibromatosis, sickle-cell disease, Marfan's syndrome, radiation therapy, or Down's syndrome) may result in moyamoya. This syndrome is found in younger patients because moyamoya collaterals usually do not develop beyond the third decade of life.

The term *moyamoya disease* is sometimes applied to young children (usually <4 years old) who develop bilateral carotid occlusion without apparent cause. The etiology is unknown. The course is usually downhill with seizures, hemiparesis, and encephalopathy. Arterial bypass procedures are used, but their effectiveness is unknown.

Fibromuscular Dysplasia is a nonatherosclerotic and noninflammatory vasculopathy with an unknown etiology. Women appear to be affected more often than men. The renal arteries are most commonly affected (~75%) followed by the carotid arteries (~25%), but many other small and medium arteries can also be involved. The disease is often multifocal. The diagnosis is usually based on the classic angiographic appearance of a "string of beads" (Fig. 10.8).

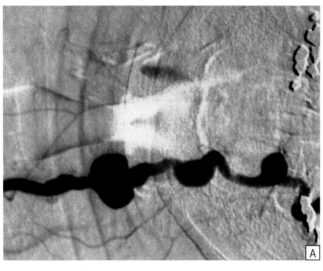
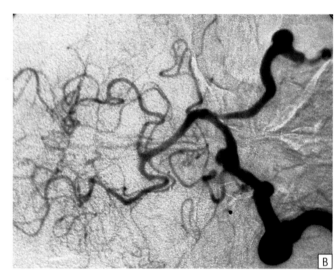
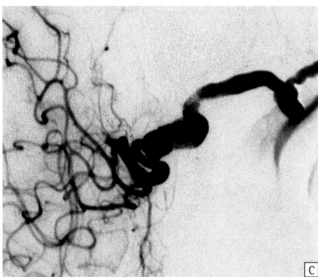
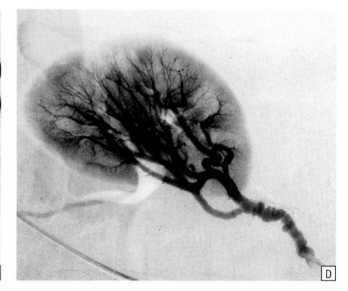

FIGURE 10.8 → Fibromuscular dysplasia in a 40-year-old woman. **A,** Segmental areas of dilatation seen in the extracranial vertebral artery (ECVA). **B,** AP view of vertebrobasilar system, with a vertebral artery (VA) aneurysm near the posterior inferior cerebellar artery (PICA). **C,** Lateral view of internal carotid artery (ICA) with alternating areas of narrowing and dilatation. **D,** Renal artery demonstrates "beaded" appearance.

Most patients with fibromuscular dysplasia are asymptomatic. However, it can result in occlusive disease of the carotid arteries. It has also been associated with cerebral embolization, dissection, intracranial aneurysms, and carotid cavernous fistulas. Patients may also have accompanying neck pain, carotid tenderness, tinnitus, or a carotid bruit. The natural history is not well established, but the rate of progression and the rate of stroke in asymptomatic cases appears to be low.

Percutaneous transluminal angioplasty has emerged as a treatment of choice in the renal arteries for those with secondary hypertension. Experience in the carotid is limited. Asymptomatic disease should not require treatment. Antiplatelet agents are often recommended.

Vasculitis. Many types of vasculitis are associated with stroke (Fig. 10.9). Infectious processes can, but rarely do, cause vasculitis.

Isolated (granulomatous) angiitis of the central nervous system can also occur. It is uncommon, but when it does occur, younger patients are often affected. The absence of systemic inflammation is a key point in the diagnosis. Although restricted to the central nervous system, the disease is often multifocal. Early symptoms include headache, confusion, intellectual decline, changes in memory, and malaise. As the disease progresses, focal signs are typical, including focal deficits (strokes), seizures, and myelopathies. Angiographic findings of multiple areas of narrowing, occlusion of vessels, and delayed emptying of vessels suggest the diagnosis. Since these changes are not specific, a biopsy is often needed. False negative biopsies are common due to the disease's segmental nature. An aggressive approach is indicated because immunotherapy may alter the progressive nature of the disease (recurrent strokes leading to death).

Infection. As mentioned above, infectious processes can be associated with vasculitic changes in the cerebral vessels in younger stroke patients. Causes include mucormycosis, tuberculosis, herpes zoster, meningovascular syphilis, and possibly HIV infection and Lyme disease.

Patients with HIV infection appear to have a higher rate of cerebral infarction than other young people. About 1% of patients with AIDS have a symptomatic stroke. In autopsy series, about 33% of patients with AIDS or ARC (AIDS related complex) have evidence of cerebrovascular disease. Approximately 85% are ischemic. Most of these strokes were not symptomatic, and were rarely the presenting syndrome. About 50% of HIV-related stroke cases are also associated with CNS infections.

The most common pathology is multifocal microvascular disease, which is associated with thickening of the intraparenchymal arterioles. Ischemic strokes in HIV-infected patients are also associated with nonbacterial thrombotic endocarditis or an inflammatory vasculopathy secondary to cryptococcal or tuberculous meningitis, lymphoma, or herpes zoster.

Patients with toxoplasmosis often have transient focal neurologic deficits. The exact mechanism for this is unclear, but toxoplasmosis should be con-

---

FIGURE 10.9 → ARTERIAL DISEASES ASSOCIATED WITH CEREBRAL INFARCTION IN YOUNG ADULTS

LARGE-ARTERY ATHEROSCLEROSIS, SMALL-ARTERY DISEASE (LACUNAR), NONATHEROSCLEROTIC DISEASE/ARTEROPATHIES

INFLAMMATORY (SEE ALSO VASCULITIS CLASSIFICATION)	NONINFLAMMATORY	VASOSPASM ASSOCIATED WITH:
Takayasu's disease	Dissection (spontaneous	Migraine
Allergic (Churg-Strauss) and	or traumatic)	Subarachnoid hemorrhage
granulomatous angitis	Posttherapeutic irradiation	(SAH)
Infective—specific: syphilis, mucormycosis,	Fibromuscular hyperplasia	Hypertensive encephalopathy
herpes zoster, tuberculosis, malaria, AIDS,	Moyamoya and progressive	Cerebral arteriography
and neuroborreliosis	arterial occlusion syndrome	
Drugs—amphetamines, cocaine,	Congophilic (amyloid)	
and pseudoephedrine	angiopathy	
Associated with systemic disease (SLE, Wegener's, poly-	Thromboangiitis obliterans	
arteritis nodosa, rheumatoid arthritis, Sjögren's,	Familial: homocystinuria, Fabry's,	
scleroderma, acute rheumatic fever, sarcoidosis,	pseudoxanthoma elasticum,	
Eale's disease, and inflammatory bowel disease)	Marfan's syndrome	
	Behçet's disease	
	Dego's disease	

sidered in the differential diagnosis of TIAs in an HIV-infected patient.

There are a few reports of Lyme disease and stroke, but a clear causal relationship has not been established. A vasculitis has been postulated. Young patients who present with predominantly cranial nerve signs should be tested for Lyme disease. This common presenting syndrome for Lyme disease otherwise may be misdiagnosed as a stroke syndrome.

CARDIAC AND EMBOLIC

In older patients, atrial fibrillation (AF) and ischemic heart disease are the most common causes of cardioembolic stroke. In younger patients, there is a much wider range of abnormalities that need to be considered (Fig. 10.10). Classic cardiac lesions associated with stroke (valvular disease, cardiomyopathy, arrhythmias, and endocarditis) occur in about 12% of young stroke patients. Recent studies have attributed 25% to 30% of ischemic strokes to cardiac embolism. As better diagnostic tests are performed prospectively, it is likely that there will be an even greater emphasis on the heart as an etiology for stroke in young patients. Transesophageal, contrast echocardiography, ultrafast computed tomography (CT), and magnetic resonance imaging (MRI) all increase the yield of cardiac abnormalities detected and are being applied to the clinical care of patients with stroke.

The diagnosis of a cardiac embolism is usually based on the presence of a potential embolic source. The two major categories of cardioembolic stroke are: 1) embologenic site within the heart, and 2) a right to left intracardiac shunt (paradoxical emboli).

Paradoxical emboli arise in the venous circulation, bypass the filtering function of the pulmonary capillary bed, and enter the systemic circulation. Clots can bypass the pulmonary arterioles either through an intracardiac shunt (e.g., patent foramen ovale) or a pulmonary fistula (e.g., pulmonary AVM).

Intracardiac shunts appear to be the more common mechanism, especially a patent foramen ovale. Other etiologies include atrial septal defect and ostium secundum. Recently, improved cardiodiagnostic tools have identified this mechanism as a potential cause of stroke in up to 25% of young stroke patients. For those who have no other identifiable cause, about 50% will demonstrate an intracardiac shunt.

Patent foramen ovale. There is strong evidence that a patent foramen ovale (PFO) is associated with stroke. The exact contribution is unknown because 2% to 10% of younger adults without stroke will have evidence of an intracardiac shunt. In addition, there is little available information on the rate of stroke in patients with a PFO. However, crude estimates are available for pulmonary fistula. Pulmonary arteriovenous malformations (PAVM) also bypass the

pulmonary capillary bed. About one third of patients with PAVM and hereditary hemorrhagic telangiectasia (Osler-Rendu-Weber disease) have radiologic evidence for previous cerebrovascular events, suggesting that the lifetime risk of a right to left shunt may be significant.

Historical points that suggest a paradoxical embolus are recent deep vein thrombosis or stroke onset associated with a Valsalva maneuver (e.g, coughing or straining). Further work is needed before rational decisions on clinical management can be made.

Valvular disease. Emboli may arise from the heart in a variety of valvular diseases. Congenital valvular disease, such as aortic stenosis, usually presents before adulthood. Other forms of valvular disease occur in stroke patients for all ages. There is little difference in the diagnostic evaluation or therapeutic recommendation for young adults. Mitral valve prolapse is one form of valvular disease that has been cited more commonly as a cause of stroke in younger populations.

Mitral valve prolapse. Case control studies have suggested that mitral valve prolapse (MVP) is associated with an increased risk for stroke. Although this may be true, the implications for managing the individual patient with stroke remain unclear. In a control population, about 20% of women and 5% to 10% of men will be found to have mitral valve prolapse. The estimated risk of stroke for those with mitral valve prolapse is less than 0.01% per year.

The finding of mitral valve prolapse should not imply that an etiology for the stroke has been found. Even when MVP is the only abnormality in a complete evaluation, associating it as the etiology of a stroke will require further studies and the establishment of additional diagnostic criteria.

The mechanism of stroke in patients with MVP is unknown. Possibilities include emboli arising from the valve, associated arrhythmias, or conditions possibly associated with MVP (e.g., increased platelet aggregability).

Arrhythmias. The etiologic and therapeutic implications for cardiac arrhythmias in younger stroke patients is similar to those in older adults. Atrial fibrillation is seen in less than 4% of young stroke patients in most clinical series. These patients should be managed as any other patient with AF and stroke. Warfarin is usually favored for secondary prevention.

Evidence for cardiac arrhythmias is obtained on history, an ECG, or Holter monitor. All are part of the routine evaluation of stroke in younger patients. If these are normal, other evaluations for cardiac arrhythmias need not be done.

Infective endocarditis should be considered in stroke patients who present with a fever and a heart murmur. Endocarditis is also suggested by the presence of systemic signs of emboli such as petechiae of skin and mucous membranes, splinter hemorrhage under the finger- or toenails, Roth spots, Osler's nodes, or Janeway lesions. Streptococci, staphylococci, and enterococci are the most common infective organisms. Patients at highest risk for infective endocarditis include those with congenital or acquired heart disease, prosthetic valves, intravenous drug use, hemodialysis, and immunosuppresion. The mechanism of stroke is a septic embolus, which can cause cerebral infarction or a mycotic aneurysm, leading to SAH or intracerebral hemorrhage (IH).

Nonbacterial (Marantic) thrombotic endocarditis. This diagnosis is usually reserved for patients without bacterial endocarditis, who have fibrin or platelet vegetations on the heart valves and cerebral emboli from these vegetations. Up to 75% of cases are associated with an occult tumor. Although associated with many tumor types, it is most commonly reported in association with lung, gastrointestinal (esp. pancreatic), ovarian, and prostatic carcinomas. There is often a history of other embolic events, congestive heart failure, or pneumonia.

Myxomas are cardiac tumors that rise from endothelial or subendothelial cells. Although rare, they are most often found in the left atrium. Stroke is caused by emboli (e.g., tumor or clot). There may be other symptoms of obstructive cardiac disease and nonspecific symptoms such as fatigue, weight loss, fever. The sedimentation rate is often elevated. On cardiac auscultation, a "plop" may be heard. Surgical treatment is usually curative. Follow-up is needed to monitor for recurrent tumor growth or aneurysmal dilatation from tumor emboli to the brain.

HEMATOLOGIC
Hematologic disorders are usually implicated in 5% to 10% of stroke in younger patients (Fig. 10.11). This is probably a low estimate. Few studies have screened for the full spectrum of known disorders, and new

---

FIGURE 10.10 → EMBOLISM AND STROKE IN THE YOUNG

CARDIAC SOURCE
Atrial fibrillation (AF) and sick-sinus syndrome (SSS)
Valvular (mitral stenosis, prosthetic valve, infective endocarditis, marantic endocarditis, Libman-Sacks endocarditis, mitral annulus calcification, mitral valve prolapse, calcific or aortic stenosis, and rheumatic heart disease)
Acute myocardial infarction and/or left ventricular aneurysm
Intracardiac tumors and myxomas
Cardiomyopathy

PARADOXICAL EMBOLISM AND PULMONARY SOURCE
Pulmonary arteriovenous malformation (including Osler-Weber Rendu syndrome)
Atrial and ventricular septal defects with shunt
Patent foramen ovale
Pulmonary vein thrombosis
Pulmonary and mediastinal tumors

OTHER
Cardiac procedures
Aortic cholesterol embolism
Transient embologenic aortitis
Emboli distal to unruptured aneurysm
Fat embolism syndrome
Foreign body emboli (iatrogenic or drug use)
Tumor embolus

FIGURE 10.11 → HEMATOLOGIC DISEASE AND COAGULOPATHIES

Thrombotic thrombocytopenia purpura
Chronic diffuse intravascular coagulation
Paroxysmal nocturnal hemoglobinuria
Oral contraceptive use/peripartum/pregnancy
Thrombocythemia
Sickle-cell or hemoglobin SC disease
Antiphospholipid antibody or lupus anticoagulant
Dysfibrinogenemia
Nephrotic syndrome
C2 deficiency
Protein C or protein S deficiency
Antithrombin III deficiency
Heparin cofactor II deficiency
Fibrinolytic insufficiency
Increased factor VIII
Decreased factor XII
Vitamin K or antifibrinolytic therapy
Alcohol intoxication
Disseminated intravascular coagulation
Platelet hyperaggregability
Hyperviscosity syndromes (dysproteinemias [myeloma, Waldenstrom's, cryoglobulinemia], polycythemia and myeloproliferative disorders)

associations are being made between hematologic abnormalities and stroke (see Chapter 3). Differentiating associated hematologic changes from clear etiologic factors has also been difficult. This field is likely to yield many new associations with stroke over the coming decade.

Hematologic etiologies should be considered in younger patients, especially those without evidence for atherosclerosis and a normal cardiac evaluation, even more so if there is a family or personal history of thrombotic events. Most hematologic disorders are associated predominantly with venous thrombosis. The number of abnormalities reported with ischemic stroke is growing rapidly. Little information is available on which of the associated abnormalities are the most important in clinical practice.

Enhanced Clot Formation

Platelet disorders: thrombocytosis/platelet abnormalities. Increased platelet counts accompanied by myeloproliferative disorders are associated with microvascular thrombosis. Strokes are common. An increase in platelets alone does not appear to significantly increase the risk of stroke (e.g., thrombocytosis following splenectomy). Both primary and secondary platelet abnormalities probably contribute to stroke in younger patients. The difficulty in obtaining blood samples for platelet function testing and the lack of clinically useful markers has limited the number of stroke patients diagnosed with platelet disorders. Even when platelet abnormalities are detected following a stroke, many are likely to be secondary to the stroke or to associated vascular risk factors.

Red cell disorders: sickle-cell disease. Sickle-cell disease is associated with stroke, especially in children. Those with hemoglobin SS, S-thalassemia, and SC disease are all at increased risk. Both large- and small-vessel strokes can occur. Large-vessel strokes are probably the result of endothelial damage with secondary hyperplasia leading to intracranial occlusive disease. The mechanism of small-vessel stroke is less well understood. The risk of stroke may also be increased by the associated anemia. Resistance vessels in the brain dilate to compensate for the decreased oxygen carrying capacity of the blood, resulting in high flows. This probably increases endothelial damage and is associated with decreased vasomotor reserve. Because the resistance vessels are already dilated, the individual may be at higher risk for distal field (watershed) infarctions. Transfusion therapy is used both to treat an acute stroke and for secondary prevention. The vascular damage associated with these hemoglobinopathies also places the patient at increased risk for intracerebral hemorrhage.

Patients with sickle-cell trait are usually asymptomatic. When stroke or other vascular problems do occur, they usually appear in young adults, and are associated with severe physiologic stress.

Polycythemias. Polycythemia vera is a primary myeloproliferative disorder resulting in increased red cell mass. The usual neurologic syndrome is related to increased viscosity and globally decreased brain perfusion (headache, lethargy, dizziness). Ischemic stroke does occur in about 10% to 20% of patients. Risk parallels the hematocrit. The risk of stroke appears to be less for the secondary polycythemias (e.g., young adults with congenital cyanotic heart disease and compensatory polycythemia).

Paroxysmal nocturnal hemoglobinopathy. In this rare acquired stem-cell disorder, the erythrocyte membrane becomes sensitive to complement lysis, resulting in hemolytic anemia. Platelets and granulocytes are often mildly reduced. Only a minority of patients have the characteristic nocturnal hemolysis and hemoglobinuria.

This disorder occurs in young adults and may result in venous thrombosis in the brain and liver. Arterial occlusion has been postulated, but is rare. The diagnosis is made by testing for red cell lysis with complement activation (Ham's test) or osmotic stress (sucrose gradient test).

Impaired Clot Regulation

The most commonly reported disorders of clot regulation are deficiencies of coagulation inhibitors. Reductions in activity of 20% to 30% are probably associated with an increased risk. Both low levels and altered functional activity have been reported.

Although they can be hereditary, most regulatory disorders are probably acquired, as a consequence of other disease states or medications. Alterations in clot regulation may interact with traditional vascular risk factors (such as smoking) to further increase the risk of thrombotic events.

Protein C/Protein S Deficiency. Both of these are vitamin K-dependent plasma proteins. Activated Protein C, in conjunction with Protein S, inhibits coagulation by inactivating factors Va and VIIIa and also inhibits platelet aggregation. Protein C is activated when thrombin mixes with thrombomodulin on the vascular endothelium. Deficiencies of either Protein C or Protein S can lead to increased clot formation.

Most clinically recognized Protein C deficiencies are probably acquired. (Heterozygotes are rarely symptomatic and are found in about 1/200–300 unselected blood donors.) Low levels are also associated with malignancies, liver disease, hemodialysis, antiphospholipid antibodies, postoperative states, disseminated intravascular coagulation, and some medications such as antibiotics containing an N-methyl thiotetrazole ring and coumadin. A few cases of stroke associated with Protein S have also been reported.

Antithrombin III normally inactivates thrombin when it is bound to heparin on the vascular endothelium. When levels are low, more activated thrombin is present, leading to an increased tendency to clot. Heparin receives its anticoagulation effect through an increase in antithrombin III activity. Resistance to anticoagulation with heparin suggests an antithrombin III deficiency.

The hereditary form of antithrombin III deficiency is an autosomal dominant trait with variable penetrance. It is estimated to occur in about 1 in 2000 people. Both alterations in the functional activity and low levels of normal antithrombin III have been reported. Most cases are probably acquired. This deficiency is associated with severe hepatic disease, renal disease, and oral contraceptive use.

Other Factors. Although alterations in the concentrations of other coagulation factors have been reported in ischemic stroke in young patients, etiologic evidence is lacking in most cases. Evaluation for these factors is usually not indicated in the diagnostic evaluation of a young patient with ischemic stroke.

Alterations in Clot Dissolution

Abnormalities of fibrinolysis have been linked to thrombosis and, in a few cases, ischemic stroke. These disorders appear to be rare and inherited (e.g., plasminogen deficiency, plasminogen activator deficiency, dysfibrinogenemia, and factor XII/prekallikrein deficiencies).

RHEUMATOLOGIC/AUTOIMMUNE

Antiphospholipid antibody syndrome is a condition with recurrent thrombotic events and the presence of antibodies directed against negatively charged phospholipids. The associated vascular events include most types of arterial and venous ischemic stroke. A subgroup of those with antiphospholipid antibodies will have a lupus anticoagulant. This antibody also interferes with the phospholipid activation in determining an activated partial thromboplastin time (aPTT). Although the laboratory result would seem to indicate an anticoagulated state, this is an artifact of the testing procedure because lupus anticoagulant is associated with thrombotic events in vivo. The aPTT does not correct with normal plasma (indicating that this is not a factor deficiency).

Cardiolipin is a phospholipid commonly used in screening for this syndrome. About 70% of patients with the antiphospholipid antibody syndrome will have an antibody directed against cardiolipin (anticardiolipin antibody).

The exact mechanism of thrombosis is unknown. Changes in endothelial function, platelet aggregation, altered prostacyclin synthesis, reduced levels of coagulation proteins, and depressed fibrinolysis have all been reported.

Although initially described in association with patients with systemic lupus erythematosis (SLE), most stroke patients with antiphospholipid antibodies do not have SLE. Antiphospholipid antibodies have been associated with other autoimmune diseases, the use of medications (phenytoin, phenothiazines, and procainamide), puerperium strokes, strokes during pregnancy, spontaneous abortions, thrombocytopenia, AIDS, Lyme disease, Behçet's syndrome, and Sneddon's syndrome (livedo reticularis and ischemic stroke). Familial antiphospholipid antibodies also occur.

Antiphospholipid antibody is found in about 2% to 5% of the normal population, implying that in the absence of other strongly suggestive signs (e.g., spontaneous abortions, livido reticularis), the diagnosis of an antiphospholipid antibody-related stroke should be made only after a thorough evaluation for other causes.

Although most experts recommend some form of stroke prevention therapy, there is no data from controlled clinical trials. Most recommend aspirin or coumadin. Experience with steroids and immunosuppressives has been disappointing.

Systemic lupus erythematosis. An association with antiphospholipid antibodies as well as vascular and valvular lesions has implicated systemic lupus erythematosis (SLE) as a cause of stroke. If SLE is quiescent at the time of the stroke or the full criteria for SLE is not met, then a full diagnostic evaluation is indicated. Even when the diagnosis is clear, the presence of several vascular risk factors can lessen its certainty.

Miscellaneous. A variety of other rheumatologic diseases have been associated with stroke, including Behçet's syndrome, rheumatoid arthritis, scleroderma, Sjögren's syndrome, polymyositis, cryoglobulinemia, Henoch-Schönlein purpura, Takayasu's disease, and necrotizing vasculitides (e.g., polyarteritis nodosa, Wegener disease). Stroke is usually not the presenting symptom, and a specialized work-up in the absence of signs or symptoms suggesting these conditions is usually not indicated.

OTHER CAUSES OF STROKE IN THE YOUNG

Drug Use

A variety of drugs have been associated with both ischemic and hemorrhagic strokes. In some series, up to 25% of strokes in young adults are drug related, nearly 50% in those under 35 years old.

Commonly associated drugs include cocaine and sympathomimetics such as phenylpropanolamine, amphetamines, and pseudoephedrine. The sympathomimetics are more strongly associated with intracranial hemorrhages. Cocaine HCl (used IV or intranasally) and alkaloid cocaine (crack cocaine) have been associated with both ischemic and hemorrhagic strokes.

There are a variety of mechanisms by which these and other substances may be associated with stroke, including foreign body emboli, spasm, vasculitis, immune complex disease, enhanced platelet aggregation, alterations in thromboxane production, decreased fibrinolytic activity, enhanced plasminogen activity, transient hypertension, cardiac dysfunction, and cardiac arrhythmias.

Moderate to heavy drinking (both acute and chronic) has been implicated in cardiovascular disease and probably contributes to the risk for cerebral infarction. Alcohol can cause stroke through induction of cardiac arrhythmias, cardiac wall motion abnormalities, hypertension, enhanced platelet aggregation, activation of coagulation, stimulation of vascular smooth muscle (leading to vasoconstriction), and altered cerebral metabolism.

Migraine Headaches

Migraine headaches occur in about 30% of young women and 15% of young men. A large number of stroke patients give a history of migraine. Although most agree that migraine is associated with an increased risk for stroke, the relative contribution is unknown.

Migraine could be associated with stroke, either as part of a migraine attack (i.e., cerebral vasoconstriction) or through associated abnormalities, such as serotonergic pathways that are also involved in platelet aggregation. Migraine has been associated with ischemic stroke in 5% to 15% of most series of young strokes. A definitive diagnosis is difficult because of the lack of reliable diagnostic criteria. Headache alone is not sufficient. Up to 30% of patients with ischemic stroke will report the presence of head pain at the time of the stroke.

Migrainous stroke most commonly occurs in women with a prior history of complicated migraine and a previous TIA-like episode preceding a headache. Most migraine-related strokes occur in the distribution of the posterior cerebral artery (PCA). Most neurologists restrict the diagnosis of migrainous stroke to those with a history of classic migraine with aura. Some additionally require that the deficit be similar to the usual aura of the migraine.

The predilection of migrainous stroke for women may be related to the increased frequency of migraine in premenopausal women, or to the possible contribution of estrogens to both migraine and ischemic stroke. Estrogen is a vasodilator. Rapid drops in serum levels, which occur before menstruation, can trigger vasoconstriction. This is thought to be associated with the trigger for catamenial migraines, microvascular angina, and possibly stroke.

Although the mechanism of migrainous stroke remains obscure, most studies report favorable outcomes and low recurrence rates. The diagnosis should be made only after a full evaluation for other etiologies (Fig. 10.12).

Birth Control Pills

Case control and cohort studies have implicated oral contraceptives as a risk for ischemic stroke, and possibly for SAH. There may be a greater risk in those who also smoke or have migraine.

Birth control pills and most hormonal replacement regiment cycle the level and ratio of estrogen and progesterone during the month. As with menstrual migraine, one of the most common times for stroke associated with the use of birth control pills that contain no estrogen is just prior to menstruation. Hypercoagulable states have also been postulated as an associated mechanism.

Originally, birth control pills contained high levels of both estrogen and progesterone, and strong evidence linked these preparations to stroke. However, no studies have shown an association with current pills, which contain less than 50 μg of estrogen. The role of progestins as a risk for stroke is not known. Even with high estrogen dose preparations, the increased risk associated with the use of oral contraceptives is less than the risk of stroke associated with pregnancy.

Pregnancy

Pregnancy, peripartum, and postpartum periods have all been associated with stroke, although the overall incidence of stroke during pregnancy (approximately 5/100,000) is not significantly different from other young women.

In addition to the etiologies discussed elsewhere in this chapter, other mechanisms may be involved in pregnancy-related stroke. Eclampsia and hypertension are associated with intracranial hemorrhage. Ischemic strokes may be caused by emboli from cardiomyopathies, amniotic fluid, or air. Vascular hyperplasia and hypercoagulable states also occur. Anemia, sepsis, or dehydration may predispose to stroke. Trauma associated with delivery has been reported with cervical dissection.

Management is based on the etiology, but is often complicated by concerns for the fetus.

Homocyst(e)ine

Several autosomal recessive enzyme deficiencies are associated with homocystinuria and stroke. The most common defect is cystathionine β-synthase deficiency, or impaired conversion of homocysteine to cystathionine. Plasma levels of homocysteine levels are increased. Homocysteine is metabolized into several forms that are collectively known as homocyst(e)ine. The homozygous state has long been associated with stroke in children. This error of methionine metabolism is associated with a marfanoid body type, lens dislocation, and mental retardation. It may cause stroke through secondary abnormalities in the vascular endothelium with an increased tendency for thrombosis.

Recent evidence suggests that the heterozygous and acquired disorders of methionine metabolism are associated with an increased risk for stroke. A gene for homocystinuria may be present in as many as 1 in 70 people. Modest elevations of homocystine levels may occur in up to 25% of young stroke patients. Testing for the heterozygote state—that is, measuring homocyst(e)inemia response to methionine loading—is difficult and not widely available. Homocystinuria and elevated levels of homocyst(e)ine often respond to dietary manipulation and treatment with folic acid or vitamin B$_6$.

Cancer and Paraneoplasm

Cerebrovascular complications are often found in patients with cancer and are the second leading cause of CNS disease in cancer patients. Symptomatic stroke is reported in 7% of those dying from cancer; evidence for cerebrovascular disease is found in about 15% of autopsies.

Cancer can be associated with stroke mechanisms such as direct effect of tumor (embolus), coagulopathies, septic infection, and reactions to thera-peutic interventions. The mechanism and type of stroke vary with each cancer. Leukemia is usually associated with hemorrhage; carcinomas are more likely to cause infarction. Many of the cancers associated with cerebrovascular disease affect young patients. Some of the most important types are presented in Fig. 10.13.

MELAS

Mitochondrial myopathy, encephalopathy, lactic acidosis, and strokelike episodes (MELAS) is a distinct syndrome associated with mitochondrial myopathies. Patients present in childhood. They typically have short stature, seizures, hemparesis, hemianopia, or cortical blindness. Ragged red fibers (typical for mitochondrial myopathies) are seen on muscle biopsy. Ischemic stroke has been associated with this syndrome; however, many of the "strokelike episodes" in MELAS syndrome do not correspond to a single vascular territory. Imaging on MR clearly shows changes that cross vascular territories. It is likely that at least some of the "strokes" that occur with MELAS syndrome are metabolic, not ischemic.

Venous Thrombosis

Venous occlusion, whether from intravascular or extravascular occlusion, can cause infarction or hemorrhage (Fig. 10.14) and is a common cause of stroke in young women. In early reports, many patients were septic. This is now rare when appropriate antibiotics are used.

Thrombosis of intracranial veins has been associated with pregnancy, puerperium, oral contraceptives, ulcerative colitis, congestive heart failure, diabetes, dehydration, sepsis, and a variety of hematologic disorders (sickle-cell disease, thrombocytopenia, polycythemia, and disseminated intravascular coagulation). Patients often present with headaches

---

FIGURE 10.12 → CRITERIA FOR MIGRAINOUS CEREBRAL INFARCTION*

Patient has history of migraine with neurologic aura (classic migraine)

Present attack is similar to previous attack, but symptoms do not resolve within 7 days or neuroimaging studies demonstrate ischemic infarction in the relevant area

Other causes of infarction have been excluded by appropriate investigations

* From the Headache Classification Committee, 1988.

FIGURE 10.13 → MECHANISMS OF STROKE ASSOCIATED WITH NEOPLASMS

DISEASE/THERAPY	MECHANISM	EFFECT
	DIRECT EFFECTS OF TUMOR ON THE BRAIN	
Germ cell tumors	Tumor emboli	Ischemic infarction
Cardiac myxomas		Neoplastic aneurysms
Many types (esp. lung, breast, and lymphoma)	Dural metastases	Sagittal sinus thrombosis
		Subdural hematoma
Many types (esp. germ cell tumors and melanoma)	Metastatic brain tumors	Intracerebral (tumor) hemorrhage
Many types (esp. astrocytomas, oligodendrogliomas, meningiomas, and pituitary adenomas)	Primary brain tumors	Intracerebral (tumor) hemorrhage
	SEPSIS-RELATED PROBLEMS	
Leukemia and lymphoma	Septic embolus (esp. fungal)	Ischemic embolic infarction
	COAGULOPATHY	
Leukemia, breast carcinoma, and lymphoma	Disseminated intravascular coagulation	Intracranial hemorrhage
Leukemia, carcinomas, lymphomas, myelomas	Coagulopathy	Intracranial hemorrhage
Adenocarcinoma of the lung, breast, or G.I. tract; lymphoma and leukemias	Nonbacterial thrombotic endocarditis	Ischemic embolic infarction
Lymphoma, breast cancer	Hypercoagulable state	Venous thrombosis
	EFFECTS OF THERAPY	
L-asparaginase (used in treating lymphoblastic leukemia)	Coagulopathy (reduction in coagulation proteins)	Parenchymal hemorrhage, ischemic infarction, and venous thrombosis
Lung cancer, neuroblastoma, lymphoma	Venous thrombosis, venous infiltration or compression	Venous occlusion
Head and neck irradiation	Large vessel occlusive disease	Ischemic infarction

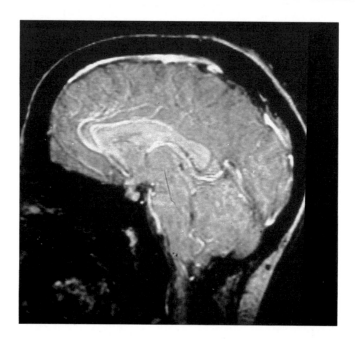

FIGURE 10.14 → A sagittal sinus thrombosis on MRI.

and focal seizures. The clinical syndromes associated with venous thrombosis are usually less specific than for arterial occlusion. Occlusion of the larger cortical veins and sinuses is often associated with increased intracranial pressure.

PROGNOSIS

For young patients who present with TIA, making reliable prognostic predictions for an individual is even more difficult than in older stroke patients. Transient neurologic deficits are common in young people and most are apparently benign. In cases where the syndrome suggests a single vascular distribution, concern is higher. Within this group of young patients with typical TIAs, the likelihood of subsequent stroke depends on the TIA's mechanism. The long term prognosis is strongly influenced by traditional vascular risk factors. For example, in young patients with a TIA associated with atherosclerotic vascular disease (i.e., vascular risk factors or atherosclerosis on angiography), the risk for stroke, myocardial infarction, and death is high. For those with TIAs, a negative work-up, and a history of migraine, the risk of serious recurrent events is low.

The prognosis for recovery and the rate of recurrent stroke or death are better in younger patients. The mortality for younger stroke patients is about 5% and the overall incidence of recurrent stroke is less than 1% per year. In most series, more than 75% of patients show significant improvement or return to normal. This more favorable outcome may be due to higher frequency of migraine, trauma, and

nonatheromatous etiologies in younger stroke patients. The prognosis, and the need for secondary prevention, will vary widely with the stroke's etiology; therefore a thorough evaluation for the underlying etiology is essential.

WORK-UP

The diagnosis and management of stroke needs to be tailored to the individual patient. This is especially true in young patients, where a great variety of medical diseases may be related to a stroke. Given the large number of possible tests, and the associated risks and expense, a systematic approach is often useful. Valuable clues are often present in the history and clinical examinations.

GENERAL COMMENTS

History
The evaluation of all stroke patients begins with three diagnostic questions: 1) Is this a stroke? 2) Where is the lesion? and 3) What type of process is involved? The first step in the initial evaluation is to consider nonvascular etiologies for the stroke syndrome. Up to a third of all patients who present with a stroke syndrome will be found to have another process that is responsible for the syndrome. The diseases in Figure 10.15 should be considered in all patients who present with a stroke.

Although cerebrovascular disease can be caused by a wide variety of diseases, it is often not the presenting symptom. A careful history, with a view

---

FIGURE 10.15 → CAUSES OF FOCAL NEUROLOGIC DEFICITS

Migraine	Orthostatic hypotension
Seizure (partial)	Cardiac arrhythmia
Hypoglycemia	Amnestic syndrome
Subdural hematoma	Narcolepsy
Intracerebral hematoma	Cataplexy
Subarachnoid hemorrhage	Intracranial inflammation
Cerebral infarction	Periodic paralysis
Tumor	Pressure neuropathy
Arteriovenous malformation	Dizziness of uncertain etiology
Demyelinating disease	Anxiety
(multiple sclerosis)	Hyperventilation
Incipient syncope	Labyrinthine disease
Encephalitis	
(esp. early herpetic infection)	

toward diseases associated with stroke, can help focus the initial diagnosis and management. Figure 10.16 highlights historical points that may suggest diseases associated with stroke.

Physical and Neurologic Examinations
The neurologic evaluation in young stroke patients helps localize the vascular territory and size of the

stroke. A general physical examination can provide important clues to diseases associated with stroke (Fig. 10.17).

General Diagnostic Evaluation
The basic evaluation for young stroke patients includes a core of diagnostic tests such as those listed in Figure 10.18. All patients should have some form of

---

FIGURE 10.16 → PATIENT HISTORY: CLUES TO THE CAUSE OF A STROKE

HISTORICAL FACT	SIGNIFICANCE
Neck trauma or manipulation	Carotid or vertebral artery dissection
Migraine	Predisposed to stroke, especially if complicated migraine
IV drug use	Endocarditis, HIV infection, vasculitis, paradoxical emboli, vasospasm, foreign body emboli
Bacterial infection	Endocarditis, septic emboli, coagulopathies
Deep venous thrombosis or pulmonary embolism	Antiphospholipid antibody syndrome, coagulopathy
Sickle cell disease	Occlusive vascular disease, subdural hematomas, SAH
Bruisability	Coagulopathy, Ehlers–Danlos syndrome, Henoch-Schönlein purpura, cryoglobulinemia
Family history of risk factors for accelerated atherosclerosis (young myocardial infarct, vascular death)	Genetic premature atherosclerosis
Pregnancy and peripartum	Coagulopathies, dissections, emboli, hemorrhage
Cancer	Nonbacterial thrombotic endocarditis
	Venous thrombosis
	Hemorrhage into tumor (esp. melanoma, germ cell tumor)
	Hemorrhage associated with myelogenous tumor or DIC
	Tumor emboli

FIGURE 10.17 → PHYSICAL EXAMINATION: CLUES TO THE CAUSE OF A STROKE

PHYSICAL FINDING	SIGNIFICANCE
Asymmetric arm blood pressures	Coarctation of aorta, aortic dissection, Takayasu's disease
Skin: needle tracts	Intravenous drug abuse, HIV infection
Skin: livedo reticularis	Sneddon's syndrome, systemic lupus erythematosis
Skin: xanthoma or xanthalasma	Hyperlipidemia
Adenopathy	HIV infection, sarcoidosis, Tangier disease
Heart murmur	Endocarditis, MVP, ventricular septal defect, asymmetric septal hypertrophy, myxoma, hamartoma (tuberous sclerosis)
Vessels: diminished pulses	Premature atherosclerosis, coarctation of the aorta, aortic dissection, Takayasu's disease
Vessels: bruit	Premature atherosclerosis, fibromuscular dysplasia, arterial dissection, homocystinuria
Extremities: venous thrombosis	Hypercoagulable state
Neurologic: multifocal deficits	Emboli, vasculitis

FIGURE 10.18 → INITIAL TESTS IN EVALUATION OF YOUNG STROKE

Complete blood count
Platelet count
Blood glucose
Serum electrolytes
Liver function tests
Blood urea nitrogen and creatinine
Prothrombin and partial thromboplastin time
Erythrocyte sedimentation rate

Serological test for syphilis (VDRL)
Hemoglobin electrophoresis (in blacks)
Electrocardiogram (EKG)
Transthoracic echocardiogram
CT scan or MR image
Chest X-ray
Cerebral angiography
Drug screen

anatomic brain imaging (CT or MRI). Although these studies may demonstrate an infarction, they are performed in the acute stage to exclude hemorrhage and nonvascular etiologies for the stroke syndrome (see Fig. 10.15). Further testing is usually directed toward a particular stroke mechanism (Fig. 10.19). Highlights of the diagnostic evaluation are outlined below.

VASCULOPATHY

As a group, diseases affecting the cranial vessels are the most common cause of stroke. In addition, the detection of emboli by demonstrating intracranial branch occlusion of the cerebral arteries can provide important diagnostic, therapeutic, and prognostic clues. Imaging of the vasculature should be part of the evaluation of almost all young patients with stroke unless an etiology is clear from the initial evaluation.

Angiography remains the standard for imaging the vessels in stroke patients. It can demonstrate the etiology of an ischemic stroke, especially if performed early after ictus. When performed within a few days of the onset, abnormalities are seen in up to 75% of young stroke cases. This high yield, combined with a lower rate of reported complications, emphasizes the importance of angiography in the diagnostic evaluation of these young patients.

The most common abnormalities found in young patients with cerebral infarction are branch occlusion (embolus), atherosclerosis, and arterial dissections. Although often appearing as a smooth tapering away from a bifurcation, the angiographic appearance of dissection in a vessel with little atherosclerosis is not specific. Less commonly, a double lumen, totally occluded vessel, or a false aneurysm can be detected. If there is doubt, an MRI of the neck may be able to demonstrate blood within a false lumen.

Ultrasound of the carotids or intracranial vessels (with transcranial Doppler) can be a useful adjunct to angiography as a screen for disease or to monitor progression of disease. MRA cannot yet match the image quality of conventional angiography, especially for the intracranial circulation. Its role is yet to be defined in the management of younger patients with stroke.

Arterial biopsy. If a vasculopathy is suspected, a biopsy can be helpful in confirming the diagnosis, assessing prognosis, and selecting therapies.

FIGURE 10.19 → SELECTED TESTS IN EVALUATION OF YOUNG STROKE

VASCULOPATHY
SPECT of brain
Transcranial Doppler
MRA
Serum lipids and Lipoprotein Lp(a)

CARDIAC AND EMBOLIC
Transthoracic echocardiogram (with contrast)
Holter monitoring
Transesophageal echocardiogram
   (with contrast)
Ultrafast CT of heart
Cardiac MRI

HEMATOLOGIC
Fibrinogen
Blood cultures
Sucrose lysis test
Serum viscosity
Coagulation (including circulating platelet
   aggregates and spontaneous platelet
   aggregation, serum viscosity, antithrombin III
   levels, protein-C, protein-S, thrombin time,
   functional fibrinogen assays, fibrin degradation products, and fibrin monomers)

RHEUMATOLOGIC/AUTOIMMUNE
Antinuclear antibody
Serum immunoglobulin levels
Ham test/sucrose gradient test
Serum complement levels
Antiphospholipid antibody screening

OTHER
CSF examination
   (for infection/inflammation/arteritis)
Cystathione beta-synthetase activity
Cyanide nitroprusside test
   (for homocystinuria)
HIV testing

Lipid screening. When atherosclerosis is associated with stroke in young adults, a search should be conducted for diseases or conditions associated with premature or accelerated disease, such as lipid abnormalities. The timing of testing can influence the results of lipid screening. During an acute stroke, cholesterol and triglyceride are often depressed. Lipid abnormalities are most marked about three months after the stroke. Fasting studies for serum cholesterol, HDL, and triglycerides should be done during hospitalization. If normal, these should be repeated at three months. When abnormalities are identified, especially in a young stroke patient, aggressive intervention is usually indicated.

CARDIAC AND EMBOLIC

As mentioned above, young stroke patients with atherosclerosis should receive an evaluation similar to that for older patients. Because of the high association of cerebral atherosclerosis with coronary artery disease, these patients should also be considered to have accelerated cardiovascular disease and must be evaluated accordingly for prevention of coronary artery disease and vascular death.

Since the heart may be responsible for at least a third of ischemic strokes in the young, an aggressive diagnostic approach is often warranted, especially when embolism is suspected. The cardiac evaluation should include an ECG, a 24 h Holter monitoring for those with higher suspicion of cardioembolic embolus, and a cardiac ultrasound. The current standard for evaluation is a 2-dimensional transthoracic cardiac echocardiogram. If this study is normal or left atrial disease is strongly suspected, a transesophageal echocardiogram (TEE) is usually indicated.

During TEE, a small ultrasound probe is passed into the esophagus, immediately behind the left atrium, allowing a superb view of the left atrium, left atrial appendage, mitral valve, and atrial septa. These areas are often not well seen on a transthoracic ultrasound and are common sites of pathologies associated with cardiac emboli in young patients.

Even when conventional views are normal, a transcardiac pathway for systolic emboli may still exist (paradoxical embolus). Until recently, this has been difficult to diagnose. Many centers are now using ultrasonic contrast such as agitated saline. The microbubbles produced are easily detected by ultrasound. During the examination, they are injected intravenously and normally pass from the right side of the heart to the left through the lungs. With intracardiac shunts, an immediate jet of contrast can be seen emerging through the cardiac septa.

The sensitivity for finding a shunt from the right atrium to the left can be enhanced by having the patient perform a Valsalva maneuver during the contrast injection. This increases pressure in the right side of the heart and increases the pressure gradient between the two chambers. Using these techniques, intracardiac shunts have been detected in up to 40% of young patients with stroke.

Newer techniques with ultrafast CT and gated MR show great promise for imaging the heart and valves and for detecting cardioembolic sources.

HEMATOLOGIC

Most hematologic diseases associated with ischemic stroke do not cause abnormalities in the commonly performed laboratory tests. A specialized diagnostic evaluation for possible prothrombotic conditions is often indicated for patients with prior venous thrombosis, family history of unusual thrombosis, or unexplained recurrent strokes, and for patients where the etiology of the stroke is unknown (especially in younger patients).

Coagulopathies. Many coagulation parameters are altered by an acute stroke. Testing performed 6 to 8 weeks after the initial event is important to confirm an initial diagnoses or for complete screening for occult coagulopathies.

Initial screening for prothrombotic states should include: prothrombin time (PT), activated partial prothrombin time (aPTT), hemoglobin electrophoresis (for blacks) and a sedimentation rate. If any of the initial results are abnormal, additional testing may be indicated (e.g., plasma mixing when the aPTT is elevated to differentiate a lupus anticoagulant from a factor deficiency). More sensitive measures such as Kaolin clotting time or the Russell Viper Venom Time can be used.

If there is evidence of systemic disease, especially neoplasms, additional testing including fibrin degradation products and serum protein electrophoresis should be ordered.

Indications for more specialized testing in younger stroke patients include: 1) family history of thrombotic events; 2) personal history of recurrent thrombosis; especially if in unusual locations; and 3) no other etiology for the stroke is found. The following tests should performed: 1) serum viscosity (for dysfibrinogenemia); 2) antithrombin III levels; 3) protein-C; 4) protein-S (especially free protein S); 5) thrombin time; and 6) functional fibrinogen assays. The number of well documented cases is small and most of these abnormalities are rare.

Other measures such as tPA, tPA inhibitor-1 activity, fibrin monomers, circulating platelet aggregates, spontaneous platelet aggregation, coagulation factors VII and VIIIc, heparin cofactor II deficiency, defective release of plasminogen activator, Factor XII deficiency, and prekallikrein deficiency may be associated with stroke in research protocols, but currently have limited clinical usefulness.

RHEUMATOLOGIC/AUTOIMMUNE

These diseases usually do not present with stroke but are often accompanied by other signs or symptoms. Serologic testing is usually not helpful in making the diagnosis. For example, rheumatoid factor is positive in many diseases. An erythrocyte sedimentation rate (ESR) is usually elevated in the immunologic and rheumatologic diseases associated with stroke, but is limited because of its lack of specificity. It is useful in suggesting that further investigations be done for an atypical cause of the stroke syndrome. Conversely, a normal ESR can be seen with biopsy proven vasculitis. If there are some findings of SLE, an ANA can be useful. Without any other findings, an ANA in a young stroke patient is of unclear significance. Up to 7% of normal individuals and up to 17% of hospitalized patients have a positive ANA. If an ANA is positive, further testing with more specific assays is indicated (e.g., anti-DNA antibodies).

Antiphospholipid antibodies have emerged as a potent and common risk factor for ischemic stroke. They may be present even when the routine coagulation measures are normal. Because of therapeutic and prognostic implications, they should be ordered in all younger stroke patients without an obvious etiology for their stroke.

Lyme titers should be ordered from the serum in individuals or in regions at risk. A few cases have reported both Lyme disease and ischemic stroke. A Lyme titer is also important when considering neuroborreliosis. If suspicion is high, a cerebrospinal fluid sample should be checked.

OTHER

Drug Testing. Although the exact contribution to the overall problem of stroke in the young is unknown, drug screening should be considered in all patients. Urine screening usually has a higher yield because of the increased concentration of most drugs and metabolites in the urine.

TREATMENTS

GENERAL COMMENTS

Many of the treatments for individual diseases were briefly mentioned in the sections above. A few of the basic therapeutic options are presented in this section.

VASCULOPATHY

Atherosclerotic vascular disease. For younger patients with a stroke related to atherosclerosis, risk factor management takes on added importance. Although cigarette smoking, lipid abnormalities, and obesity have not been conclusively associated with the risk

for stroke overall, there is evidence to suggest that these risk factors contribute more to some stroke subtypes, such as large-vessel atherosclerosis. They may play an added role in younger patients with stroke. Traditional risk factors, such as hypertension and diabetes, should also be vigorously managed. Antiplatelet agents are usually recommended for secondary prevention of stroke, as well as coronary artery disease.

Risk factor modification can reduce the risk of stroke and death even in cases of genetically accelerated atherosclerosis. In these diseases, vascular disease may be related to an abnormal or excessive response to an environmental factor (e.g., cigarette smoke).

Dissection. Although there is some debate, the overall prognosis is good. The risk of recurrence is apparently small. Most authorities recommend either antiplatelet medication, anticoagulation, or a combination. There is no clear role for surgery.

Migraine. For those diagnosed with migrainous stroke, treatment usually consists of minimizing the chance for recurrence by prophylactic measures, such as avoiding environmental triggers (e.g. smoking), cessation of possibly associated medications (including high dose estrogens), and prescribing migraine medications, for instance β-blocker or calcium channel antagonist. Low-dose aspirin is often recommended for at least the first few years, both for its antimigraine and antiplatelet actions.

CARDIAC AND EMBOLIC

In patients with a cardioembolic stroke, anticoagulation is usually recommended. This may be restricted to the first year following a stroke, the period of greatest risk for recurrent stroke. For the remainder of patients, aspirin should be used in most, especially when there is atherosclerotic disease. The use of other agents for secondary prevention, such as ticlopidine, is being defined.

When an etiology for a paradoxical embolus is found, anticoagulation should be used if there is evidence for peripheral venous thrombosis. In all cases, closure of the pulmonary or cardiac conduit should be considered. Closure of the foramen ovale can be done with an "umbrella" placed through the patent foramen ovale in the cardiac catheterization laboratory. Over several months, the umbrella will be overgrown by endocardium. Clinical testing is currently underway.

HEMATOLOGIC

Coagulopathy. Treatment for many of the ongoing coagulopathies, such as deficiencies of protein C, protein S, or antithrombin III, is usually with warfarin. Heparin should be used at the beginning of warfarin therapy to reduce the chances for the complication of warfarin-induced skin necrosis, which is more common in these patients.

RHEUMATOLOGIC/AUTOIMMUNE

Antiphospholipid antibodies. Most authorities recommend therapy for stroke patients with an antiphospholipid antibody. Usually this is aspirin, but coumadin or ticlopidine is often used in patients where stroke occurred while taking aspirin or with recurrent vascular events. The role of immunosupression is unknown in patients with an antiphospholipid antibody. Immunosupression or plasmapheresis may

have a role in the treatment of patients with underlying rheumatologic disease.

OTHER

The therapies associated with the other and miscellaneous causes of stroke in younger patients vary with the individual disease. A key principle remains for all aspects of stroke management of younger patients: given the low acute mortality, long life expectancy, and generally good recovery, an aggressive approach toward diagnosis and treatment of underlying diseases is strongly recommended.

REFERENCES

Adams HP, Butler MJ, Biller J, Toffol GJ. Nonhemorrhagic cerebral infarction in young adults. *Arch Neurol.* 1986; 43:793–796.

Graus F, Rogers LR, Posner JB. Cerebrovascular complications in patients with cancer. *Medicine.* 1985; 64:16–35.

Hart RG, Kanter MC. Hematological disorders and ischemic stroke. *Stroke.* 1990; 21:1111–1121.

Hart RG, Miller VT. Cerebral infarcion in young adults: a practical approach. *Stroke.* 1983; 14:110–114.

Headache Classification Committee of the International Headache Society. Classification and diagnostic criteria for headache disorders, cranial neuralgias, and facial pain. *Cephalagia.* 1988; 8:27–54.

Lisovoski F, Pousseaux P. Cerebral infarction in young people. A study of 148 patients with early cerebral angiography. *J Neurol Neurosurg Psychiatry.* 1991; 54:576–579.

Natowicz M, Kelley RI. Mendelian etiologies of stroke. *Ann Neurol.* 1987; 22:175–192.

Pavlakis SG, Gould RJ, Zito JL. Stroke in children. *Adv Pediatr.* 1991; 38:151–179.

Roach ES, Riela AR. Pediatric cerebrovascular disease: a diagnostic approach. *Int Pediatr.* 1992; 7:161–172.

Stern BJ, Kittner S, Sloan M, et al. Stroke in the young. *Md Med J.* 1991; 40:453–462 (Part I); 565–570 (Part II).

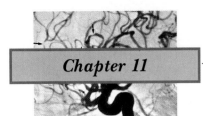

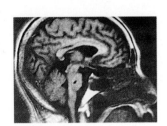

Chapter 11

EDWARD FELDMANN

Intracerebral Hemorrhage

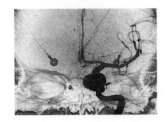

INTRACEREBRAL HEMORRHAGE (IH) is defined as bleeding

within the brain parenchyma. Although IH is responsible for

about one tenth of all strokes (Fig. 11.1), its role as a cause of

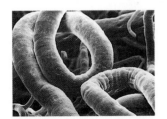

stroke depends on the racial, medical, and geographic features

of the population under study. An increasingly aging popula-

tion and more widespread recreational drug abuse have con-

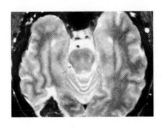

tributed to dramatic changes in the etiologic spectrum of

intracranial hemorrhage.

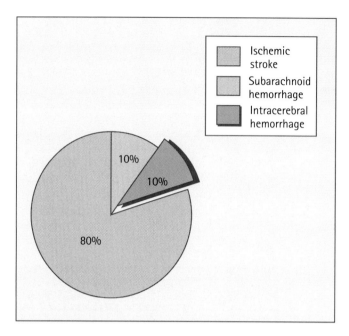

FIGURE 11.1 → Percentage of strokes attributable to intra-cerebral hemorrhage (IH).

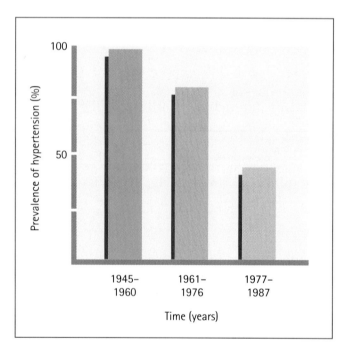

FIGURE 11.2 → The declining role of hypertension as a cause of IH. The ordinate displays the prevalence of hypertension in patients with IH from the particular era designated on the abscissa.

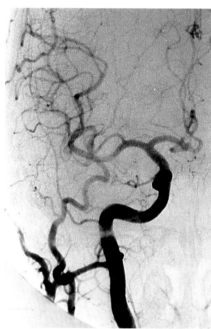

FIGURE 11.3 → In this cerebral angiogram, threadlike penetrating arteries branch off from large intracerebral vessels. These small arteries are believed to be responsible for IH.

ETIOLOGY

HYPERTENSION

High blood pressure remains the most common risk factor associated with IH, but its importance declined during the last several decades as physicians became more adept at quickly recognizing and controlling hypertension in their patients (Fig. 11.2). At present, high blood pressure is believed to be primarily responsible for about half of all IH cases.

Clinical and radiologic criteria are used to establish hypertension as the cause of IH. The patient should, of course, have a history of hypertension. Common locations of bleeding that are typical for hypertensive IH include the putamen, thalamus, cerebellum, and pons. History, physical examination, and laboratory data should not suggest another possible cause such as trauma, drug abuse, or amyloid angiopathy.

Neurologists and pathologists have not agreed on the mechanism of hypertensive IH. Most physicians believe that hypertension chronically damages the small arteries in the brain that range from 50 to 200 µm in diameter (Fig. 11.3). These weakened vessels are thought to bleed if blood pressure or blood volume rises abruptly. Pathologic support for this hypothesis lies in the detection of lipohyalinosis and microaneurysms of small penetrating arteries in the brains of patients with hypertensive IH (Figs. 11.4, 11.5). The

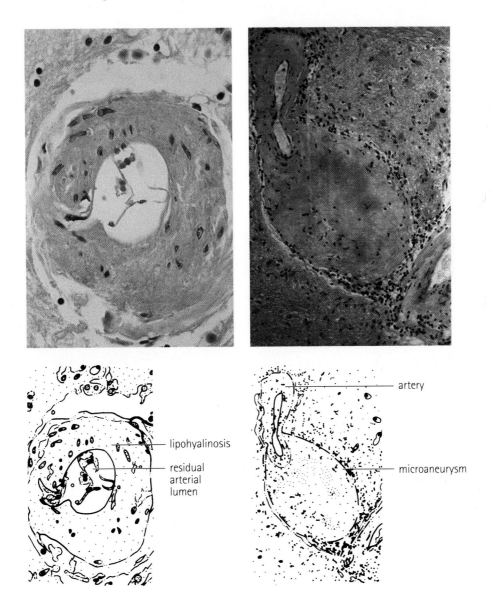

FIGURE 11.4 → Lipohyalinosis partially obliterates the lumen of a small penetrating artery in the brain.

FIGURE 11.5 → Microaneurysm of a small penetrating artery in the brain.

distribution of these vascular lesions throughout the central nervous system mirrors the predominant sites of IH occurrence (see Fig. 11.17). It remains unclear whether lipohyalinosis or microaneurysm is the most important pathologic substrate that leads to bleeding in chronic hypertension.

In acute IH, symptoms are produced as the enlarging hematoma compresses neural tissue, rendering it dysfunctional (Fig. 11.6). The neurologic deficit becomes permanent if necrosis occurs. Alternatively, the deficit may worsen transiently if edema develops around the hematoma. With very deep parenchymal hemorrhages, such as those located in the thalamus, the hemorrhage commonly extends into the ventricular system (Fig. 11.7). Over time the blood is resorbed by white blood cells and the space left behind fills with cerebrospinal fluid (see Fig. 11.19F).

The actual period of bleeding in hypertensive IH is a brief and self-limited process that probably lasts only minutes. In certain patients, however, the volume of the hematoma may increase dramatically over the first several hours. These patients experience deterioration in focal neurologic function and level of consciousness within hours of hemorrhage onset. It is unclear why some patients continue to bleed for longer periods of time than others. Some neurologists believe that extreme and persistent elevations in blood pressure may be responsible. Patients who experience a decline in neurologic function days after hemorrhage onset are likely to be suffering from raised intracranial pressure secondary to edema around the hematoma or, possibly, systemic metabolic derangements that can exacerbate any existing neurologic disorder.

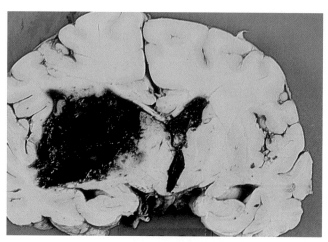

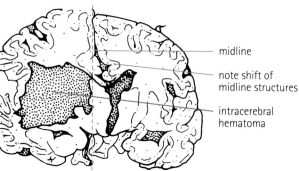

midline

note shift of midline structures

intracerebral hematoma

FIGURE 11.6 → Intracerebral hematoma produces mass effect on surrounding nerve tissue.

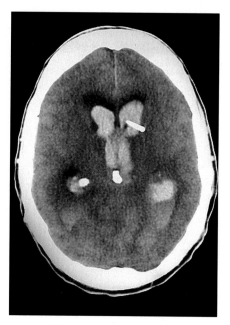

FIGURE 11.7 → CT scan illustrates intraventricular blood and a shunt in the left lateral ventricle.

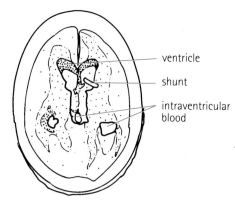

ventricle

shunt

intraventricular blood

NONHYPERTENSIVE INTRACEREBRAL HEMORRHAGE

Early diagnosis and successful management of hypertension has clearly reduced the role that it plays in the etiology of IH. Neurologists are thus encountering greater numbers of patients with IH secondary to amyloid deposition in cerebral vessels, anticoagulants and thrombolytic agents, neoplasms, prescription and illicit drugs, aneurysms and vascular malformations, as well as other miscellaneous causes (Fig. 11.8).

Cerebral Amyloid Angiopathy

Cerebral amyloid angiopathy (CAA) causes lobar hemorrhages in elderly patients who typically do not have hypertension. The disease is marked by a high risk of recurrent hemorrhage and, in familial forms, by the appearance of IH in patients as young as their twenties or thirties (Fig. 11.9). The prevalence of CAA in the brains of normal persons increases dramatically with age, appearing in more than half of people over 90 years of age. Surgical biopsy and autopsy data estimate the prevalence of CAA in patients with IH to be approximately 12%. CAA is also found in the brains of many patients with nonhemorrhagic neurologic disorders such as degenerative dementia.

The amyloid of CAA has a tendency to deposit in medium and small superficial cortical and meningeal arteries, sparing the peripheral vasculature. Any of the major lobes of the cerebral hemispheres may be affected. As illustrated in Figure 11.10, these deposits exhibit yellow-green birefringence under polarized light. The amyloid deposits typically—but not invariably—coexist with numerous

---

FIGURE 11.8 → CAUSES OF IH*

Hypertension	50%
Cerebral amyloid angiopathy	12%
Anticoagulants	10%
Tumors	8%
Prescription and street drugs	6%
AVMs and aneurysms	5%
Miscellaneous	9%

* The data reflect approximations based on literature reports.

FIGURE 11.9 → CLUES TO THE PRESENCE OF CEREBRAL AMYLOID ANGIOPATHY IN IH PATIENTS

- Elderly patient or young patient with family history of IH
- Lobar location
- Hypertension absent
- History of recurrent hemorrhage

other pathologic brain changes (e.g., senile plaques and neurofibrillary tangles). In addition, abnormalities occur in the vessel walls of arteries that contain the amyloid deposits, including fibrinoid necrosis and small aneurysm formation. The latter vascular changes are known as CAA-associated vasculopathy.

The familial form of CAA is inherited as an autosomal disorder in some Icelandic and Dutch families. The composition of the deposited amyloid subunit differs in the two familial subtypes. The amyloid subunit found in the Dutch form is also found in the brains of Alzheimer patients and the sporadic form of CAA. The relationship between subunit type and bleeding risk remains unclear. Preliminary data suggests that the presence of certain subunits confers a particularly high risk for fatal hemorrhage.

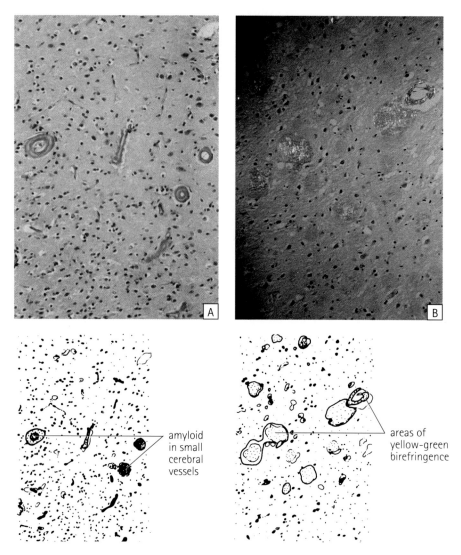

FIGURE 11.10 → **A,** Hematoxylin-eosin stain of small cerebral vessels that contain amyloid. **B,** Amyloid exhibits yellow-green birefringence under polarized light.

The mechanism responsible for hemorrhage in patients with CAA is unknown. Elucidation of the mechanism has been hampered by the lack of animal models. Moreover, some patients harbor coexistent hypertension, making it difficult to identify the exact cause of bleeding. CAA-associated vasculopathy is suspected to occur in patients with severe amyloid deposition, which weakens the vessel walls and presumably enhances the risk of rupture. However, not all patients with CAA and hemorrhage harbor the CAA-associated vasculopathy.

Anticoagulation
Nearly one out of every 100 patients treated with anticoagulants suffers intracerebral bleeding. Approximately one in ten cases of IH may be attributed to conventional anticoagulants. The risk of IH increases when the underlying brain parenchyma is diseased (e.g., after acute ischemic stroke) or when the degree of systemic anticoagulation is high. Currently available epidemiologic data do not precisely identify what degree of prothrombin or partial thromboplastin time elevation begins to increase the risk of IH, although low dose chronic oral anticoagulation is less risky than standard therapy.

Patients with warfarin-related IH are typically on anticoagulation for years before the hemorrhage occurs. Their relative risk of IH is estimated to be increased nearly eightfold when compared to non-anticoagulated patients. Most neurologists would agree that the risk increases in proportion to the degree of anticoagulation. Compared with IH caused by hypertension, the duration of bleeding in anticoagulation-associated IH may last hours rather than minutes (Fig. 11.11). The cellular or vascular events that lead to bleeding and the precise artery that bleeds have not been identified.

Thrombolytic Agents
IH related to the administration of agents such as urokinase, streptokinase or tissue plasminogen activator has been documented in nearly 1% of patients who received them for treatment of acute myocardial infarction. The hemorrhages are lobar and more frequent as the dose of thrombolytic agent is increased. Studies of IH in patients treated with thrombolytic agents for acute ischemic cerebral infarction are difficult to interpret because hemorrhagic transformation of infarcts occurs spontaneously in these patients as well.

Neoplasms
Approximately one out of every 15 patients with IH harbors an underlying neoplasm responsible for the hemorrhage, but less than one out of every 100 brain tumors will bleed at some point in its course. Even fewer brain tumors will present with IH as the initial symptom. The responsible lesions are commonly high grade astrocytomas or metastases from primary sites of renal, lung, or melanoma tumors (Fig. 11.12). The diagnosis of underlying tumor causing IH should be suspected in patients with systemic cancer (Fig. 11.13) or a history of progressive, focal neurologic symptoms preceding the hemorrhage. Radiologic signs suggestive of neoplasm include massive early edema, multiple lesions or abnormal enhancement, and bleeding into sites atypical for hypertensive IH.

FIGURE 11.11 → FEATURES OF ANTICOAGULATION-RELATED IH

- Bleeding may last hours
- Systemic bleeding uncommon
- Lobar location common
- Anticoagulation excessive
- Underlying lesion increases risk (infarction, tumor)

Illicit Drug Abuse and Prescription Drugs

A significant proportion of stroke in young persons can be attributed to the abuse of illicit drugs. One fourth of these strokes are hemorrhagic. One out of every 16 IH cases is believed to be related to drug abuse. Street drugs linked to IH include cocaine, amphetamine ("speed"), and phencyclidine (PCP). Prescription drugs documented to cause IH include phenylpropanolamine (in Dexatrim), Talwin-pyribenzamine, and methylphenidate (Ritalin) (Fig. 11.14). In most patients the hemorrhage occurs soon after that drug is used, regardless of whether the patient habitually takes the drug or is ingesting it for the first time.

Cocaine-related IH is becoming more common in emergency rooms across the country. Any route or form of cocaine abuse can lead to IH, but the use of "crack" is particularly risky. The clinical features of cocaine-related IH are indistinguishable from typical hypertensive IH, except for the fact that most of the patients are young and male.

Phenylpropanolamine (PPA) is a popular sympathomimetic appetite suppressant available in over-the-counter diet pills. Its use has been linked to IH in young females. Patients often have taken excessive amounts of the drug, but IH may occur in a first-time user ingesting conventional doses. Simultaneous ingestion of other sympathomimetics increases the risk of IH.

Neurologists do not agree on the mechanism of IH in patients using sympathomimetics. The most widely accepted hypothesis suggests that IH occurs after sudden blood pressure elevations following drug use in patients who harbor underlying vascular brain lesions or whose brain vessels have been damaged by chronic abuse of the drug. Underlying vascular lesions found in some of these patients include aneurysms and vascular malformations. Neurologists have identified vasculitis, arterial "beading," or drug-induced vasospasm as other vascular disorders that predispose to IH in other patients who take these drugs. Often no underlying lesion is detected.

The link between vasculitis and drug-related IH is controversial. While vascular lesions such as AVMs are frequently detected in patients with cocaine-related hemorrhage, pathologically proven vasculitis has not been documented. Vasculitis has been demonstrated in very few cases of IH related to the use of other sympathomimetics, such as PPA. Often vasculitis is deemed to be the underlying vascular pathology because "beading"—a segmental narrowing and dilatation of intracranial vessels—is demonstrated on arteriography, but this is a nonspecific radiologic finding. Beading may be found in infectious brain illnesses or after subarachnoid hemorrhage, as well as in vasculitis. Animals have been demonstrated to develop beading within minutes of catecholamine infusion. Moreover, the occurrence of IH within minutes after a drug is first used is inconsistent with vasculitis as the cause. Vasculitis is more likely in patients who abuse a drug chronically or resume a drug after a period of abstinence (Fig. 11.15). Meningeal biopsy should provide pathologic support for the diagnosis. Immunosuppressive therapy can be initiated, but some physicians treat patients merely by discontinuing exposure to the offending agent.

Ethanol

IH has been documented in patients who chronically abuse alcohol. This drug can have profound effects on the coagulation system and platelets, and may significantly increase the risk of bleeding by acutely elevating blood pressure (Fig. 11.16).

FIGURE 11.12 → TUMORS COMMONLY RESPONSIBLE FOR IH

METASTASES FROM SYSTEMIC CANCER: Lung
Renal
Melanoma
Choriocarcinoma

PRIMARY BRAIN TUMOR: Glioblastoma

FIGURE 11.13 → CLUES TO DIAGNOSING TUMOR-RELATED IH

- Focal neurologic symptoms precede hemorrhage
- Known systemic cancer that metastasizes to the nervous system
- CT shows unusual bleeding site, multiple lesions, excessive edema, or abnormal enhancement

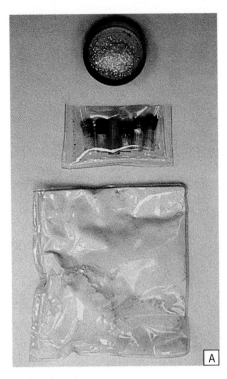
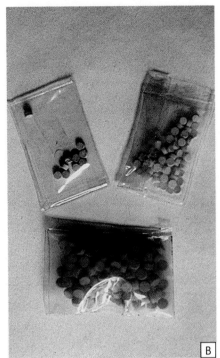
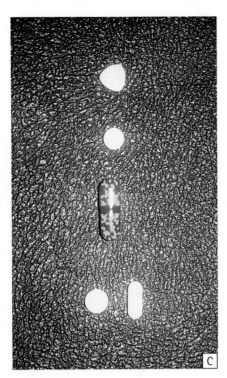

FIGURE 11.14 → Drugs known to cause IH. **A,** Street drugs, from top: pharmaceutical cocaine, crack vials, street cocaine. **B,** Variously colored examples of PCP. **C,** Prescription drugs, from top: dextroamphetamine sulfate (Dexedrine, 5 mg); methylphenidate hydrochloride (Ritalin, 5 mg); phenyl-propanolamine hydrochloride (Dexatrim); pyrobenzamine (PBZ, 50 mg) (left); pentazocine (Talwin, 50 mg) (right).

FIGURE 11.15 → CRITERIA FOR DIAGNOSING DRUG-RELATED VASCULITIS CAUSING IH

- Drug use is chronic or recurrent following a period of abstinence
- Angiography may reveal "beading"*
- Histologic proof obtained by meningeal-cortical biopsy
- Dramatic response to immunosuppressive therapy

* Beading on angiography, in isolation, is not diagnostic of vasculitis.

FIGURE 11.16 → ALCOHOL-RELATED RISK FACTORS FOR IH

- Platelet dysfunction
- Impaired hepatic synthesis of coagulation factors
- Chronic hypertension
- Acute, binge-related hypertension
- Alcohol-induced cerebral vasospasm
- Impaired sympathomimetic (e.g., cocaine) metabolism

Arteriovenous Malformations (AVMs) and Aneurysms

Parenchymatous hemorrhage, in addition to sub-arachnoid hemorrhage, occasionally occurs in patients with aneurysms and AVMs. Because AVMs are located within brain parenchyma, while aneurysms lie in the subarachnoid space, IH occurs more commonly with the bleeding of AVMs. These vascular lesions account for about one in 20 instances of IH. Clues to the diagnosis of AVM-associated IH include presentation early in life, lobar hemorrhage, a history of inherited vascular malformations, or radio-logic features suggestive of an underlying vascular lesion. Angiography usually confirms the diagnosis, but angiographically occult lesions require MRI or surgical exploration for diagnosis. In young patients with typical clinical presentations, surgical explo-ration can also be curative if the offending lesion is removed, thereby preventing recurrence of IH.

DIAGNOSIS

CLINICAL FEATURES

The neurologic deficit of IH is focal and rapid in onset. Most patients attain their maximal deficit over a

---

FIGURE 11.17 → CLINICAL FEATURES OF IH BY SITE

PUTAMEN (35%)*	Hemiparesis, hemisensory loss, visual field cut, dysphasia in left hemisphere and neglect in right, headache uncommon
LOBE (30%)	Headache common, hypertension uncommon 　　Frontal: hemiparesis 　　Parietal: hemisensory loss 　　Temporal: dysphasia and visual field cut 　　Occipital: visual field cut
CEREBELLUM (15%)	Headache, vomiting and inability to walk; less common are limb ataxia, cranial nerve palsies, gaze palsy without hemiparesis; progression to coma unpredictable
THALAMUS (10%)	Hemisensory loss, hemiparesis, eye movement abnormalities (downward gaze, upgaze palsy, small unreactive pupils, ptosis), vomiting; headache uncommon, hydrocephalus common with large hemorrhage
PONS (5%)	Large: coma, quadriplegia, tiny reactive pupils Small, tegmental: gaze palsy, ataxia, contralateral motor and sensory deficit
CAUDATE (5%)	Cognitive abnormalities, hemiparesis, gaze palsy, hydrocephalus common

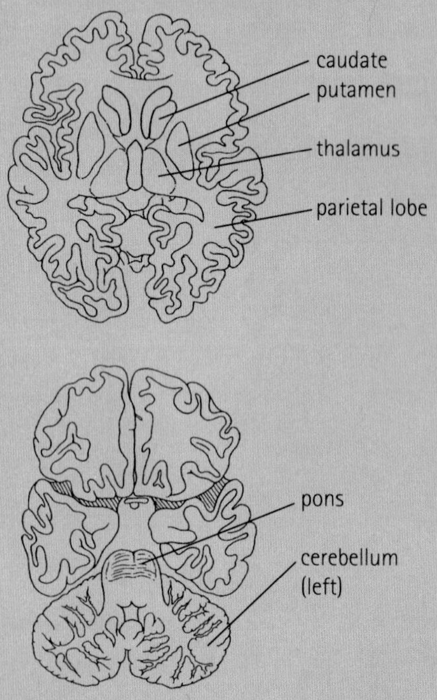

caudate
putamen
thalamus
parietal lobe

pons
cerebellum (left)

* Values in parentheses reflect the percentage of hemorrhages occurring at that site.

---

period of minutes to hours. The most common sites of bleeding in order of declining frequency are putamen, hemisphere, cerebellum, thalamus, pons, and caudate. Each site has a typical clinical presentation (Fig. 11.17) that suggests a clinical syndrome.

The specific symptoms associated with each syndrome depend on the location and volume of the hemorrhage. Small intracerebral hemorrhages mimic the clinical presentation of ischemic stroke, but usually have distinguishing features (Fig. 11.18). Although cerebral infarction may be heralded by transient ischemic attacks (TIAs), it is rarely attended by headache, vomiting, or early impaired arousal—features more often seen with IH. These rules do not always distinguish ischemia from infarction, however. The clinical course of a TIA, with resolution of deficit within minutes to hours, is virtually never seen with IH. The acute decline of unstable or progressing cerebral infarction is also rare because IH patients almost never experience acute recurrence of the hemorrhage.

Major advances in computed tomography (CT) and magnetic resonance (MR) resolution have resulted in the discovery that small IHs can mimic the clinical presentation of small vessel or "lacunar" infarction. In some series, as many as 10% of patients with IH present with a recognized lacunar syndrome. Any of the classic lacunar syndromes other than pure sensory stroke may be mimicked by IH, including pure motor stroke, ataxic hemiparesis, dysarthria–clumsy hand, and sensorimotor stroke. These syndromes have been seen with small bleeds into the internal capsule, putamen, pontine tegmentum, thalamus, and midbrain.

Hypertension is common but headache is rare in these patients. Rapid recovery of neurologic deficits is the rule. Astute clinicians suspect the diagnosis of hemorrhage when a patient whose presentation is otherwise typical for ischemic lacunar stroke exhibits undue nausea or vomiting, a history of transient diplopia, or another symptom inconsistent with small vessel infarction.

IH occasionally presents like a tumor, with a relentlessly progressive course over days or weeks attended by convulsions and radiologic features that suggest a neoplastic lesion. CT scan usually reveals a low-density lesion with ring-enhancement and surrounding edema. Surgical removal is curative, demonstrating old blood surrounded by a neovascular capsule. Such clinical presentations are not seen with hypertensive IH.

One fourth of IH patients experience seizures, more than half of which occur within the first two days of hemorrhage. The risk of seizures increases dramatically when the blood lies closer to the cortex, but is almost nonexistent with deep, thalamic bleeds. It is difficult to predict which patients with IH will develop a chronic seizure disorder, especially because antiepileptic drugs are frequently administered to patients at hemorrhage onset, even in the absence of seizures. Consequently, there are no well established guidelines for the acute or chronic use of antiepileptic drugs in patients with IH.

Lobar hemorrhages have distinctive clinical features. Only with lobar IH does headache occur at onset in most patients. Moreover, hypertension is a rel-

---

FIGURE 11.18 → FEATURES DISTINGUISHING IH AND ISCHEMIC STROKE

HEMORRHAGE
- No prior TIAs
- Headache, vomiting, lethargy*
- No resolution in 24 h
- Acute rebleeding with clinical decline is rare

ISCHEMIA
- Prior TIAs common
- Vomiting, lethargy rare
- Resolution in 24 h with TIA
- Acute decline can occur with unstable stroke

* The absence of these symptoms does not rule out IH.

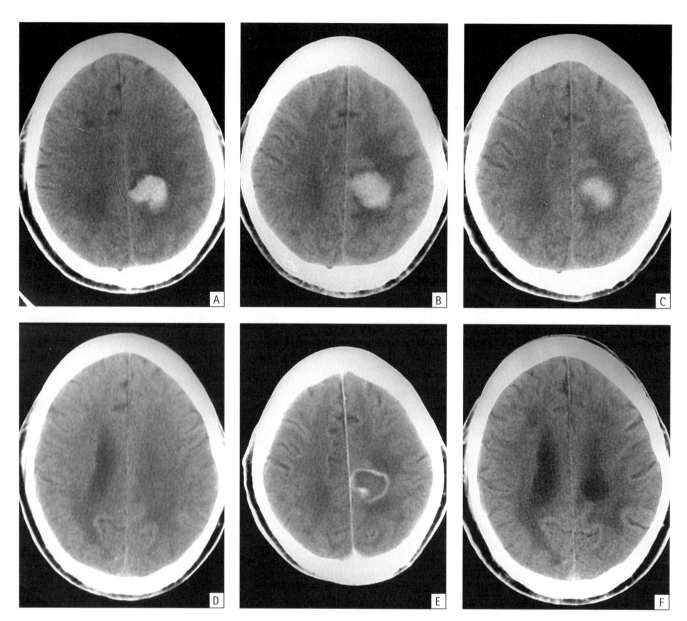

FIGURE 11.19 → Sequential CT scans illustrate radiologic evolution of IH. **A,** Day 1: High-density hematoma without edema. **B,** Day 9: Less dense blood, but increasing low-density edema around the hematoma. **C,** Day 16: Even less dense blood, slightly less edema compared with **B. D,** Day 46: Subtle hypo-density revealed without dye contrast. **E,** Dye-enhanced scan reveals ring enhancement. **F,** Five years later: CSF-filled cleft is the only sign of the prior hemorrhage.

FIGURE 11.20 → MRI FINDINGS IN IH			
TIME AFTER BLEED	HEMOGLOBIN	T1-WEIGHTED IMAGE	T2-WEIGHTED IMAGE
First several hours	Intracellular, oxygenated	Minimal hypointensity	Minimal hyperintensity
12 hours	Intracellular, deoxygenated	Minimal hypointensity	Clearly visible Hypointensity
3 days	Intracellular, methemoglobin	Hyperintensity	Hypointensity
1 week	Extracellular, methemoglobin	Hyperintensity	Hyperintensity + black rim from macrophage formed hemosiderin

atively uncommon cause of bleeding at this site. Identified etiologies include vascular malformations, tumors, anticoagulation, and cerebral amyloid angiopathy. More than one fourth of lobar hemorrhages have no identifiable predisposing cause.

Bleeding into the ventricular system occurs in many cases of IH, especially if the hemorrhage is large or the primary parenchymal site is close to the midline. Primary bleeding into the ventricles without associated parenchymal hemorrhage, however, is rare.

LABORATORY TESTING

Intracerebral hemorrhage appears as a high-density lesion on CT scanning. In the subacute period following hemorrhage, CT scan without dye contrast enhancement reveals edema surrounding the lesion, while an enhanced scan often shows a ring-enhancing area surrounding the hematoma (Fig. 11.19). An enhanced scan may reveal an unsuspected lesion responsible for the hemorrhage, such as an AVM or tumor. As the hemorrhage is resorbed over a period of weeks, it becomes increasingly hypodense, ultimately leaving in its wake a hole containing CSF density material. CT scan detects virtually all cases of IH.

When the diagnosis remains in doubt, the next test of choice is magnetic resonance imaging (MRI). Lumbar puncture is rarely performed because it is dangerous in the presence of mass effect, especially with posterior fossa hemorrhages.

The appearance of hemorrhage on MRI depends heavily on the time between bleeding and the performance of imaging (Fig. 11.20). In the week that follows the bleeding, hemoglobin evolves from an intracellular oxygenated form to an extracellular methemoglobin form. The latter is ingested by macrophages and turned into hemosiderin. The hemosiderin, which appears black, is a permanent finding on future MRIs, marking the occurrence of prior hemorrhages. This sequential change in hemoglobin is responsible for the varied appearance of blood on MRI over time (Fig. 11.21). Neither T1- nor T2-weighted images may be diagnostic in the first several hours after bleeding. It is also difficult to schedule and perform MRI rapidly in acutely ill IH patients. Thus, in most hospitals CT scan remains the primary diagnostic modality for patients with suspected IH. MRI, in contrast, offers superb sensitivity in detecting angiographically occult AVMs that cause IH. Because

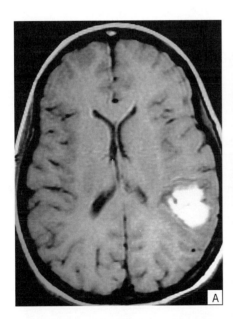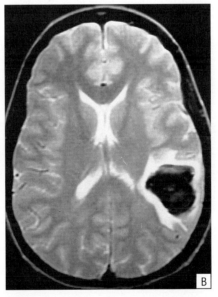

FIGURE 11.21 → MRI of intracerebral hematoma. **A,** Hyperintensity on T1-weighted image suggests hematoma is at least 3 days old. **B,** Corresponding T2-weighted image shows hypointense lesion with no surrounding black rim (hyperintensity surrounding lesion is edema), suggesting that the lesion is less than one week old.

these lesions bleed repeatedly over a period of time, their MRI appearance is defined by a small lesion with evidence for acute, subacute, and chronic bleeding (Fig. 11.22). True AVMs are larger, show similar changes due to bleeding and also reveal areas of slow blood flow.

Cerebral angiography is not usually performed while evaluating patients with IH. Indications generally include a presentation atypical for hypertensive IH or other unusual features (Fig. 11.23). Angiography is most likely to identify an underlying lesion such as an AVM or tumor in a normotensive patient with a lobar IH. However, angiography is often unrevealing because occult AVMs and amyloid angiopathy are common causes of IH in this setting and cannot be identified by angiography. Moreover, a mass of obscuring blood may make angiographic interpretation difficult. The availability of noninvasive, high-resolution MRI has resulted in the perfor-

mance of fewer angiograms for IH patients. Magnetic resonance angiography may also prove increasingly useful in the near future.

THERAPY FOR INTRACEREBRAL HEMORRHAGE

MEDICAL THERAPY

The first steps in the management of IH are protection of the airway as well as recognition and treatment of life-threatening raised intracranial pressure (Fig. 11.24). If the patient appears to be compressing vital midline structures due to intracranial hypertension, hyperventilation and mannitol should be instituted immediately. There is no established role for the immediate use of corticosteroids, barbiturates, or intracranial pressure monitoring; corticosteroids are potentially harmful in this setting.

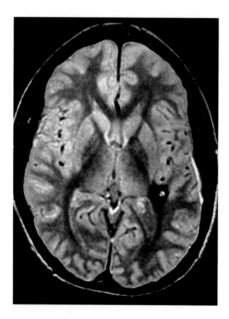
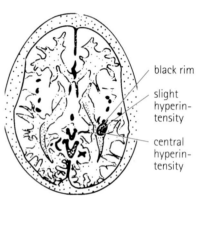

black rim

slight hyperintensity

central hyperintensity

FIGURE 11.22 → MRI of angiographically-occult AVM. The central hyperintensity surrounded by a black rim suggests evidence for chronic bleeding on T2-weighted image. The slight area of hyperintensity suggests acute bleeding.

FIGURE 11.23 → INDICATIONS FOR CEREBRAL ANGIOGRAPHY IN IH PATIENTS

- Hypertension not present
- Hemorrhage site is lobar
- Multiple hemorrhages present

The next step involves reducing significant elevations in blood pressure. Blood pressure that enters the range encountered in malignant hypertension is likely to exacerbate bleeding. However, less severe hypertension should not be dramatically reduced. The vasculature surrounding the hematoma has no autoregulatory capacity. Thus, a sudden drop in perfusion pressure can result in ischemia, with a worsening in the patient's neurologic condition.

The patient must have any coagulopathy reversed as soon as possible. Fresh frozen plasma and vitamin K are used in patients on warfarin, while protamine is administered to patients with IH who are on heparin. Patients with platelet disorders, elevated bleeding times, or persistent bleeding receive platelet transfusions. They are virtually never required in IH patients who have been taking aspirin or other non-steroidal anti-inflammatory drugs. Hemophiliacs must receive adequate amounts of their deficient coagulation factor. Protamine and epsilon-aminocaproic acid are administered to patients with hemorrhage occurring in the setting of thrombolysis.

As discussed above, there are few guidelines for the use of antiepileptic drugs in IH patients. These agents appear to be unnecessary for patients with deep hemorrhages who have not had a seizure. Many patients with superficial hemorrhages are treated even if they have not had a convulsion, although this approach is of unproven benefit.

Therapy varies for patients who harbor cerebral vasculitis underlying the hemorrhage. Some physicians simply force the patient to withdraw from the offending agent (e.g., cocaine) if it can be identified. Others institute therapy with corticosteroids or, if steroids fail, more powerful immunosuppressants are used.

SURGICAL THERAPY

The role of craniotomy with surgical removal of IH is controversial. In one of the rare randomized trials of surgery for supratentorial IH, survival improved with surgery but functional recovery was poor. Other studies have not shown a benefit from surgery. Thus, most neurologists and neurosurgeons would exhaust all medical efforts prior to considering surgery for deep, inaccessible hemorrhages. Surgery becomes a more realistic option if the hemorrhage is superficial or if the patient exhibits progressive intracranial hypertension refractory to medical therapy. Surgery in this setting may be life-saving, but the functional outlook remains poor. Surgery is often performed on cerebellar hemorrhage patients because of their propensity to suffer unpredictable dramatic declines and because the hematoma is usually superficial. Ventricular drainage and emergent shunting are employed in IH patients who develop acute hydrocephalus, but these techniques are indirect, leaving the hematoma undisturbed.

When a diagnosis is necessary and physicians suspect an underlying cause other than hypertension for IH, surgery with exploration and biopsy are performed. Neoplastic lesions, AVMs, amyloid, or an unsuspected lesion such as an abscess have been found when hemorrhage sites are biopsied, especially in lobar hemorrhages. Surgery has not been established as the only possible method of diagnosis. Information obtained through surgery may not significantly improve functional outcome or survival. These doubts should be kept in mind, as the complications of surgery and biopsy include recurrent hemorrhage and infection. There are no controlled studies to guide clinicians in their decisions regarding surgery for patients with IH.

FIGURE 11.24 → STEPWISE MEDICAL MANAGEMENT OF IH

- Protect airway
- Recognize and treat life-threatening intracranial hypertension: administer hyperventilation and mannitol as needed
- Reduce hypertension if extreme (e.g., > 200/120 mm Hg), but no further than into the high-normal range (e.g., 180/95 mm Hg)
- Correct any coagulopathy present
- Administer antiepileptic drugs as needed

Stereotactic techniques offer an alternative to craniotomy for removing an intracerebral hemorrhage. Because the technique is less invasive it offers a lower morbidity (Fig. 11.25). CT scanning can be used to guide a cannula through a burr hole into the mass of blood. A silicone tube is passed through the track left by the cannula and urokinase is inserted into the hemorrhage to help it dissolve and aspirate easily. Studies have not shown that this method results in superior functional recovery when compared with conventional craniotomy. Moreover, the stereotactic method does not allow for examination of the hemorrhage site and biopsy when an underlying secondary cause of the hemorrhage is suspected. Studies using stereotaxy that employs a device combining an endoscope, laser, and video camera have shown good outcomes in patients with IH, but the studies were not blind. Clearly, new methods for the surgical therapy of IH are promising, but more data are needed before the role of stereotactic surgery for this disease is well defined.

PROGNOSIS

The size of the hemorrhage is paramount for predicting survival and functional recovery. The overall mortality of IH is approximately 40%. This figure increases dramatically to nearly 90% if the hematoma is larger than 60 cc in volume. Alternatively, survival with good functional recovery can be expected with hematomas that are less than 20 cc in volume. The effect of underlying lesions such as tumor or amyloid angiopathy on survival and functional outcome is unclear. Many physicians formerly believed that the presence of intraventricular extension of the hematoma was an especially ominous prognostic sign. However, studies have shown that intraventricular blood in a patient with IH merely reflects the hematoma's large size. It is not an independently useful predictor of outcome. In general, lobar hemorrhages have a better prognosis than deep hemorrhages.

Recent studies employing multivariate analysis to identify prognostic variables for the outcome of IH have found that initial neurologic deficit, in addition to size of the hemorrhage, is a helpful predictor. The combination of admission Glasgow Coma Score (GCS), hemorrhage size, and pulse pressure have been shown to be more than 90% accurate in predicting 30 day mortality after IH. Actual clinical outcomes in 82 patients substantiated the accuracy of this probability model. Probability for survival at 30 days exceeded 90% if the hemorrhage was less than half a lobe in size, admission GCS was more than 9, and pulse pressure was less than 40 mm Hg. In contrast, the probability for 30 day survival with coma, a hemorrhage larger than a lobe, and a pulse pressure greater than 65 mm Hg was less than 10%.

IH almost never recurs as long as hypertension is treated. Since physicians are now more aggressive about lowering high blood pressure, IH recurrence is rare.

The long-term functional outlook for medically treated survivors of IH is good. In most studies, only about one in five patients is left with a permanent severe neurologic deficit. The remainder either make a nearly complete recovery or are able to resume independent lives with a mild neurologic deficit. Acute neurologic care and aggressive rehabilitation efforts should therefore be directed at the IH patient who survives the initial stages of the illness.

FIGURE 11.25 → A stereotactic device allows precise localization and invasion of an intracerebral lesion.

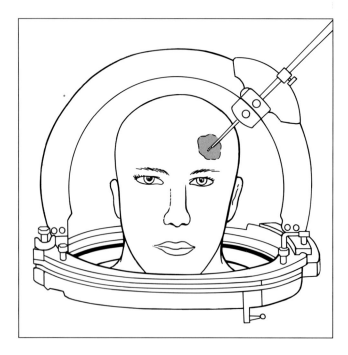

REFERENCES

Caplan LR. Intracerebral hemorrhage revisited. *Neurology.* 1988; 38:624–627.

Kase CS. Intracerebral hemorrhage: non-hypertensive causes. *Stroke.* 1986; 17:590–594.

Kase CS, Mohr JP. General features of intracerebral hemorrhage. In: Barnett HJM, Mohr JP, Stein BM, Yatsu FM (eds). *Stroke.* New York: Churchill Livingstone. 1986; 497–523.

Tanaka Y, Furuse M, Iwasa H, et al. Lobar intracerebral hemorrhage: etiology and long-term follow-up study of 32 patients. *Stroke.* 1986; 17:51–57.

Tuhrim S, Dambrosia JM, Price TR, et al. Prediction of intracerebral hemorrhage survival. *Ann Neurol.* 1988; 24:258–263.

Young WB, Lee KP, Pessin MS, et al. Prognostic significance of ventricular blood in supratentorial hemorrhage: a volumetric study. *Neurology.* 1990; 40:616–619.

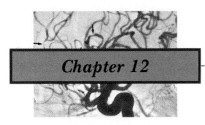

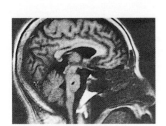

Chapter 12

J. PHILIP KISTLER

DARYL R. GRESS

ROBERT M. CROWELL

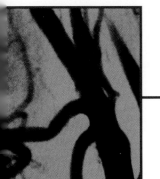

Subarachnoid Hemorrhage Due to a Ruptured Saccular Aneurysm

RUPTURE OF AN INTRACRANIAL saccular aneurysm is the

most common cause of subarachnoid hemorrhage (SAH).

Although autopsy studies estimate that 5% of the population

harbor aneurysms, the incidence of ruptured saccular

aneurysm is about 4 to 10 per 100,000 each year. It is a devas-

tating disease because it occurs at all ages—from the teenage

years through the eighth decade. Its greatest incidence is in the

fifth, sixth, and seventh decades. As many as 25% of SAH

patients die within the first 24 hours. Nearly half die within the

first year following rupture.

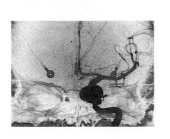

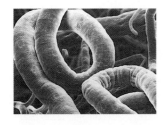

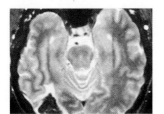

A team approach to managing these patients is evolving, due to the advent of the operating microscope, interventional neuroradiologic techniques, and neurologic intensive care units. Neurosurgery, interventional neuroradiology, neuromedicine, and nursing often confer about when to time surgery, whether surgery or interventional neuroradiologic techniques should be chosen to obliterate aneurysms, as well as what kind of bedside monitoring and management is proper for patients with vasospasm and hydrocephalus. The following discussion outlines the diagnosis and management of these patients with a team approach in mind.

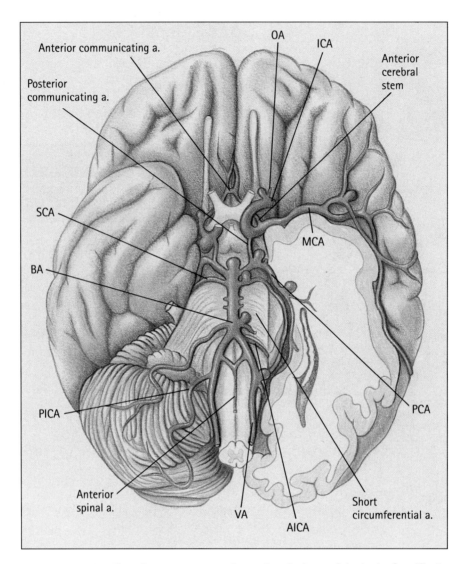

FIGURE 12.1 → Saccular aneurysms are located at the base of the brain. Specifically, the aneurysms form at the takeoff of one of the branch arteries. Saccular aneurysms do not occur past the first major bifurcation of the arteries and their primary branches at the base of the brain. (ACA = anterior cerebral artery; SCA = superior cerebral artery; BA = basilar artery; PICA = posterior inferior cerebellar artery; OA = ophthalmic artery; ICA = internal carotid artery; PCA = posterior cerebral artery; AICA = anterior inferior cerebellar artery; VA = vertebral artery)

PATHOPHYSIOLOGY

Most saccular aneurysms occur at the bifurcations of the large arteries at the base of the brain and rupture into the subarachnoid space of the basal cisterns (Fig. 12.1). Less commonly, they rupture into the brain or ventricular system or both, resulting in intracerebral hemorrhage (IH) or acute hydrocephalus. Mycotic aneurysms, in contrast, occur at distal branch points of the middle, anterior, posterior cerebral, vertebral, or basilar arteries. They rupture into the subarachnoid space over the cortical surface rather than into the basal cisterns. Complications such as vasospasm and hydrocephalus are uncommon. The size and sites of the saccular (Berry) aneurysm and of the subsequent subarachnoid, intraventricular, or intracerebral clot determine the clinical features of the initial rupture as well as the subsequent development of symptomatic vasospasm and hydrocephalus. The most common sites of saccular aneurysms include the junction of the anterior communicating artery and the anterior cerebral artery (ACA), the junction of the posterior communicating artery and the internal carotid artery (ICA), the bifurcation of the middle cerebral artery (MCA), and the top of the basilar artery (BA) (see Fig. 12.1). Approximately 85% of cases occur in the anterior circulation; 12% to 31% of patients have multiple aneurysms; 9% to 19% have bilateral, identical locations.

As an aneurysm grows, it often develops a neck with a dome. The neck's length and the size of the dome vary greatly. Their dimensions are important in planning microsurgical obliteration. The internal elastic lamina disappears at the base of the neck, the media thins, and connective tissue replaces smooth muscle cells. At the site of rupture—most often the dome—the wall thins to less than 0.3 mm; the rent is often no more than 0.5 mm long.

It is impossible to determine which aneurysms are likely to rupture, but limited data suggest that size is an important variable. Those larger than 7 mm may warrant prophylactic microsurgical obliteration.

CLINICAL PRESENTATION AND EVALUATION

PRODROMAL SYMPTOMS

Prodromal symptoms may betray the location of an unruptured aneurysm and, at times, suggest progressive enlargement. The onset of a third cranial nerve palsy—particularly when associated with pupillary dilation, loss of light reflex, and/or focal pain above and behind the eye—points to an expanding aneurysm at the junction of the posterior communicating artery and the ICA. Focal pain occurs as the aneurysm grows. The aneurysm must be 7 mm or greater before the third cranial nerve becomes involved. Hence, the pain may warn of the aneurysm prior to its involvement with the third cranial nerve. Prompt surgical intervention is indicated whenever a suspected expanding aneurysm is subsequently diagnosed by angiography. Sixth cranial nerve palsy suggests a cavernous sinus aneurysm. Visual field defects may point to an expanding supraclinoid carotid aneurysm. Occipital and posterior cervical pain suggest a posterior/inferior cerebellar artery (PICA) or anterior/inferior cerebellar artery (AICA) aneurysm. Pain in or behind the eye and in the low temple may indicate an expanding middle cerebral aneurysm.

Whether an aneurysm can cause small, intermittent leakage of blood in the subarachnoid space (the warning leak) is an unresolved issue. However, the clinical correlates of a small aneurysmal rupture or leak must be documented. Sudden unexplained headache at any location should arouse the suspicion of SAH and be investigated by a computed tomography (CT) or magnetic resonance imaging (MRI) scan to search for blood in the basal cisterns. Up to 25% of the time, the CT scan fails to detect SAH. If the clinical suspicion is high, a lumbar puncture may be necessary.

ACUTE MAJOR SUBARACHNOID HEMORRHAGE

For the brief moment of aneurysmal rupture, when acute major subarachnoid hemorrhage occurs, intracranial pressure approaches the mean arterial pressure and cerebral perfusion pressure falls. These changes may account for the sudden transient loss of consciousness that occurs in 45% of cases. A brief moment of excruciating headache may precede the blackout, but most patients first experience headache on regaining consciousness. In 10% of patients, aneurysmal bleeding may be severe enough to cause loss of consciousness for several days. About 45% of patients present with severe headache, usually associated with exertion but without loss of consciousness. The patient often calls the headache "the worst of my life." Words like "explode" or "burst" may be used. It is commonly described as "all over" or "in the back of the head and neck." Whatever the onset, vomiting is a prominent symptom. Vomiting with sudden headache should raise the possibility of acute SAH.

Although sudden, severe headache in the absence of focal neurologic symptoms is the hallmark of aneursymal rupture, neurologic deficits sometimes emerge. Unilateral third cranial nerve palsy strongly suggests a posterior communicating artery aneurysm. Sixth nerve palsy is common, but does not have great significance as a localizing sign, although it often corresponds to an infratentorial aneurysmal rupture. A middle cerebral bifurcation aneurysm may rupture into the subdural space and present as a subdural hematoma. Anterior communicating aneurysms sometimes rupture into the basal cisterns of the subarachnoid space, forming a clot that is large enough to produce a localized mass effect. Both, however, may rupture into the brain parenchyma, resulting in intracerebral hemorrhage (IH) (Figs. 12.2, 12.3). Common resultant deficits include hemiparesis, aphasia of the dominant hemisphere, and anosognosia (hemineglect) of the nondominant hemisphere for middle cerebral bifurcation aneurysm (see Fig. 12.2). Memory loss and abulia are caused by anterior communicating artery aneurysm ruptures (see Fig. 12.3A). Cerebral edema often follows IH and results in a progressive deterioration that sometimes requires emergency surgical intervention. Acute hydrocephalus, which can occur independently of acute cerebral edema, may

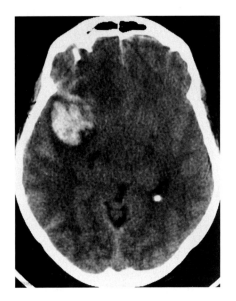
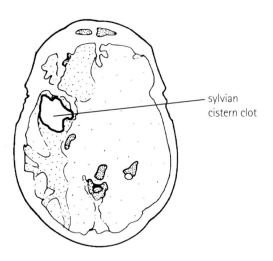

sylvian cistern clot

FIGURE 12.2 → Middle cerebral stem bifurcation aneurysm ruptured into the temporal lobe. Clot is noted specifically in the sylvian cistern and insular cistern. This was mistakenly diagnosed as an intracerebral hemorrhage (IH). Any hemorrhage that connects with the sylvian cistern should be suspected as being caused by the middle cerebral bifurcation aneurysm.

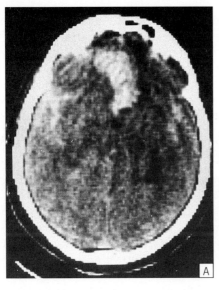

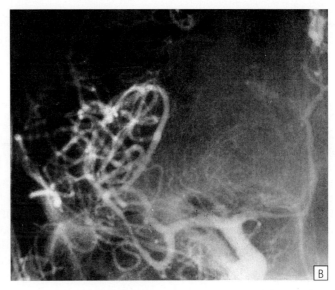

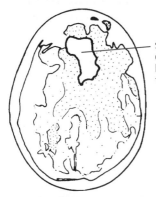

subarachnoid clot in inter-hemispheric fissure

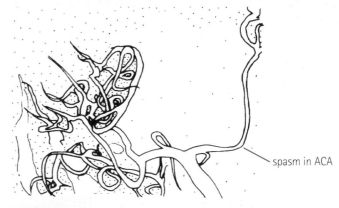

spasm in ACA

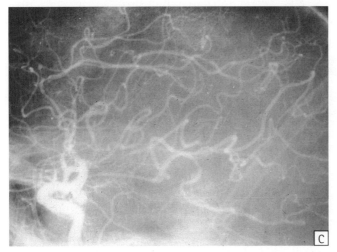

FIGURE 12.3 → A, Anterior communicating artery aneurysm rupture into the basal frontal interhemispheric fissure and into the frontal lobe. Clot is also noted in the sylvian cistern on the right. Diffuse blood is noted in the sylvian cistern on the left, extending into the insular cistern. Severe vasospasm is predicted for the anterior communicating complex and for the right middle cerebral artery (MCA) bifurcation branches, but not the middle cerebral stems or the left middle cerebral bifurcation. **B,** Severe spasm is seen in the anterior communicating complex, in particular the left distal A1 anterior cerebral artery (ACA). There is no signifi-cant spasm in the left MCA bifurcation or the MCA stem. **C,** Severe spasm at the proximal M2 branches of the right MCA corresponds to the clot in the right syl-vian cistern that extends into the insular cistern on day 2 (CT scan).

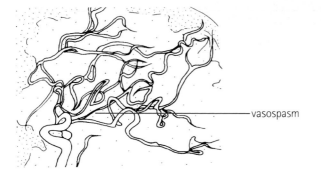

vasospasm

account for the persistence of a stuporous or comatose state (Fig. 12.4). Often there is no adequate explanation for the initial neurologic deficits. In most cases, they gradually improve over a matter of days.

Careful documentation of the *initial neurologic deficit,* attempting to establish its cause, and closely following its course is of utmost importance for managing patients and recognizing the onset and evolution of *delayed neurologic deficits.* While a clinical grading system was once widely used to categorize the status of patients, it does not adequately quantitate the clinical deficit or describe its pathophysiologic nature. Diagnostic and therapeutic decisions regarding these patients are best made with accurate, serial, quantitative documentation.

INITIAL EVALUATION

Documentation of subarachnoid blood on CT scan remains the cornerstone of the initial evaluation. However, if the diagnosis is suspected and no blood is seen on CT scan, a lumbar puncture is necessary to exclude SAH. Since the advent of early surgery (see below), early angiography has been recommended. If no aneurysm is found, then the chance for repeat SAH is low. Nonetheless, angiography is generally repeated at 1 to 3 weeks to further exclude the possibility of an aneurysm missed on the initial study.

Baseline electrolytes are valuable because hyponatremia may develop, due either to inappropriate antidiuretic hormone (ADH) secretion or, more often, to an unknown factor that causes loss of salt and water in the urine with subsequent volume depletion and dilutional hyponatremia. Platelet count, bleeding time, and other clotting parameters should also be documented. Serum viscosity increases when the hematocrit is above 40% or when the serum fibrinogen levels are above 250 mg. Adjustment of the serum viscosity becomes important if the patient is likely to develop symptomatic cerebral vasospasm.

DELAYED NEUROLOGIC DEFICITS

There are three major causes of delayed neurologic deficits (i.e., those following stabilization or improvement of the initial neurologic symptoms and signs): hydrocephalus, rerupture, and cerebral vasospasm. Recognizing the onset and severity of each of these deficits depends on knowing precisely the cause and extent of the initial neurologic findings. An early CT scan (24–48 h after the hemorrhage or immediately after early surgery) that accurately assesses ventricular size in addition to the extent and location of subarachnoid blood is invaluable for diagnosing the three complications.

HYDROCEPHALUS

Hydrocephalus after SAH is most appropriately divided into three categories: acute, subacute, and delayed (see Fig. 12.4). Each category has its own characteristic mechanism of production, timing of onset, symptomatology, and management.

Acute hydrocephalus usually develops after intraventricular hemorrhage or when an excessive amount of blood is deposited in the basal cisterns of

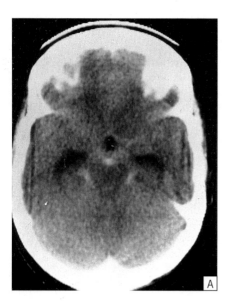 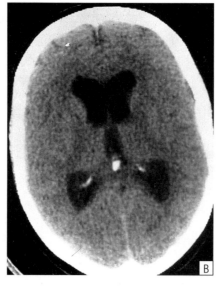 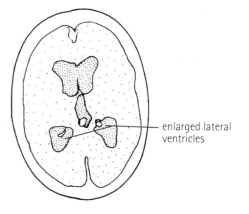

enlarged lateral ventricles

FIGURE 12.4 → Hydrocephalus secondary to subarachnoid hemorrhage (SAH) is seen on day 3, as evidenced by enlarged lateral ventricles. **A:** Inferior plane. **B:** Superior plane.

the posterior fossa. It is most commonly associated with ruptured anterior communicating artery aneurysms or top of the BA aneursyms. It occurs in the first 24 hours and can be seen immediately following aneurysmal rupture. The abrupt onset of stupor or the persistence of coma after the initial rupture suggests its presence. It must be treated immediately by ventriculostomy. Frequently, bilateral ventriculostomies need to be placed because of a thick clot in the third ventricle that may block either or both foramina of Monro. Occasionally, this maneuver results in dramatic improvement. At other times, improvement after ventricular drainage may be gradual. If the intraventricular clot is too extensive, ventriculostomy may not help. The risk of infection increases significantly when the ventriculostomy drainage continues for longer than a week. If the cerebrospinal fluid (CSF) drainage is still bloody at that time, ventricular drainage should be continued either by removing the original drain and replacing it at a second site or by installing an internal drain (ventriculoperitoneal shunt).

A subacute form of communicating hydrocephalus may develop in the first few days to a week following SAH. Although it too may present with the precipitous onset of coma, it usually develops slowly. Progressive drowsiness accompanied by inability to look up are suggestive findings. The quiet abulic state that is associated with the onset of symptomatic cerebral vasospasm in the anterior communicating artery complex is often difficult to distinguish from this subacute form of hydrocephalus. Comparing the length (in mm) of the ventricular span at the level of the frontal horns to a previous CT may help make the diagnosis. Similarly, enlargement of the temporal horns may also suggest hydrocephalus. However, a change as small as 1 mm in the ventricular span may be all that is required to produce a stuporous state. Fortunately, in many instances, this form of hydrocephalus gradually resolves. Ventricular or lumbar drainage, which may not be required, can theoretically precipitate rerupture by acutely decompressing the ventricles. Therefore, when the level of stupor mandates ventricular drainage, the pressure should be relieved gradually. To avoid excessive lowering of the intracranial pressure, the drainage system should drain above a gradient approximately 5 cm higher than the level of the forehead.

Delayed hydrocephalus may appear 10 or more days after the hemorrhage, as the patient seems to be recovering well from surgery. Gait difficulty and trouble getting out of bed then appear along with a quiet behavior. The CT scan documents hydrocephalus. The lumbar pressure is normal, but often lumbar puncture will result in improvement. Ventriculoperitoneal drainage is almost always needed in this setting and is associated with a high rate of improvement.

RERUPTURE

Rerupture of an aneurysm, which is generally heralded by a sudden severe increase in headache, may be associated with nausea and vomiting, loss of consciousness, as well as a new neurologic deficit or death. A moderate to severe increase in headache alone, however, is not diagnostic. Only a repeat CT scan demonstrating an increase in the amount of blood in the subarachnoid space or a lumbar puncture showing new blood can reliably confirm the diagnosis. However, repeating a lumbar puncture in patients who have had an increase in headache is hazardous and should only be done if the diagnosis will change the therapy.

Antifibrinolytic therapy has been associated with a decrease in the incidence of rerupture. Fortunately, the trend for early surgery precludes the consideration of antifibrinolytic therapy and its inherent risks of systemic thrombosis, either venous or arterial, with subsequent embolism. If surgery is to be delayed, antifibrinolytic therapy can be recommended but it has also been associated with an increasing incidence of symptomatic cerebral vasospasm. Therefore, it is only recommended if the extent and location of blood on the CT scan does not suggest that symptomatic cerebral vasospasm will occur.

CEREBRAL VASOSPASM

Narrowing of the arteries at the base of the brain following SAH from ruptured saccular aneurysm (cerebral vasospasm) can lead to cerebral ischemia and infarction (symptomatic cerebral vasospasm). As such, it is the major cause of delayed morbidity or death, occurring in approximately 30% of patients. Most patients seem to improve or are stable during the period between the aneurysmal rupture and the onset of infarction. Signs usually appear 4 to 14 days after the initial SAH, peaking at 7 days.

If the neurologic deficit and the clinical cause of the initial aneurysmal rupture have been clearly delineated, delayed neurologic deficits from severe cerebral vasospasm are usually recognizable. These delayed deficits correspond to ischemia in specific arterial territories. The location and severity of vasospasm determine whether cerebral infarction will develop.

In order for ischemia to occur, severe vasospasm must be accompanied by narrowing of the artery, as seen on selective cerebral angiography, to less than 2 mm diameter for the distal ICA, less than 1 mm for the A1 segment (precommunal) of the ACA or the M1 segment (stem) of the MCA, and less than 0.5 mm of the A2 segment of the ACA and the M2 segment of the MCA or PCA.

Clinical evidence suggests that the extent and location of clotted blood found by CT scan in the basal cisterns and fissures of the subarachnoid space can be used to predict the incidence, location, and severity of cerebral vasospasm in patients after SAH. A high incidence of symptomatic cerebral vasospasm was found in patients whose early CT scans showed globular subarachnoid clots larger than 5 mm × 3 mm in the basal cisterns, or layers of blood 1 mm thick or greater in the cerebral fissures (Fig. 12.5). In addition, the location of the clot in the subarachnoid space correlates almost perfectly with the location of the spasm in the artery lying in the subarachnoid space. However, this correlation only applies to blood in the supratentorial basal cisterns. CT scan cannot reliably detect significant clots in the posterior fossa.

Furthermore, an accurate prediction requires that a CT scan be obtained 24 to 96 hours after SAH. Blood that appears on a CT scan obtained within the first hours following SAH may disappear from a scan taken after 24 hours, presumably because it "washes away." Time diminishes the x-ray attenuation values of subarachnoid clotted blood; its full extent and location cannot be reliably detected after 96 hours. The three patients presented below illustrate this vasospasm predictive CT scan methodology.

Patient One: A Healthy Middle-Aged Male

On Day 2 following the SAH, the patient was slightly drowsy with a severe headache but was otherwise normal neurologically (see Fig. 12.5). Extensive amounts of clot that were noted in the stem of the sylvian fissure, the sylvian cisterns, and the basal frontal interhemispheric fissure led to a prediction of severe vasospasm in each MCA stem distally, at both

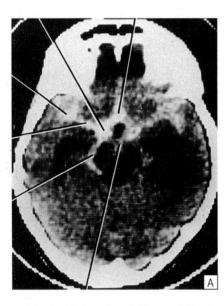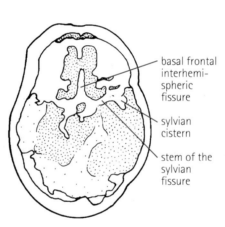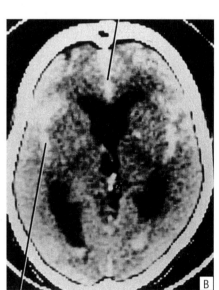

basal frontal interhemispheric fissure

sylvian cistern

stem of the sylvian fissure

FIGURE 12.5 → Day 2 CT scan following SAH. The basal cisterns are depicted. Clot is noted in the right and left suprasellar cistern, the right and left stem of the sylvian fissure **(A)**, the right and left sylvian cistern **(B)** as well as the basal frontal interhemispheric fissure. Based on the extensive amount of clot, spasm was predicted in the middle cerebral stems bilaterally, at the bifurcation of both MCAs and in the anterior communicating complex (see patient 1).

middle cerebral bifurcations and at the anterior communicating artery complex. On Day 7, the patient developed a bihemispheric ischemic state with progressive bilateral hemiparesis, dysphasia, abulia, and stupor. Coma and death ensued on Day 10, due to extensive bilateral middle and anterior cerebral tentorial infarction and edema.

Patient Two: A Healthy Middle-Aged Female

On Day 2, a clot in the left sylvian cistern with dissection into the temporal lobe was noted (Fig. 12.6). The patient was alert, speaking clearly, and had a minor headache. A middle cerebral bifurcation aneurysm was suspected. Severe vasospasm was predicted only at the bifurcation of the MCA stem in the immediate

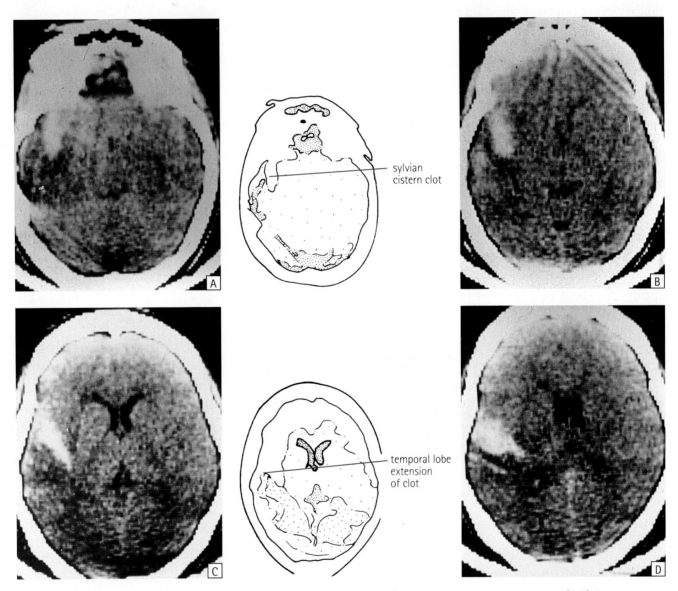

FIGURE 12.6 → Day 2 CT scan shows a clot in the left sylvian cistern **(A,B)** extending into the temporal lobe **(C,D)** from a ruptured middle cerebral bifurcation aneurysm.

proximal MCA branches (M2). Figure 12.6A shows the angiogram on Day 2 without severe vasospasm. On Day 8, the patient became dysphasic. The angiogram shows proximal middle cerebral M2 branch vasospasm (Fig. 12.7). The angiogram did not disclose spasm in other locations. The spasm cleared and the patient went on to successful aneurysmal surgery.

Patient Three: A Healthy Middle-Aged Male

A clot in the basal frontal interhemispheric fissure dissecting into the frontal lobe and in the left sylvian cistern was seen on Day 2 (see Fig. 12.3A). The patient, as predicted, developed severe symptomatic vasospasm in the anterior communicating complex and at the middle cerebral bifurcation on the left, but not in the middle cerebral stem on the left or right.

Comments on the Patients On occasion, especially in younger patients, clot in the stem of the sylvian fissure around the MCA stem or at the sylvian cistern

near the bifurcation of the MCA may give rise to severe spasm, but symptoms may not follow. Blood can flow up through the ACA and the cortical surface anastomotic channels to supply the MCA territory. However, when extensive clot exists around the MCA stem or bifurcation and around the anterior communicating complex, severe vasospasm will occur in both places. Devastating infarction of the hemisphere may follow.

Early surgery with subsequent washing out of threatening subarachnoid blood may be the only effective way to prevent spasm. Once it occurs and symptoms of ischemia develop, its treatment consists only of methods to improve cerebral perfusion. Should that not be enough, cerebral angioplasty can be successful. Therefore, it becomes important to predict vasospasm by CT scan and to follow the patient neurologically to detect the earliest signs of symptomatic vasospasm. Most recently, transcranial Doppler assessment of flow in the middle and anterior cere-

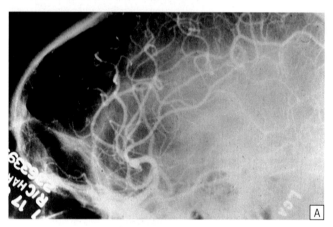
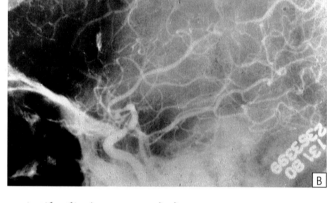
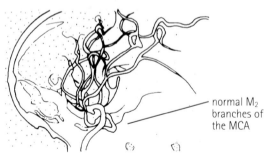

normal M₂ branches of the MCA

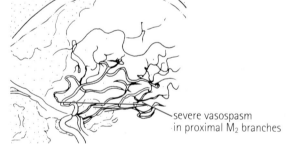

severe vasospasm in proximal M₂ branches

FIGURE 12.7 → A, Day 2 angiogram of the middle cerebral bifurcation with normal size vessels. **B,** Day 8 angiogram following the onset of dysphasia. Note the severe spasm that decreas- es the caliber of the proximal M2 branches of the left MCA. The vasospasm was predicted from the day 2 CT scan showing clot in the left sylvian cistern.

bral stems, the BA, and the posterior cerebral stems has been effective in documenting the onset and progression of vasospasm at these locations (Fig. 12.8). Given these facts, patient management must include clinical and neuroradiologic assessment in relation to the temporal course of the rupture and surgical or interventional neuroradiologic repair.

ACUTE MEDICAL MANAGEMENT

Once the diagnosis of SAH is made, appropriate urgency must be focused on evaluation and management (Fig. 12.9). Hypertension must be controlled acutely in an effort to prevent rebleeding. Intravenous medications such as nitroprusside with continuous monitoring are often appropriate. While seizure is not common, the risks of convulsion with increased blood pressure and intracranial pressure justify the routine use of intravenous phenytoin. Since early obliteration

of the aneurysm is preferred, most patients will require angiography to plan definitive therapy.

Subsequent care in the intensive care unit depends on close monitoring, not only of physiologic parameters, but also of neurologic status. Treatment with a calcium antagonist, nimodipine, may be associated with fewer stroke deficits attributed to vasospasm and improved outcome. However, no difference in the severity of vasospasm, as judged by reliable angiographic data, could be demonstrated in the nimodipine studies. The site and mechanism of action are uncertain. Nimodipine treatment is now considered routine, but it cannot relieve vasospasm. Transcranial Doppler studies should be performed routinely to assess developing vasospasm. Severity of vasospasm correlates with velocity of flow in the narrowed arterial segments. As the flow velocities increase, medical treatment for spasm can be intensified (Fig. 12.10). Intravascular volume must be maintained and hyperv-

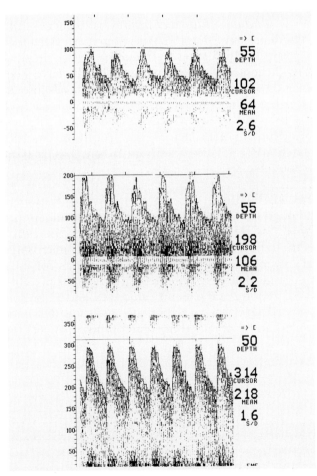

FIGURE 12.8 → Transcranial Doppler study showing normal flow in the MCA stem on Day 1 following SAH (top). On Day 5 (middle), the peak systolic flow velocity increased from 102 cm/s to 198 cm/s, indicating the onset of moderate vasospasm in the MCA stem. On Day 7, the patient became symptomatic in the cerebral territory supplied by that MCA. The peak systolic flow velocity in the MCA stem had increased to 314 cm/s (bottom). This is consistent with severe vasospasm where the residual lumen diameter of the MCA stem at that point is less than 1 mm.

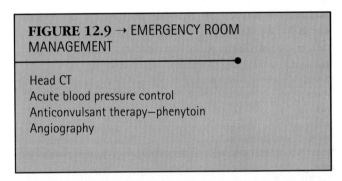

FIGURE 12.9 → EMERGENCY ROOM MANAGEMENT

Head CT
Acute blood pressure control
Anticonvulsant therapy—phenytoin
Angiography

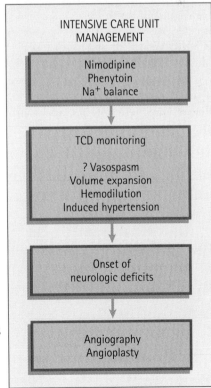

FIGURE 12.10 → Flow chart for intensive care management of SAH.

INTENSIVE CARE UNIT MANAGEMENT

Nimodipine
Phenytoin
Na⁺ balance

TCD monitoring

? Vasospasm
Volume expansion
Hemodilution
Induced hypertension

Onset of
neurologic deficits

Angiography
Angioplasty

olemic therapy can sometimes improve cerebral perfusion. A decrease in hematocrit is commonly associated with intravascular volume expansion, thereby improving whole-blood viscosity. Attention must also be given to electrolyte balance. Some patients with SAH will develop hypo-natremia; free water restriction is important in their management. Free water should also be minimized to avoid cerebral edema. However, as vasospasm worsens, increasing blood pressure becomes the most useful technique. Medications such as neosynephrine can raise systolic blood pressure to levels of 180 to 220 mm/Hg. Early treatment of the aneurysm allows safer application of induced hypertension, improving the ability to treat vasospasm. Information from transcranial Doppler and neurologic examination allows adjustments in therapy as conditions change (see Fig. 12.8). If neurologic deficits attributable to vasospasm occur despite maximal medical therapy, consideration must be given to urgent angiography and angioplasty.

SURGICAL MANAGEMENT OF INTRACRANIAL ANEURYSMS

Rebleeding is the most devastating complication that can occur after SAH from an intracranial aneurysm. Prompt obliteration of the aneurysm, therefore, is a logical step to protect the patient. Cerebral angiography to obliterate the lesion is usually warranted as soon as SAH has been diagnosed. Since the introduction of microsurgery for intracranial aneurysms in the 1970s, copious data support surgical treatment of aneurysms to prevent recurrent SAH.

MICROSURGICAL TECHNIQUE

Modern neuroanesthesia, which provides tight control of blood pressure, prevents a hypertensive episode that might lead to rebleeding. The use of hyperventilation, inhaled anesthetic agents, and mannitol will relax the brain for safe surgical exposure of the aneurysm.

The operating microscope provides up to 40 × magnification, permitting visualization and preservation of normal structures while the aneurysm is obliterated. An array of dissectors, bipolar coagulators, and aneurysm clips has been developed for this purpose. When an aneurysm clip cannot be safely applied, a ligature or muslin wrapping may be appropriate.

Recent data indicates that intraoperative rupture triples morbidity and mortality. To prevent this serious problem, *temporary clipping* of parent vessels to soften the aneurysm permits safe final preparation and clipping. Measures for cerebral protection that can prevent stroke include mannitol, hypothermia, and barbiturates.

Postoperative angiography is warranted in many cases. If an aneurysmal remnant ("dog ear") is demonstrated, the patient should be considered for possible retreatment or follow-up angiography at 6 months to 1 year. In the postoperative period, prophylactic anticonvulsants are administered, usually for 3 months.

Endovascular techniques have successfully obliterated some intracranial aneurysms. A balloon may effectively destroy an aneurysm in certain situations. Recently, very encouraging results have been obtained with tiny thrombogenic metallic coils inserted through a catheter to fill the aneurysm. Such methods may be considered, in experienced centers, if there are adverse patient factors (e.g., recent myo-cardial infarction) or adverse aneurysm factors (basilar trunk location, etc.).

SPECIAL FEATURES

Although the proper timing of aneurysm surgery is a subject of debate, prompt aneurysm obliteration seems to best prevent rebleeding. Modern microsurgical experience confirms improved results for most aneurysms that were operated on as soon as possible.

Poor grade patients (grades IV and V) present a special case. Recent experience indicates that good results can be obtained in some of these patients (up to 50% of grade IV cases). Our current practice is to place an external ventricular drain. If intracranial pressure (ICP) can be controlled (under 20–30 cm CSF), prompt operation is recommended. In grade V cases where ICP cannot be controlled, the hopeless outlook does not warrant surgery.

SPECIAL ANEURYSM TYPES

Giant aneurysms pose a special challenge for treatment. Sometimes temporary clipping, cardiopulmonary bypass, or endovascular treatment can permit safe aneurysm obliteration. Giant aneurysms at the top of the BA are particularly difficult, but can be surgically obliterated with a reasonable morbidity (Fig. 12.11). However, an operating microscope and neurosurgeons experienced in this technique are essential for success.

Multiple aneurysms occur in approximately 15% of patients with intracranial aneurysm. When a patient presents with SAH in this setting, obliterating the bleeding lesion is the top priority. In some cases, other lesions can be obliterated during the same operation. When unruptured multiple aneurysms are inaccessible through the craniotomy approach, a later operation may be necessary for their removal.

Unruptured aneurysms represent a problem area. Every ruptured aneurysm was once an unruptured aneurysm. Obliteration, therefore, is tempting. However, because most of the estimated 3 to 5 million aneurysms in the general population will never bleed, widespread application of intervention does not seem warranted. The question becomes which aneurysms are likely to hemorrhage. Current data strongly indicate that lesions 1 cm or larger carry a high risk of bleeding and, therefore, are candidates for surgical obliteration. Smaller aneurysms warrant careful follow-up; if they enlarge, surgery should be considered.

Approximately 5% of all cases of aneurysm are *familial*. In this situation, at least 2 primary blood relatives (parents, siblings, and children) have aneurysms. Discussion with family members as to risk is appropriate, as is screening by magnetic reasonance angiography (MRA).

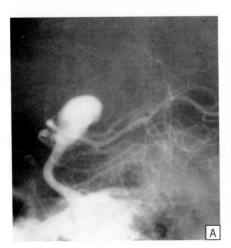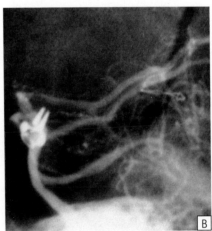

FIGURE 12.11 → **A,** Giant aneurysm at the top of the basilar artery (BA). **B,** Postsurgical obliteration of the same aneurysm.

REFERENCES

Botterell EH, Lougheed WM, Scott JW, et al. Hypothermia, and interruption of carotid and vertebral circulation, in the surgical management of intracranial aneurysm. *J Neurosurg.* 1956; 13:1-42

Davis KR, Kistler JP, Heros RC, et al. Neuroradiologic approach to the patient with a diagnosis of subarachnoid hemorrhage. *Radiol Clin North Am.* 1982; 20:87-94.

Drake CG. Management of crebral aneurysm. *Stroke.* 1981; 12:273-283.

Fisher CM. Clinical syndromes in cerebral thrombosis, hypertensive hemorrhage, and ruptured saccular aneurysm. *Clin Neurosurg.* 1975; 22:117-147.

Fisher CM, Kistler JP, Davis JM. Relation of crebral vasospasm to subarachnoid hemorrhage visualized by computerized tomographic scanning. *Neurosurgery.* 1980; 6:1-9.

Kistler JP, Ropper AH, Martin JB. Cerebrovascular diseases. In: Braunwald E, Isselbacher KJ, Petersdorf RG, et al. (eds). *Harrison's Principles of Internal Medicine,* 12th ed. New York: McGraw-Hill. 1960; 1977-2002.

Mohr JP, Kistler JP, Zabromski JM, et al. Intracranial aneurysms. In: Barnett HJM, Mohr JP (eds). *Stroke: Pathophysiology, Diagnosis and Management.* London: Churchill Livingstone. 1985; 643-677.

Ojemann RG: Management of the unruptured intracranial aneurysm. *N Engl J Med.* 1981; 304:725-726.

Ojemann RG, Cromwell RM. Intracranial aneurysms and subarachnoid hemorrhage: incidence, pathology, clinical features, and medical management. *Surgical Management of Cerebrovascular Disease.* Baltimore: Williams & Wilkins. 1983; 128-140.

Ropper AH, Zervas NT. Outcome one year after subarachnoid hemorrhage from cerebral aneurysm. *Neurosurg.* 1984; 60:909-915.

Soni RC: Aneurysm of the posterior communicating artery and oculomolar paresis. *Neurol Neurosurg Psychiatry.* 1974; 37:475-484.

Sundt TM, Whisnant JP: Subarachnoid hemorrhage from intracranial aneurysms. *N Engl J Med.* 1978; 299:116-122.

Wiebers DO, Whisnant JP, O'Fallon WM. The natural history of unruptured intracranial aneurysms. *N Engl J Med.* 1981; 304:696-698.

Wijdicks EFM, Vermeulen M, Hijdra A, etal. Hyponatremia and cerebral infarction in patients with ruptured intracranial aneurysms: is fluid restriction harmful? *Ann Neurol.* 1985; 17:137-140.

Petruk KC, West M, Mohr G, et al. Nimodipine treatment in poor-grade aneurysm patients. Results of a multicenter double-blind placebo controlled trial. *Neurosurg.* 1988; 68:505-517.

Pickard JD, Murray GD, Illingworth R, et al. Effect of oral nimodipine on crebral infarction and outcome after subarachnoid hemorrhage: British aneurysm nimodipine trial. *BMJ.* 1989; 298:636-642.

Ohman J, Servo A, Heiskanen O. Long-term effectts of nimodipine on cerebral infarcts and outcome after aneurysmal subarachnoid hemorrhage and surgery. *Neurosurg.* 1991; 74:8-13.

Kistler JP, Heros RC. Subarachnoid Hemorrhage Due to a Ruptured Saccular Aneurysm. *Neurological and Neurosurgical Intensive Care.* 2nd ed. Rockville, Md:

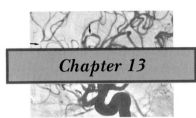

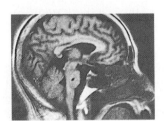

Chapter 13

GUSTAVO C. ROMÁN

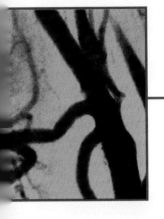

Vascular Dementia

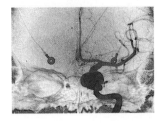

ONE OF THE MAJOR TRAGEDIES of old age is dementia, the progressive loss of the intellectual fund of knowledge and cognitive capacities acquired during a lifetime. With the increasing longevity of large segments of the population, age-associated dementias are becoming a major medical and social problem worldwide. Stroke, which is also a common disorder in the aged, may be thought to be an important cause of dementia. However, it has been difficult to determine in any given patient if stroke is the cause of the dementia, an element that worsened a preexisting degenerative dementia, or is simply an incidental finding. Furthermore, advances in brain imaging—particularly high-resolution computerized tomography (CT), magnetic resonance imaging (MRI), and cerebral blood flow (CBF) techniques—as well as observations from neuropsychology and neuropathology studies, have demonstrated that dementia may result not only from multiple strokes, but also from a single, strategically located ischemic infarction, or from extensive small-vessel lesions of the white matter in the absence of large-vessel strokes. Diagnostic criteria have been defined only recently, but for years the lack of case-definition and diagnostic criteria hampered the determination of the magnitude of dementia caused by cerebrovascular disease (CVD).

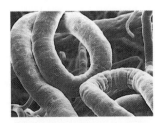

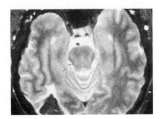

HISTORICAL ASPECTS

Psychiatry and neurology have grown closer together in the study of dementia. In 1903, Emil Kraepelin (Fig. 13.1), the famous "Linnaeus of psychiatry," brought together at the Deutsche Forschungsanstalt für Psychiatrie in Munich neuroanatomists of the stature of Brodmann and Nissl, as well as clinicians and neuropathologists such as Alfons Jakob, Spatz, Spielmeyer, and Alzheimer (Fig. 13.2). A solid histopathologic basis thus became available for classifying clinical disorders with preponderant behavioral and cognitive manifestations. Kraepelin coined the name "Alzheimer's disease" (AD) for what is now recognized as the most common form of degenerative dementia with typical neurofibrillary tangles and neuronal loss. Another psychiatrist with extensive training in neuropathology, Otto Binswanger (Fig. 13.3), described in 1894 the entity he called *encephalitis subcorticalis chronica progressiva*, a subcortical ischemic

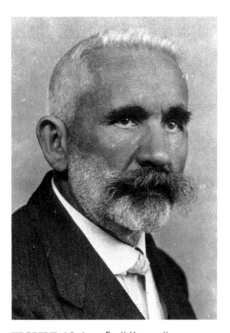

FIGURE 13.1 → Emil Kraepelin (1856–1926). Under his classification, the group of "senile psychoses" included presenile and senile mental disturbances. He separated *arteriosclerotic dementia* from *senile dementia*. Arteriosclerotic dementia was further divided into apoplectiform (dementia apoplectica) and insidious forms. Senile psychoses also included senile melancholia and organic psychoses (e.g., syphilitic general paresis, alcoholic Korsakoff psychosis), and other causes such as brain tumors. Kraepelin considered Alzheimer's disease to be a presenile form of dementia. (Portrait courtesy of the National Library of Medicine, Bethesda, MD)

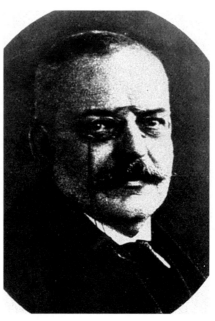

FIGURE 13.2 → Alois Alzheimer (1864–1915). By combining clinical and pathologic expertise, he provided definitive descriptions of dementing conditions such as general paresis, cerebral arteriosclerosis, and the form of senile dementia that now bears his name. (Portrait courtesy of the National Library of Medicine, Bethesda, MD)

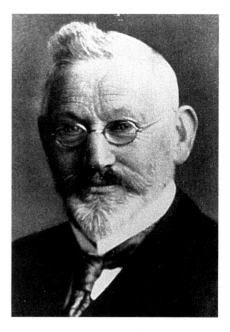

FIGURE 13.3 → Otto Binswanger (1852–1929). As a medical student in Strasbourg he became interested in pathology under von Recklinghausen; later he went to study neuropathology with Theodor Meynert at the famous Neurological Institute of Vienna. He graduated from Göttingen, obtained a position there as a resident under Ludwig Meyer, and combined pathology with clinical practice in psychiatry. In 1882, he was appointed Associate Professor of Psychiatry at the University of Jena, where he spent the rest of his career. In 1893, his book on the histopathology of syphilitic general paralysis separated this disease from other forms of dementia. In 1894, he described the subcortical leukoencephalopathy that now bears his name. His disciples included Hans Berger, Oskar Vogt, and K. Brodmann. He wrote extensively on epilepsy, hysteria (having studied with Charcot in Paris) and psychiatry. (Portrait courtesy of the National Library of Medicine, Bethesda, MD)

leukoencephalopathy, differentiating it from neurosyphilis and other forms of insanity and dementia in the aged. In turn, at the 1902 meeting of the German Society of Psychiatry, Alzheimer gave the name "Binswanger's disease" (BD) to this condition, recognized it as a vascular cause of senile dementia, and provided its histologic description.

Since Kraepelin's time, the term "cerebral arteriosclerosis" had included all patients with vascular dementia (VaD), incorrectly implying that progressive narrowing of the cerebral arteries was responsible for cortical neuronal loss and atrophy, most often due to AD. In 1974, the term multi-infarct dementia (MID) was coined as an alternative. Thereafter, MID became virtually synonymous with all forms of VaD. To counteract this misconception, the current recommendation is to use the all-inclusive term VaD, since MID is just one of several possible forms of dementia resulting from CVD.

EPIDEMIOLOGY OF VASCULAR DEMENTIA

VaD is currently defined as a complex disorder characterized by cognitive impairment that is severe enough to impede activities of daily living and results from ischemic or hemorrhagic CVD or from ischemic-hypoxic brain lesions. An estimated one-half million Americans suffer from stroke and dementia. VaD is considered the second most common cause of dementia in the elderly, accounting for almost 15% of all demented cases in clinical series (Fig. 13.4A). In autopsy-based studies, 50% of demented elderly patients have dementia of the Alzheimer type (DAT) and 25% suffer from combined vascular and degenerative dementia; 20% have pure VaD, and the remaining 5% have other forms of dementia (Fig. 13.4B). Population-based studies of VaD in Europe have found prevalences ranging from 1.5/100 for women ages 75–79 in Cambridge, England, to 16.3/100 for men older than 80 years in Appignano, Italy. A consistent increase in prevalence with age was found. Men had a higher incidence of VaD than women in most age groups. This is similar to the predominance of atherosclerotic cardiovascular disease in men but contrasts with AD since, despite regional differences, a predominance of AD in women has been noted repeatedly. Unlike the observations in North America and Europe, VaD is more common than AD in Japan,

FIGURE 13.4A → FREQUENCY OF VASCULAR DEMENTIA IN CLINICAL SERIES		
FINAL DIAGNOSIS	N	%
Alzheimer's disease	612	45.0
Vascular dementia	*181*	*13.3*
Psychiatric disorders	130	9.5
Miscellaneous	127	9.3
Not demented	80	5.8
Alcoholic dementia	68	5.0
Metabolic conditions	39	2.8
Normal-pressure hydrocephalus	34	2.5
Neoplasms	31	2.3
Huntington's disease	16	1.2
Posttraumatic dementia	15	1.1
Infections	11	0.8
Toxic conditions	8	0.6
Parkinson's disease	6	0.5
Subdural hematoma	3	0.2
Postanoxic dementia	2	0.1
TOTAL	1363	100

N= Number of patients

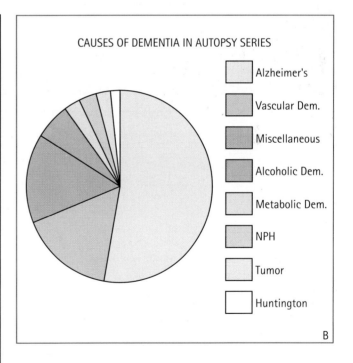

FIGURE 13.4 → Frequency of vascular dementia. **A,** Frequency in nine hospital-based clinical series of patients referred for evaluation of progressive intellectual deterioration. (Adapted from Cummings JL, Benson DF, 1992) **B,** Frequency in autopsy series (%).

China, and Russia, probably due to the higher frequency of small-vessel involvement in CVD in these countries (Fig. 13.5).

CLASSIFICATION OF VASCULAR DEMENTIA

VaD may result from a number of different types of cerebrovascular lesions, which may occur singly or in combination (Fig. 13.6).

MULTI-INFARCT DEMENTIA

MID may result from multiple, large, complete infarcts, cortical and subcortical in location. Dementia occurs in approximately 25% of all stroke survivors older than 60 years of age. Since the vast majority of patients with multiple strokes fail to develop VaD, it is obvious that factors such as the number, location, and extent of stroke lesions are important in determining whether or not dementia is the outcome. Furthermore, MRI of the brain in patients suffering from VaD demonstrated that white-matter lesions were 10 times larger in VaD patients than in non-demented patients with stroke. These findings indicate that the changes occurring in the white matter as a result of infarcts are more important than previously recognized in the production of the dementing syndrome. White-matter changes encircling infarcts often extend well beyond the limits of the vascular territory

---

FIGURE 13.5 → REGIONAL VARIATIONS IN FREQUENCY OF VASCULAR DEMENTIA

		TYPES OF DEMENTIA			
AUTHORS	OVERALL PREVALENCE	VD	SDAT	MIXED	MISC
Schoenberg, 1985 (USA)	2.2	15.0	55.0	–	30.0
Kase, 1989 (USA)	2.0	9.0	56.0	6.0	29.0
Sulkava, 1985 (Finland)	6.7	39.0	50.0	–	11.0
Molsa, 1982 (Finland)	2.0	36.1	51.8	–	12.1
Karasawa, 1982 (Japan)	4.6	36.4	12.6	–	51.0
Kawano, 1990 (Japan)	6.7	50.0	25.0	14.6	10.4
Li, 1990 (China)	1.1	42.9	28.6	14.3	14.3

FIGURE 13.6 → CLASSIFICATION OF VASCULAR DEMENTIA

I. MULTI-INFARCT DEMENTIA
Multiple large complete infarcts, cortical and subcortical, usually with perifocal incomplete infarction

II. STRATEGIC INFARCT DEMENTIA
Restricted few infarcts in functionally critical brain regions (angular gyrus, thalamus, basal forebrain, PCA and ACA territories)

III. SMALL-VESSEL DISEASE WITH DEMENTIA
Subcortical:
    Binswanger's disease
    Lacunar state
    Multiple small complete lacunar infarcts with large perifocal incomplete infarctions
Cortical and subcortical:
    Hypertensive and arteriosclerotic angiopathy
    Amyloid angiopathy with hemorrhages
    Collagen-vascular disease with dementia

IV. ISCHEMIC-HYPOXIC DEMENTIA (HYPOPERFUSION)
Diffuse anoxic-ischemic encephalopathy
Restricted injury due to selective vulnerability
Incomplete white-matter infarction
Border-zone infarction

V. HEMORRHAGIC DEMENTIA
Traumatic subdural hemorrhage
Subarachnoid hemorrhage
Cerebral hematoma

VI. OTHER MECHANISMS

Adapted from Brun A, 1992.

affected by the initial ischemia. These changes are called incomplete white-matter infarctions, and take place in the border zone between the normal tissue and the completed infarction (Fig. 13.7). Border zones of incomplete infarction are characterized by partial loss of myelin, axons, and oligodendroglial cells, and by the presence of macrophages and reactive astrocytic gliosis. In nonhuman primates with experimental middle cerebral artery (MCA) occlusion, areas of incomplete ischemic necrosis have been observed with a moderate decrease in flow, whereas coagulative necrosis resulted from a marked reduction of CBF or from complete ischemia. White-matter lesions may disconnect extensive cortical areas, leading to cognitive loss that is clinically manifested as a subcortical dementia.

STRATEGIC SINGLE-INFARCT DEMENTIA

A number of clinical dementing syndromes may occur from localized ischemic damage in cortical and subcortical areas that are functionally important for higher cerebral functions (Fig. 13.8).

Posterior Lesions and Temporal Lobe Lesions

Association areas of the posterior cerebrum, such as the angular gyrus at the temporoparietal border, are

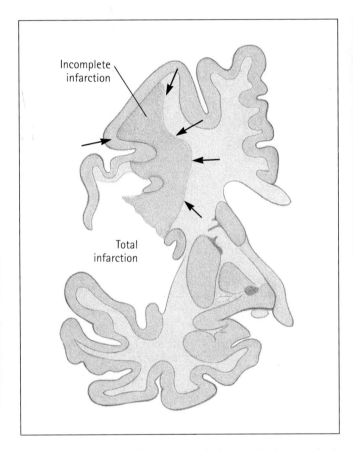

FIGURE 13.8 → LOCATIONS OF STRATEGIC STROKES THAT MAY RESULT IN VASCULAR DEMENTIA

1. Posterior association areas (e.g. gyrus angularis)
2. Posterior cerebral artery territories:
   - Paramedian thalamic artery territory
   - Inferomedial temporal lobes
3. Watershed carotid artery territories:
   - Superior frontal
   - Parietal regions
4. Bilateral anterior cerebral artery territories:
   - Basal forebrain lesions
5. Frontal white-matter lacunes

FIGURE 13.7 → Senile leukoencephalopathy is characterized by areas of incomplete white-matter infarction, histologically similar to the changes occurring in areas surrounding an ischemic stroke between zones of total necrosis and healthy tissue (between arrows). (Courtesy of Escourelle R, Poirer J, 1971)

important for integrating somatosensory information with visual and auditory information (Fig. 13.9). Strokes involving the angular gyrus present with acute onset of fluent Wernicke's aphasia, alexia with agraphia, memory disturbance, spatial (right–left) disorientation, acalculia, difficulty with spelling words and understanding spelled-out words, finger agnosia, and constructional disturbances. Memory loss, which is considered the *sine qua non* of dementia syndromes, can occur with vascular lesions involving the mesial temporal lobes bilaterally. Lesions in the left temporal lobe predominantly impair verbal memory, while right temporal lesions affect the storage of nonverbal information, such as geometric or tonal patterns. Posterior cerebral artery (PCA) infarctions may present with an amnestic syndrome often accompa-

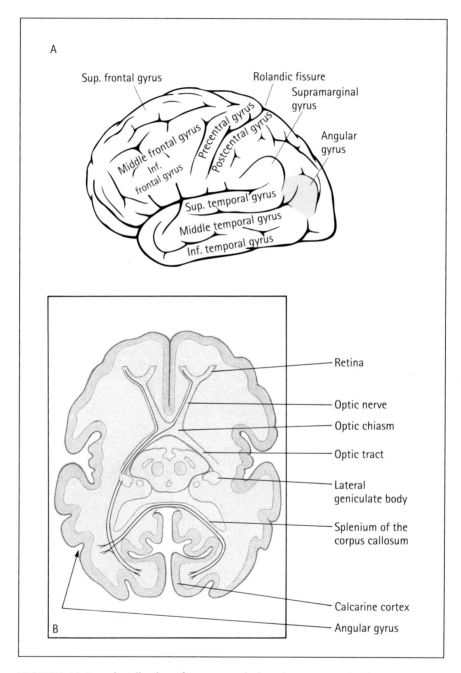

FIGURE 13.9 → Localization of *gyrus angularis* at the cross-roads of somatosensory, visual, and auditory information. **A,** Lateral view of the cerebral hemisphere. **B,** Cross-section diagram indicating the location of the visual pathway. (Adapted from Brazis PW, et al. 1990)

nied by psychomotor agitation, visual hallucinations, confusion, and visual impairment. MCA occlusions presenting with severe aphasia are excluded from the VaD group since appropriate evaluation may be impossible. Confusional episodes and psychosis may follow right MCA infarctions and bilateral carotid artery occlusions. Some patients with parietal lobe infarctions may present with substantial cognitive and behavioral abnormalities beyond disordered spatial perception.

Border-Zone Infarcts

Bilateral frontal watershed or border-zone infarctions (Fig. 13.10) may cause dementia in approximately 10% of VaD cases. These lesions are usually due to episodes of severe hypotension or critical reduction

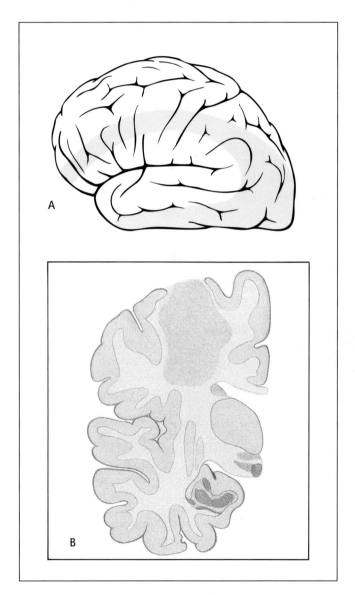

FIGURE 13.10 → **A,** The location of watershed or boundary-zone infarcts involving mostly the border zones between the ACA and MCA territories, posterior to the interparietal sulcus. (Adapted from Cummings JL, Benson DF, 1992) **B,** Watershed lesion involving the white matter between the ACA and MCA territories. (Courtesy of Escourelle R, Poirer J. 1971)

of CBF (i.e., cardiac arrest or shock), showers of emboli, or hemorrheologic alterations such as increased blood viscosity or polycythemia.

Thalamic Dementia

The neural tract that links the hippocampus to the mamillary bodies via the fornix (Fig. 13.11), and continues from the mamillary bodies to the anterior thalamic nuclei (also called the hippocampo-mamillothalamic tract of Vicq d'Azyr), is of major importance in memory functions. The complete neural circuit projects from the thalamus to the cingulate gyrus, then to the presubiculum, the entorrhinal area, insula, then back to the hippocampus. This is the "limbic circuit" described in 1937 by James Papez at Cornell University in Ithaca, New York, as the basic "mechanism of emotion" (Fig. 13.12). Lesions involving the medial temporal lobes or the cingulate gyrus produce memory disturbances along with loss of mechanisms involved in what Mesulam calls "channeling drive toward the appropriate object and imparting affective coloring to thought and perception."

Bilateral cingulate gyrus lesions and unilateral forebrain lesions such as those seen with anterior cerebral artery (ACA) infarctions present with abulia, transcortical motor aphasia, memory impairment, and dyspraxia. Basal forebrain lesions may result from vasospasm secondary to ruptured ACA aneurysms, presenting with severe amnesia and behavioral changes. Likewise, infarctions involving the medial (or dorsomedial) and anterior thalamic nuclei present with memory disturbances, apathy, disinterest, and abulia or, rarely, with agitated confusion. Infarction of the paramedian territory of the thalamus, often irrigated by a single pedicle that originates in one of the basilar communicating arteries or the posterior cerebral artery (PCA), may give rise to a bilateral butterfly-shaped lesion of the intralaminar formations of the thalamus and the paramedian region of the midbrain (Fig. 13.13). The resulting syndrome ("thalamic dementia") presents with transient loss of alertness, frontal lobe behavior, vertical gaze and convergence deficits, blepharospasm, tremor or asterixis, eventually leading to dementia or severe memory loss.

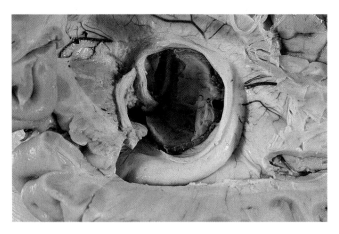

FIGURE 13.11 → Anatomic dissection of hippocampus, fornix, and mamillary body, which form the initial portion of the limbic circuit. External surface of temporal lobe has been removed for visualizing these structures.

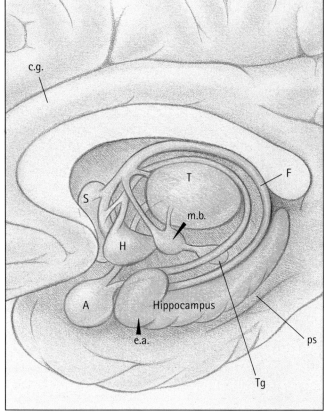

FIGURE 13.12 → The limbic system. (Adapted from Mesulam M-M, 1985) (A=amygdala, H=hypothalamus, F=fornix, m.b.=mamillary body, S=septum, T=thalamus, c.g.=cingulate gyrus, e.a.=entorhinal area, p.s.=presubiculum, Tg=midbrain tegmentum)

These findings are often seen in the top-of-the-basilar syndrome, caused by emboli or thrombosis of the distal basilar artery (BA). Relatively small thalamic strokes have also been associated with extensive decrease of CBF in frontal regions. The importance of the latter mechanism in the pathogenesis of VaD remains to be determined.

SMALL-VESSEL DISEASE WITH DEMENTIA

Lesions due to small-vessel disease may be cortical or subcortical in location, including the basal ganglia and the white matter.

Cortical Lesions

The main cortical small-vessel lesions are laminar necrosis and granular atrophy. *Laminar necrosis* presents with neuronal loss and gliosis in cerebral or cerebellar cortices following neuronal ischemic changes, presumably as a consequence of transient global ischemic injury (i.e., after cardiac arrest). It affects layers or segments of the cortex in border zones selectively vulnerable to changes in blood perfusion. These changes are commonly observed in association with border-zone infarcts. *Granular atrophy* indicates multifocal punched-out foci of tissue destruction or scarring situated entirely in the cortex

(Fig. 13.14). These foci are accompanied by focal gliosis and are found in the crests of the gyri along the arterial border zones.

Subcortical Lesions

The main subcortical small-vessel lesions include lacunes of the basal ganglia and white-matter lesions. *Small-vessel lesions of the white matter* are probably ischemic-hypoxic in origin and are frequently observed in the brains of elderly subjects; hence the name "senile leukoencephalopathy." The clinical syndrome produced by extensive white-matter lesions has been called "subcortical dementia" or senile dementia of the Binswanger type and is characterized by memory deficits, abnormal executive function, and psychomotor retardation—frequently accompanied by personality and mood alterations. A subcortical dementia syndrome, however, may also result from lesions affecting dorsomedial thalamic nuclei, caudate nuclei, dorsolateral frontal cortex, and the white-matter connections between these structures.

Lacunes

In 1901, Pierre Marie provided a complete neuropathologic description of lacunes and the clinical features observed in elderly patients affected by mul-

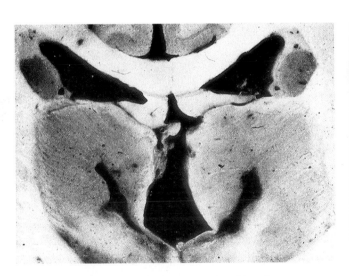

FIGURE 13.13 → Thalamic dementia resulting from a "butterfly-shaped" bilateral infarction of the intralaminar formations of the thalamus. (Courtesy of the late Prof. R. Escourelle, Hôpital de la Salpêtrière, Paris, France)

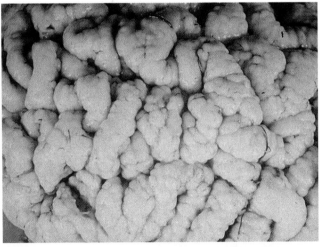

FIGURE 13.14 → Extensive granular atrophy in the brain of a centenarian producing pseudo status verrucosus. (Courtesy of Prof. G. Toro, Bogotá, Colombia)

tiple lacunar strokes (Fig 13.15A). He called this condition *état lacunaire* (lacunar state). *Lacunar infarcts* (or lacunes) are small cavitary lesions that result from brain infarcts and measure less than 1.5 cm in maximum diameter. Most of these lesions are located in the thalamus and basal ganglia, pontine base, and cerebral white matter. A small number of lacunes may represent healed or reabsorbed minute brain hemorrhages, as well as localized dilatation of the perivascular space. Lacunes are found in the distal territories of both small lenticulostriate arteries and pontine penetrating arterioles. The anatomic structure of these arteries is partly responsible for the relatively high rate of lacunar strokes in hypertensive subjects. These small arteries lack the progressive branching and ramification commonly observed in other arterial territories. Also, they originate at right angles from a large-caliber parent vessel being directly exposed to the physical stresses of arterial hypertension (Fig. 13.15B). This results in progressive degeneration of the vessel wall, infiltration by hyaline substance and lipids (lipohyalinosis), and eventual formation of the so-called microaneurysms of Charcot and Bouchard (Fig. 13.16). Rupture of these microaneurysms in the basal ganglia or pons has been assumed to explain the typical anatomic location of hypertensive intra-

cerebral hemorrhages in the basal ganglia and pons. Moreover, this process of arteriolosclerosis of small, penetrating vessels may also lead to progressive narrowing of the lumen, finally resulting in occlusion and ischemic lacunar stroke in their distal territories. Reabsorption of these minute infarctions leaves the typical cavities characteristic of lacunes.

A number of clinical syndromes have been associated with lacunes, including pure motor hemiplegia, pure sensory stroke, ataxic hemiparesis, the dysarthria–clumsy hand syndrome, sensorimotor stroke, and abnormal movements syndromes. The cause of the dementia that afflicts some patients with the lacunar state (or lacunar dementia) remains controversial, but it is probably due to the common association of basal ganglia lacunes with white-matter lacunes as well as with more extensive subcortical white-matter lesions.

It has been proposed that a single lacune destroying the genu of the internal capsule, and interrupting the inferior and anterior thalamic peduncle, may result in a dementing frontal lobe syndrome. Multiple lacunar strokes of the basal ganglia and pons often present with pseudobulbar palsy. The latter is defined as a supranuclear paralysis of the muscles of the face, tongue, and pharynx, manifested by asym-

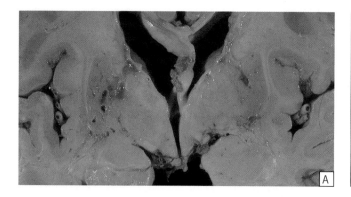
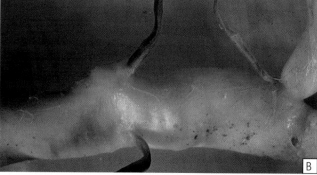

FIGURE 13.15 → **A,** Multiple lacunar strokes involving basal ganglia and internal capsule *(etat lacunaire)*. **B,** Vascular lesions involving penetrating branches of the basilar artery. (Courtesy of Prof. D.P. Perl, New York)

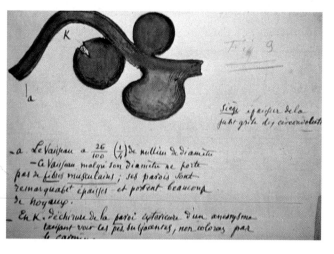

FIGURE 13.16 → Drawing from Charcot's laboratory notes illustrating a microaneurysm stained with carmine red (the so-called "aneurysm of Charcot and Bouchard"). The legend translates as: "Fig. 9. *Situation:* inside the thin portion of the convolutions. -a. The vessel has a diameter of 26/100 (1/4) mm. This vessel, despite its diameter, has no *muscle fibers*, its walls are remarkably thick and carry numerous nuclei. -In K. tear of the external wall of an aneurysm permits visualization of the underlying wall, not colored by carmine red." (Courtesy of the late Prof. R. Escourolle, Hôpital de la Salpêtrière, Paris, France)

metric weakness of the perioral facial muscles, with automatic-voluntary dissociation of facial movements, swallowing difficulties, spastic dysarthria, and loss of emotional control with pathologic or spasmodic laughing, crying, and weeping (emotional incontinence). Frontal white-matter lacunes may produce a clinical dementia syndrome with prominent frontal lobe signs that is neuropathologically indistinguishable from Binswanger's disease.

SENILE DEMENTIA OF THE BINSWANGER TYPE

Binswanger's disease (BD) is a form of chronic cerebrovascular disease that affects patients 50 years of age and older. Hypertension, diabetes, cardiovascular disease, and often recurrent hypotension are known risk factors. A history of repeated small strokes, commonly lacunes, with discrete neurologic deficits is obtained. The exquisite sensitivity of modern imaging techniques in detecting white-matter changes has prompted a sudden increase in the reported incidence of BD, despite the fact that hypertension is under better control in the general population. Although the results of most neuropathologic studies have confirmed the hypoxic-ischemic nature of the radiologic periventricular lesions observed in BD, some white-matter lesions in the elderly may have a different etiology, as mentioned below.

Clinical Aspects

The essential clinical features of BD include pseudobulbar signs, abulia, mood and behavioral changes (agitation, irritability, depression, euphoria), bilateral pyramidal signs, inattention, memory disorder, psychomotor retardation, as well as other subcortical features, including gait disturbances, urinary incontinence, and Parkinsonian signs (mainly rigidity and akinesia). The presence of gait disturbances, urinary incontinence, and dementia resembles normal-pressure hydrocephalus. The form of dementia observed in BD is classified clinically as a subcortical dementia.

Neuropathology

Complete neuropathologic study, preferably of whole brain sections, is mandatory for the definite diagnosis of senile dementia of the Binswanger type (SDBT). Lesions consist of extensive, homogeneous, or spotty demyelination of the centrum semiovale, predominantly periventricular in distribution, usually sparing the U fibers, optic radiations, corpus callosum, internal and extreme capsules, and often the axis of the temporal lobes (Fig. 13.17). Microscopically, variable degrees of myelin loss range from rarefaction of oligodendrocytes to severe demyelination with partial axonal preservation, invariably accompanied by astrocytic gliosis. The most severe lesions consist of

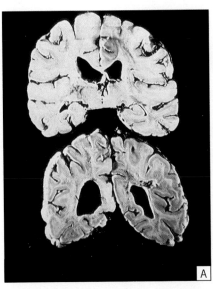
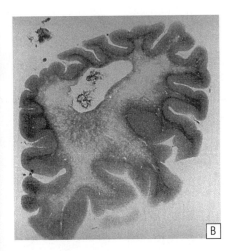
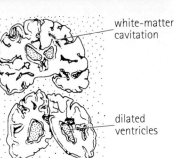
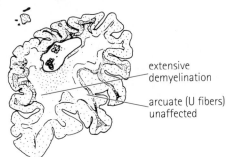

FIGURE 13.17 → Brain lesions in Binswanger's disease. **A,** Extensive white-matter lesions. Notice the presence of multiple lacunes. **B,** Myelin stain showing cavitation and extensive white-matter necrosis, with sparing of arcuate U fibers.

white-matter cavitation

dilated ventricles

extensive demyelination

arcuate (U fibers) unaffected

necrotic foci with cavitation, including white-matter lacunes as well as more extensive foci of leukomalacia. Prominent and constant thickening, sclerosis, and hyalinization of arterioles in the white matter and basal ganglia are also seen. The perivascular spaces may be dilated *(état criblé)*. Lacunes are almost invariably found in the basal ganglia, white matter, and pons. The cortical mantle is usually normal.

Radiologic Aspects

The white-matter changes suggestive of BD appear on CT as symmetrical or nearly symmetrical areas of hypodensity that involve the periventricular white matter of the centra semiovalia (Fig. 13.18A,B). These lesions show no contrast enhancement. Ventricular dilatation and features of nonobstructive hydrocephalus may also occur. The MRI pattern described

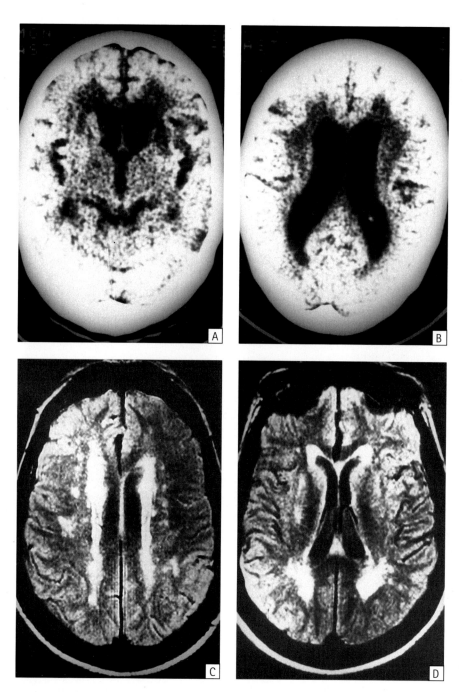

FIGURE 13.18 → **A, B:** Areas of decreased attenuation in the periventricular frontal and parietal white matter (so-called leukoaraiosis) in the CT scan of an elderly demented patient. **C, D:** Periventricular hyperintensity in MRI T2 in a case of Binswanger's disease.

in BD is an intense halo of hyperintensity of variable thickness with patchy distribution and irregular margins observed on spin-echo images, indicating a prolonged T2 relaxation time of the type associated with edema or destruction of myelin (Fig. 13.18C,D). Lacunes are frequently visualized in the centrum ovale and basal ganglia. Most of the lacunes demonstrated on postmortem exam are too small to be visualized by CT.

The differential diagnosis of these radiologic images includes other obvious causes of diffuse white-matter changes such as edema, metastases, stroke, or trauma. In addition, myelin diseases of adult and elderly patients, including multiple sclerosis and uncommon late-onset variants of adrenoleukodystrophy, globoid cell leukodystrophy, and other unusual forms must also be differentiated. Multiple sclerosis and most leukodystrophies show diffuse white-matter hyperintensity that extends from the ventricular wall to the corticomedullary junction, involving arcuate fibers. Lack of enhancement of the lesions is another important feature that differentiates BD.

Other forms of dementia, such as Pick's disease, progressive subcortical gliosis, and presenile glial dystrophy, may show subcortical lucencies. Although clinically distinct from senile dementia, postanoxic apallic syndrome with secondary wallerian degeneration, postradiation lesions, methotrexate-induced and other treatment-related leukoencephalopathies, progressive multifocal leukoencephalopathy, and the encephalitis of the acquired immunodeficiency syndrome (AIDS) could be included in the radiologic differential diagnosis.

The most difficult differential diagnosis of BD, both clinically and radiologically, is with normal-pressure hydrocephalus (NPH). The triad of ataxia, dementia, and incontinence, which is typical of NPH, is also seen in patients with BD. Diagnosis is further complicated when BD presents with massive ventricular dilation. Both entities disclose periventricular hypodensities on CT, as well as extensive hyperintensities on cerebral MRI. In normal pressure hydrocephalus (NPH), however, the lesions are smooth, symmetric, and fail to extend as dorsally as those of BD. Isotope cisternography, low CSF outflow, a positive CSF tap test, and a positive response to a shunt procedure may also help in the differential diagnosis of NPH.

OTHER MECHANISMS

Ischemic-Hypoxic (Hypoperfusion) Dementia

Dementia may result from global brain ischemia secondary to cardiac arrest or profound hypotension with extensive cortical and white-matter lesions, or from restricted ischemia in watershed territories.

Hemorrhagic Dementia

Hemorrhagic lesions, including chronic subdural hematoma, sequelae of subarachnoid hemorrhage (SAH), and cerebral hematomas—often due to amyloid angiopathy in the elderly—may produce VaD.

Combinations of the above lesions and other factors yet unknown may also play a role in the pathogenesis of VaD.

RISK FACTORS FOR VASCULAR DEMENTIA

A number of well-known risk factors for vascular disease probably also apply to VaD. These include increasing age, male sex, hypertension, smoking, and hypercholesterolemia. The frequency of all types of dementia increases with age, with rates doubling every 5.1 years. In contrast with AD—which predominates in women—VaD is more common in men. However, elderly women with a history of myocardial infarction were found to be 5 times more prone to dementia than men.

HYPERTENSION

Hypertension is the most important risk factor for vascular disease. The incidence of VaD increases significantly in subjects with risk factors for stroke (hypertension, heavy cigarette smoking, heart disease, diabetes mellitus) in comparison with age-matched controls without these risk factors. Several studies have shown impaired memory and other cognitive dysfunctions among hypertensive patients when compared with normotensive controls. The Framingham Heart Study recently reported that inadequate treatment of hypertension was associated with poor cognitive performance.

TRANSIENT ISCHEMIC ATTACKS AND STROKES

Transient ischemic attacks (TIAs) are a risk factor for stroke and also perhaps for VaD, although this has not been confirmed. The notion that the volume of brain loss from stroke determined the dementia outcome was based on a correlation found in 1963 by Tomlinson, Blessed, and Roth. They observed that infarcts larger than 20 mL were more frequent in demented patients than in controls; a marked difference between the two groups was present beyond 50 mL. However, although the volume of ischemic injury from stroke remains an important predictor of VaD, the location and bilaterality of the vascular lesions in specific brain regions, the extent of white-matter damage, and the presence of lacunes are also important determinants. Small focal lesions in critical brain regions, such as the thalamus, may lead to memory dysfunction and other cognitive deficits that result in dementia, while numerous large-vessel strokes in areas that are relatively "silent" from the cognitive viewpoint may fail to produce significant cognitive deficits.

SENILE LEUKOENCEPHALOPATHY

With the arrival of MRI, it became possible to diagnose intracranial and intraspinal lesions with higher precision and at earlier stages, but a number of unsuspected lesions also began to be observed in the brains of elderly subjects. The nature and significance of these white-matter lesions (WMLs) was initially unknown. They were called unidentified bright objects (UBOs), incidental subcortical lesions, periventricular hyperintensity, or white-matter lucencies. In the CT literature, these images have been described under the neologism *leukoaraiosis* (Greek for "white rarefaction") (see Fig. 13.18A,B). From the MRI viewpoint, these white-matter lesions have been classified as: 1) rims, 2) caps, 3) punctiform lesions, and 4) confluent periventricular WMLs (Figs. 13.18, 13.19). Several correlative radiologic-neuropathologic studies have demonstrated the probable nature of these images.

Rims

A pencil-thin line of hyperintensity along the walls of the lateral ventricle is seen in most MRI studies (see Fig. 13.19), probably representing normal characteristics of the tissue density in these areas.

Caps

Caps are areas of increased signal intensity on T2-weighted MRI images around the frontal and occipital poles of the lateral ventricles (see Fig. 13.19). Normally, there is less myelin anterior to the frontal horns, and focal zones of ependymal breakdown in elderly brains are usually present, resulting in higher fluid concentration in these areas. These factors could prolong the T2 constant, resulting in hyperintensity. Caps, therefore, probably are also normal, age-associated changes.

Punctiform Lesions

Punctiform lesions are well-circumscribed WMLs, usually located deep in the centrum ovale (see Fig. 13.19). Punctiform hyperintense lesions on MRI have been associated with a variety of neuropathologic changes, including small lacunar infarctions, vascular ectasia, and small plaques of demyelination. However, a large proportion of these patients probably have *état criblé*. This term refers to the dilatation of Virchow-Robin perivascular spaces (Fig. 13.20), usually with thinning and pallor of the perivascular myelin, in addition to shrinkage, atrophy, and isomorphic gliosis of the parenchyma around the blood vessel. Arteries and arterioles in *état criblé* are generally thickened, ectatic, have sclerotic walls that show changes of fibrohyalinosis (Fig. 13.20C), and fail to stain with Congo red—indicating absence of amyloid angiopathy. Damage of the blood-brain barrier occurs with an increase in the water content of perivascular tissues and astrocytes, which may explain the increase in MR signal intensity. Although *état criblé*

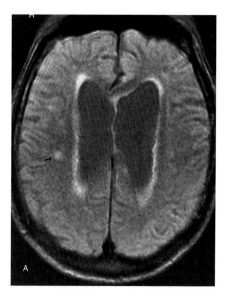

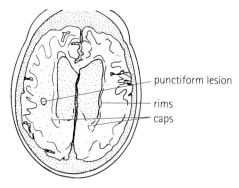

FIGURE 13.19 → MRI T2 lesions of the white matter in the elderly.

was originally thought to represent late effects of arterial hypertension as a result of recurrent bouts of "cerebral congestion," most likely these changes are due to the elongation, twisting, and formation of loops in cerebral arterioles during normal aging. Five or fewer punctiform lesions are considered normal in the aging brain.

Confluent Periventricular Lesions

Extensive periventricular lesions, confluent in appearance (see Fig. 13.18), most likely correspond to areas of incomplete necrosis of the white matter in the elderly brain. This change is denominated "senile leukoencephalopathy" since a strong correlation exists between advancing age and the presence and magni-

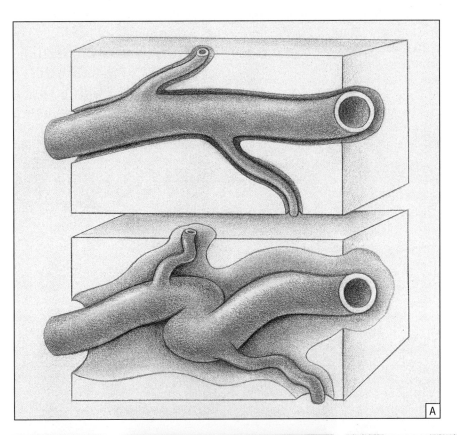

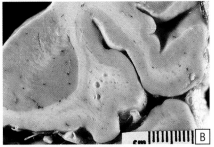

FIGURE 13.20 → *État criblé.* **A,** Dilatation of perivascular space resulting from vascular ectasia due to elongation of blood vessels with age. (Adapted from Awad IA et al, 1986 with permission of the American Heart Association, Inc.) **B,** Macroscopic appearance. Notice dilatation of perivascular spaces in the white matter. **C,** Histologic appearance. Notice extensive dilatation of the perivascular spaces, loss of the normal architecture of the blood vessels, and marked rarefaction of the tissue. (Courtesy of T. del Ser, M.D., Madrid, Spain)

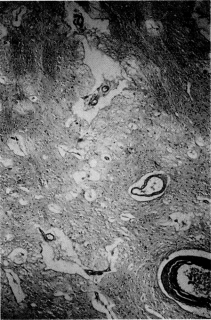

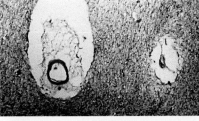

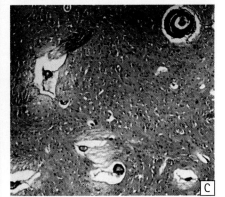

tude of these lesions on MRI in most studies. Occasional cases in young adults have, however, been reported. Neuropathologic correlation has shown that these lesions correspond to areas of incomplete infarction of the white matter, characterized, in the early stages, by pallor of myelin and gliosis. Lesions may range from incomplete infarction to necrosis and cavitation. Luxol fast blue myelin staining appears to be highly sensitive in detecting early myelin damage. These lesions are invariably accompanied by abnormalities of the blood vessels, mainly thickening of the vessel wall or arteriolosclerosis. The end stage of senile leukoencephalopathy is Binswanger's disease, a condition characterized by extensive loss of periventricular white matter, which typically spares the U fibers and other regions anatomically protected from perfusion deficits. Senile leukoencephalopathy lesions have also been described in patients with AD and in association with cerebral amyloid angiopathy. Amyloid deposits predominate in meningocortical segments of long penetrating arterioles, showing characteristic birefringence under polarized light after staining with Congo red. Fibrinoid necrosis and hyaline changes of cortical arterioles affected by amyloid may result in cortical microinfarctions. Microhemorrhages are often accompanied by one or more large lobar hematomas.

PATHOGENESIS OF SENILE LEUKOENCEPHALOPATHY AND BINSWANGER'S DISEASE

The pathogenesis of senile leukoencephalopathy and BD lesions may be correlated with a number of changes in the cerebral vasculature that occur with

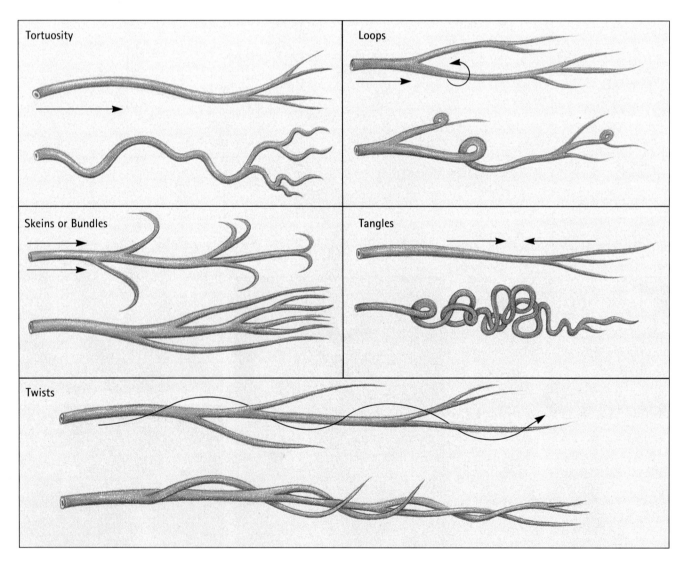

FIGURE 13.21 → Morphologic alterations of blood vessels in the elderly. (Adapted from Ravens JR, 1978)

aging, including: 1) morphologic alterations of blood vessels, 2) arteriolosclerosis resulting from effects of arterial hypertension and other conditions on cerebral arterioles, 3) territorial susceptibility to ischemia, 4) loss of CBF autoregulation, 5) hypoperfusion from hypotension or cardiac arrhythmias, and 6) interference with vascular metabolic functions at the capillary level.

MORPHOLOGIC ALTERATIONS OF BLOOD VESSELS

A number of changes have been described in the vasculature of the elderly brain (Fig. 13.21). In 1837, Tuke first noted the presence of "tortuosity and kinking" of the blood vessels in the brains of the elderly. These changes have been confirmed with new techniques such as the acid and alkaline phosphatase endothelial stainings, microangiography, and scanning electron microscopy. In the cortex, deep cortical arterial branches form fountainlike ramifications or skeins by repeated branching of a small arteriole (Fig. 13.22A). Occlusion of the parent arteriole would affect a large territory and may be important in the pathogenesis of laminar necrosis of the cerebral cortex. Arteriolar coils formed by intertwining of small branches is also common, resulting in ropelike struc-

tures. There is always clockwise rotation of these vessels and the number of these structures increases with advancing age. In the medullary arterioles, the most common findings are increasing tortuosity and formation of twists, bundles, and glomerular loops (Fig. 13.22B). According to Ravens, these changes are probably due to elongation of the blood vessels with age, along with damage of the blood-brain barrier, loss of the nutritional perivascular support leading to gliofibrillary proliferation, and adventitial proliferation of connective tissue fibers with progressive thickening of the membrana limitans gliae.

ARTERIOLOSCLEROSIS

Fibrohyaline thickening of the wall of medullary arteries begins during the fifth decade of life, increasing in frequency and severity with advancing age (Fig. 13.23). These sclerotic changes are similar to those observed in the perforating arteries of the basal ganglia (see Fig. 13.20C). Histologic lesions consist of concentric lamellar arrangements of collagen fibers with deposition of a fibrohyaline substance, mainly in the subadventitia; changes in the media are not prominent. In larger medullary arteries (>100 μm) some medial muscle fibers degenerate. Splitting and

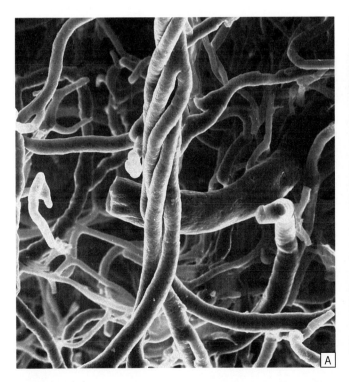

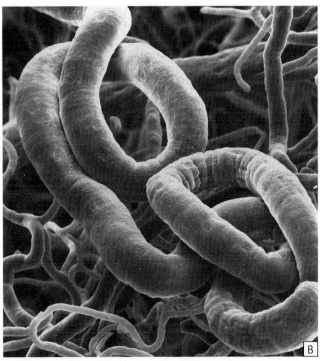

FIGURE 13.22 → Scanning electron micrographs illustrating some morphologic changes of cerebral arterioles in the elderly. **A,** Skeins or fountainlike ramifications in cortical arterioles. (Courtesy of M. Akima, M.D. Tokyo, Japan, and the editors of *Laboratory Investigation).* **B,** Arteriolar coils of medullary arterioles forming loops and twists. (Reprinted with permission from Duvornoy HM, 1981; © Pergamon Press, Ltd.)

fibroelastosis of the internal elastic lamina with normal intima is noted. On electron microscopy, these sclerotic changes are caused by proliferating collagen fibers, accumulation of cell debris, and deposition of amorphous material in the subadventitia, with thickening of the basal laminae. Arteriolosclerosis of the medullary arteries, which increases with age (Fig. 13.24), is more frequent and severe in the periventricular frontal white matter of subjects with a history of hypertension and in patients with BD.

LOSS OF CBF AUTOREGULATION

A progressive loss of cerebral vasomotor responsiveness and a decrease in CBF that occurs with aging is greatly enhanced by vascular risk factors for vascular disease, particularly hypertension. The changes of arteriolosclerosis mentioned above probably represent the morphologic substratum of this progressive loss of CBF autoregulation with aging. Striking loss of reactivity of the cerebral blood vessels in response to IV acetazolamide can be shown by single-photon emission CT (SPECT) in elderly patients (Fig. 13.25). This mechanism probably constitutes a risk factor for VaD in the elderly, especially during episodes of hypotension or cardiac arrhythmias.

TERRITORIAL SUSCEPTIBILITY TO ISCHEMIA

Depending on morphologic factors, there are regions of the white matter that are resistant to hypoperfusion and others that are susceptible. Resistant areas are

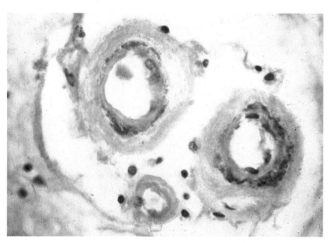

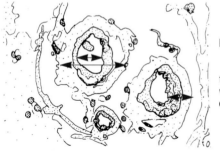

high sclerosis index

thickening of wall
with narrowing
of lumen

FIGURE 13.23 → Histologic appearance of arteriolosclerosis of medullary arterioles. (Courtesy of T. del Ser, M.D., Madrid, Spain)

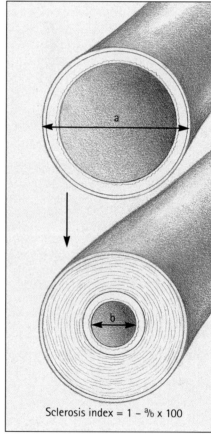

FIGURE 13.24
→ The progressive thickening of the arterioles with age and hypertension can be quantified by the sclerosis index. Occlusion of the arteriole would equal an index value of 100.

Sclerosis index = 1 – $^a/_b$ × 100

irrigated by relatively short penetrating arterioles, such as in arcuate U fibers (Fig. 13.26A) and corpus callosum (Fig. 13.27). Resistant areas may also receive dual blood supply, such as the internal capsule–claustrum–extreme capsule region. The periventricular white matter is a watershed territory that is susceptible to ischemia because of the irrigation by long penetrating medullary arteries, which originate from superficial cortical branches of the cerebral arteries. These medullary arteries, which have few or no branches, span a considerable distance, terminating in the vicinity of the dorsolateral angles of the lateral ventricles (Fig. 13.26B). Except for the choroidal arteries, there are no arteries inside the ventricles.

Therefore, the irrigation of the periventricular white matter proceeds exclusively in a centripetal pattern from the cortex to the ventricles. Because of these morphologic reasons, these distal territories are particularly susceptible to ischemia. Also, medullary arteries, such as the lenticulostriate branches that irrigate the basal ganglia, are affected preferentially by hypertension (Fig. 13.26B). In addition, elongation and loop formation in these vessels increase the resistance to flow and the risk of interrupted blood flow through the distal territories in the event of hypotension or cardiac pump failure. These *letzte Wiese* or *dernier près* (last meadow) territories constitute an area of predilection for cerebral ischemia similar to

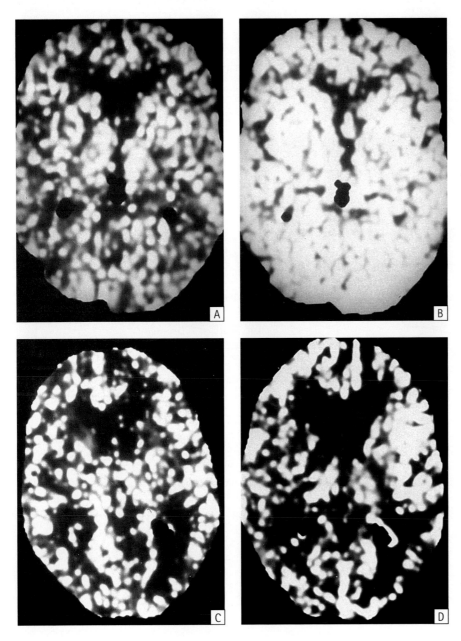

FIGURE 13.25 → Loss of autoregulation of vasoreactivity in response to IV Diamox injection in patients with leukoaraiosis, in comparison with age-matched controls. **A,** Normal, baseline SPECT. **B,** Normal, after Diamox injection. **C,** Leukoaraiosis, baseline SPECT. **D,** Leukoaraiosis, after Diamox. Notice the lack of vascular reactivity in response to Diamox in contrast with the normal subject (seen in **B**). (Courtesy of Prof. V. Hachinski, M.D., London, Ontario, Canada)

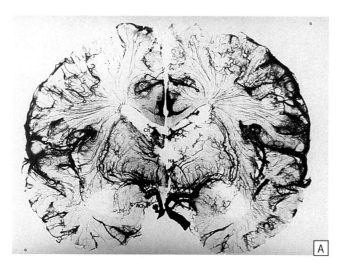

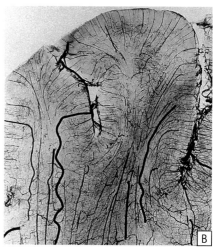

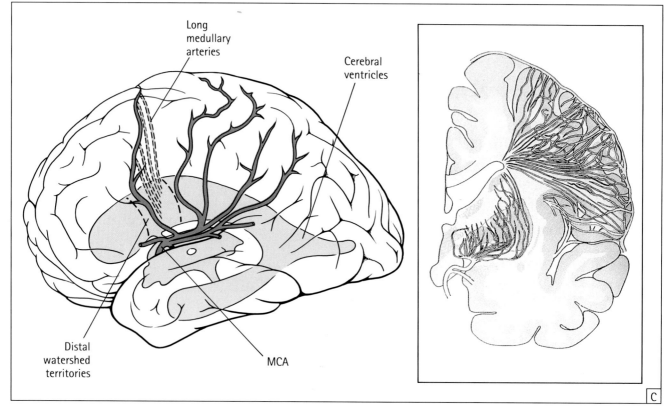

FIGURE 13.26 → **A,** Vascular supply of cortex and subcortical arcuate U fibers by short medullary arterioles. **B,** Vascular supply of periventricular white matter by long medullary arteries. (**A, B:** Courtesy of *The Journal of the American Medical Association.* Original illustrations from Prof. G. Solomon, Marseille, France) **C,** Comparison of basal ganglia and periventricular blood supply. Extensive lesions may occur along the angles of the lateral ventricles in the distal territories of long medullary arteries. Lacunar strokes are the predominant lesions in the distal lenticulostriate arterial territories. Coronal view (inset).

the arterial end zones of basal ganglia and pons affected by lacunes (Fig. 13.26C).

HYPOPERFUSION FROM HYPOTENSION OR CARDIAC ARRHYTHMIAS

Senile leukoencephalopathy may occur as a result of low cardiac output in association with arrhythmias, orthostatic hypotension due to autonomic failure, surgery, or excessive antihypertensive treatment. Despite the controversy of the term "cardiogenic dementia," it may be an important risk factor for the development of VaD in the elderly.

OTHER FACTORS

The nutritional role of the blood vessels for the surrounding oligodendroglia and myelin is often overlooked. With elongation of medullary arterioles, the arterial pressure required to maintain a constant flow in the terminal territories increases. This additional increase in blood pressure may not be met by the failing cardiovascular system of the elderly individual or it may be counteracted by the use of antihypertensive treatment. Furthermore, in the presence of a loss of autoregulation of CBF, compensatory vasodilatation of the arterial cerebral bed fails to occur simultaneously (see Fig. 13.25), resulting in additional reduction of perfusion. The net result would be a decrease in the provision of oxygenated blood to the periventricular tissues, including most prominently oligodendroglia, axons, and myelin. The problems do not cease at this point, since alterations of the blood-brain barrier and increase in the perivascular spaces *(état criblé)* may further interfere with nutritional functions.

DIAGNOSTIC CRITERIA FOR VASCULAR DEMENTIA

In 1991, the Neuroepidemiology Branch, National Institute of Neurological Disorders and Stroke (NINDS), National Institutes of Health in Bethesda, MD, USA, in cooperation with the Association International pour la Recherche et l'Enseignement en Neurosciences (AIREN) in Geneva, Switzerland, organized an international workshop to define the diagnostic criteria for research studies of vascular dementia.

PROBABLE VASCULAR DEMENTIA

Criteria

The criteria for the clinical diagnosis of probable vascular dementia include all of the following:

1. *Dementia*, defined by cognitive decline from a previously higher level of functioning, manifested by impairment of memory and two or more cognitive domains (orientation, attention, language, visuospatial functions, executive functions, motor control, praxis), preferably established by clinical examination and documented by neuropsychologic testing. Deficits should be severe enough to interfere with activities of daily living not due to the physical effects of stroke alone.

   EXCLUSION CRITERIA: cases with disturbance of consciousness, delirium, psychosis, severe aphasia, or major sensorimotor impairment precluding neuropsychologic testing. Also excluded are systemic disorders or other brain diseases (such as AD) that could, by themselves, account for deficits in memory and cognition.

FIGURE 13.27 → COMPARISON OF ANATOMIC FEATURES OF CORPUS CALLOSUM AND CENTRUM SEMIOVALE*

	CORPUS CALLOSUM	CENTRUM SEMIOVALE
CSF proximity (Virchow-Robin spaces)	++++	0/+
Blood supply	Short arterioles	Medullary art.
Length of vessels	< 8 mm long	> 20 mm long
Arteriole-venule pairs	++	0/+
Direction of arterioles	Perpendicular to axons	Parallel to axons
Companion arteriole	+++	0/+
Vascular aging changes	+	++++
Vascular hypertensive changes	+	++++
Arteriolar disease	+	++++
Hypoxemia	+	+
Hypotension	+	++++

Adapted from Moody DM, et al. 1988.
*May explain differences in susceptibility to hypoperfusion.

2. *Cerebrovascular disease*, defined by the presence of focal signs on neurologic examination (e.g., hemiparesis, lower facial weakness, Babinski sign, sensory deficit, hemianopsia, dysarthria, etc.) that are consistent with stroke (with or without history of stroke). Brain imaging (CT or MRI) should show evidence of relevant CVD, including multiple large-vessel strokes or a single strategically placed infarct (angular gyrus, thalamus, basal forebrain, PCA or ACA territories), as well as multiple basal ganglia and white-matter lacunes or extensive periventricular ischemic white-matter lesions, or combinations thereof.
3. *A relationship between the above two disorders*, manifested or inferred by the presence of one or more of the following:
   a. Onset of dementia within 3 months following a recognized stroke.
   b. Abrupt deterioration in cognitive function, or fluctuating, stepwise progression of cognitive deficits.

Clinical Features

Clinical features consistent with the diagnosis of probable vascular dementia include the following:
1. *Early presence of a gait disturbance* (small-step gait *[marche à petits-pas]*, magnetic, apraxic-ataxic, or Parkinsonian gait).
2. *History of unsteadiness* and frequent, unprovoked falls.
3. *Early onset of urinary frequency*, urgency, and other urinary symptoms not explained by urologic disease.
4. *Pseudobulbar palsy*.
5. *Personality and mood changes*, abulia, depression, emotional incontinence, other subcortical deficits (including psychomotor retardation), and abnormal executive function.

UNCERTAIN VASCULAR DEMENTIA

Features that make the diagnosis of vascular dementia uncertain or unlikely include:
1. *Early onset of memory deficit* as well as progressive worsening of memory and other cognitive functions, such as language (transcortical sensory aphasia), motor skills (apraxia), and perception (agnosia), in the absence of corresponding focal lesions on brain imaging.
2. *Absence of focal neurologic signs, other than cognitive disturbance*.
3. *Absence of cerebrovascular lesions on* brain CT or MRI.

POSSIBLE VASCULAR DEMENTIA

Clinical diagnosis of *possible* vascular dementia may be made:

In the *presence of dementia* (section 1) with focal neurologic signs, but
1. In the *absence of brain imaging* confirmation of definite CVD.
2. In the *absence of a clear temporal relationship between dementia and stroke*.
3. In patients with *subtle onset and variable course (plateau or improvement) of cognitive deficits and evidence of relevant CVD*.

DEFINITE VASCULAR DEMENTIA

Criteria for diagnosis of definite vascular dementia are:
1. *Clinical criteria for probable vascular dementia*.
2. *Histopathologic evidence of CVD* obtained from biopsy or autopsy.
3. *Absence of neurofibrillary tangles* and neuritic plaques exceeding those expected for patient's age.
4. *Absence of other clinical or pathologic disorder capable of producing dementia*.

Classification

Classification of vascular dementia for research purposes may be made on the basis of clinical, radiologic, and neuropathologic features for subcategories or defined conditions such as:
- Cortical vascular dementia
- Subcortical vascular dementia
- Binswanger's disease
- Thalamic dementia.

The term *"AD with CVD"* should be reserved to classify patients fulfilling the clinical criteria for probable AD who also present clinical or brain imaging evidence of relevant CVD. Traditionally, these patients have been included with VaD in epidemiologic studies. The term "mixed dementia" used hitherto should be avoided.

These criteria require future validation but offer a solid base for future studies of VaD.

REFERENCES

Awad IA, Johnson PC, Spetzler RF, Modak JA. Incidental subcortical lesions identified on magnetic resonance imaging in the elderly II: postmortem pathological correlations. *Stroke.* 1986; 17:1090–1092.

Awad IA, Spetzler RF, Hodak, JA, et al. Incidental lesions noted on magnetic resonance imaging of the brain: prevalence and clinical significance in various age groups. *Neurosurgery.* 1987; 20:222–227.

Brazis PW, Masdeu JC, Biller J. *Localization in Clinical Neurology.* 2nd ed. Boston: Little, Brown & Co. 1990.

Brun A, Frederiksson K, Gustafson L. Pure subcortical arteriosclerotic encephalopathy (Binswanger's disease): a clinicopathologic study. Part 2: pathologic features. *Cerebrovasc Dis.* 1992; 2:82–92.

Cummings JL, ed. *Subcortical Dementia.* New York: Oxford University Press, 1990.

Cummings JL, Benson DF. *Dementia: A Clinical Approach.* 2nd ed. Boston: Butterworth-Heinemann, 1992.

Duvornoy HM, Delon S, Vannson JL. Cortical blood vessels of the human brain. *Br Res Bull.* 1981; 7:519–579.

Englund E, Brun A, Alling C. White matter changes in dementia of Alzheimer's type. *Brain.* 1988; 111: 1425–1439.

Escourelle R, Poirer J. *Manual of Basic Neuropathology.* Philadelphia: W.B. Saunders, 1971; 96–97.

Frederiksson K, Brun A, Gustafson L. Pure subcortical arteriosclerotic encephalopathy (Binswanger's disease): a clinicopathologic study. Part I: clinical features. *Cerebrovasc Dis.* 1992; 2:82–86.

Furuta A, et al. Medullary arteries in aging and dementia. *Stroke.* 1991; 22:442–446.

Hartmann A, Kuschinsky W, Hoyer S, eds. *Cerebral Ischemia and Dementia.* Berlin: Springer-Verlag, 1991; 9–15.

Liu CK, Miller BL, Cummings JL, et al. A quantitative MRI study of vascular dementia. *Neurology.* 1992; 42:138–143.

Mesulam M-M. *Principles of Behavioral Neurology.* Philadelphia: F.A. Davis, 1985; 182.

Moody DM, Bell MA, Challa VR. The corpus callosum, a unique white-matter tract: anatomic features that may explain sparing in Binswanger disease and resistance to flow of fluid masses. *AJNR.* 1988; 9:1051–1059.

Moody DM, Bell MA, Challa VR. Features of cerebral vascular pattern that predict vulnerability to perfusion or oxygenation deficiency: an anatomical study. *AJNR.* 1990; 11:431–439.

Ravens JR. Vascular changes in the human senile brain. *Adv Neurol.* 1978; 20:487–501.

Rocca WA, Hofman A, Brayne C, et al. The prevalence of vascular dementia in Europe: Facts and fragments from 1980–1990 studies. *Ann Neurol.* 1991; 30:817–824.

Román GC, ed. Vascular Dementia. Proceedings of the NINDS/AIREN international workshop on vascular dementia. (Bethesda, MD, April 19–21, 1991) *New Issues in Neuroscience.* 1992; 4:75–196.

Román GC, Tatemichi T, Erkinjuntti T, et al. Vascular dementia: diagnostic criteria for research studies. *Neurology.* 1993; 43:250–260.

Román GC. Senile dementia of the Binswanger type. A vascular form of dementia in the elderly. *JAMA.* 1987; 258:1782–1788.

Tatemichi TK. How acute brain failure becomes chronic: a view of the mechanisms of dementia related to stroke. *Neurology.* 1990; 40:1652–1659.

Tatemichi TK, Desmond DW, Mayeux R, et al. Dementia after stroke: baseline frequency, risks, and clinical features in a hospitalized cohort. *Neurology.* 1992; 42:1185–1193.

Van Swieten JC, et al. Periventricular lesions in the white matter on magnetic resonance imaging in the elderly: a morphometric correlation with arteriolosclerosis and dilated perivascular spaces. *Brain.* 1991; 114:761–774.

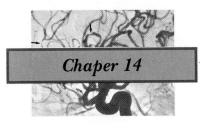

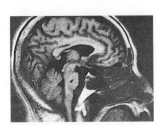

JUDY FINE-EDELSTEIN

VIKEN L. BABIKIAN

RICARDO SANCHEZ

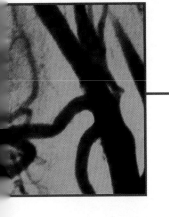

Noninvasive Evaluation of Patients with Cerebrovascular Disease

CEREBRAL ISCHEMIC EVENTS account for approximately 85% of all types of stroke, and cover a spectrum of clinical presentations that ranges from transient ischemic attacks (TIAs) to cerebral infarction. Stroke data banks have broken the diagnosis of ischemic stroke into a number of subtypes, including: 1) stroke secondary to cardiac embolism; 2) cerebral ischemia associated with stenotic lesions in large arteries such as the internal carotid, middle cerebral, or basilar arteries; 3) lacunar disease associated with lipohyalinosis or atherosclerosis of arterioles; and 4) "other"—strokes of unknown cause as well as uncommon etiologies such as hypercoagulability, inflammatory vasculitis, venous thrombosis, and migraine. Subarachnoid and intracerebral hemorrhage, and venous thrombosis are the main categories of nonischemic stroke.

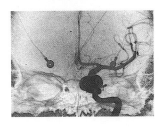

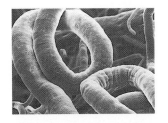

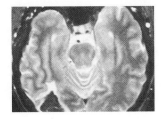

The diversity of cerebrovascular disease makes an accurate diagnosis a prerequisite to decisions regarding appropriate treatment. The diagnostic evaluation of each patient starts at the bedside and is completed with laboratory investigations tailored to verify the clinical impression. Each technique of neurovascular investigation differs in its ability to detect the presence of disease. The clinician, therefore, must be thoroughly familiar with all of them. Traditionally, these techniques have been divided into invasive and noninvasive studies. Contrast angiography remains the "gold standard" for visualizing both the intracranial and extracranial cerebrovasculature, but it has the disadvantage of being an invasive test. Noninvasive methods that image the brain include computed tomography (CT) and magnetic resonance imaging (MRI). Noninvasive techniques utilized to study the cerebral vasculature include ultrasound, Doppler, duplex scanning (DS), color flow imaging (CF), bruit analysis, transcranial Doppler sonography (TCD), oculoplethysmography (OPG), and magnetic resonance angiography (MRA). Cardiac evaluation in stroke patients is performed with noninvasive transthoracic echocardiography (TTE), and a newer minimally invasive technique known as transesophageal echocardiography (TEE).

This chapter will focus on current noninvasive methods. General principles to aid in choosing a specific diagnostic test are reviewed in the last section.

ULTRASOUND IMAGING

PHYSICAL PROPERTIES OF ULTRASOUND

The principles of ultrasound technology are based on the physical properties of sound waves, which are a form of mechanical energy that causes particles to oscillate as they move through tissue media. Oscillation frequencies ranging between 20 cycles/sec (20 Hz) and 20,000 cycles/sec (20 KHz) are audible. Sound waves greater than 20 KHz are ultrasonic—beyond the limit of human hearing.

Ultrasound imaging instruments are equipped with a transducer, which houses a piezoelectric crystal that can both transmit and receive ultrasonic waves. The generated waves travel in the form of a beam through the tissue under study, losing some of their intensity as they are absorbed and scattered. A portion of the waves that strikes an obstacle, such as the interface between the arterial endothelium and lumen, is reflected back to the probe. The strength of the

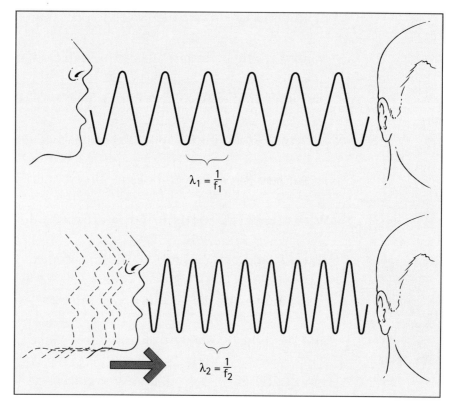

FIGURE 14.1 → A, The frequency of a stationary source as seen by the receiver produces a particular wavelength, which is equal to 1/frequency. **B,** When the source moves toward the receiver, the wavelength is reduced and the frequency is increased. The Doppler shift describes the "shifted" frequency detected, which in turn depends on the frequency emitted, the velocity of the source, the speed of sound, and the angle between the direction of motion and the receiver.

reflected echoes is proportional to the difference in density of the two tissues at the boundary interface. The signal received by the probe is then transmitted to an oscilloscope, where it can be displayed in various modes. *B-mode* technology, a popular format, generates static images, displaying the signal in terms of its brightness, which is proportional to the amplitude of the echo received. *Real-time* ultrasonography produces multiple successive action shots in a brief time period. These images are then displayed rapidly enough to give the sensation of motion. The development of high resolution real-time ultrasound permits visualization of physiologic motion, such as the contraction of the left ventricular wall, displaying a detailed image on the screen as the probe is swept over the field of interest.

While real-time B-mode ultrasonography can demonstrate anatomy, Doppler-mode imaging provides the opportunity to assess intraluminal flow characteristics. Doppler-mode imaging is based on the principles of the Doppler shift, which describes the frequency change of a sound wave in relation to motion of the emitting source, receiver, or reflecting object. (Fig. 14.1). The frequency of a wave is perceived as higher when the sound source is traveling toward the observer and lower when the motion is in the opposite direction. The magnitude of the Doppler shift is also proportional to the moving object's speed and to the cosine of the angle between the direction of motion and the ultrasonic wave. The measured Doppler shift can then be used to determine the velocity of blood flow. When ultrasonic waves are transmitted through blood vessels, they strike moving red blood cells and are reflected back to the receiver. The frequency shift is increased when erythrocytes move toward the transducer, and decreased when the movement is away from the probe. The magnitude of the measured frequency shift is proportional to the flow velocity of the red blood cells.

If blood flow in an arterial system is maintained at a steady rate, preservation of mass and incompressibility of blood demand that the product of the flow velocity and of the arterial cross-sectional area be approximately constant at different points in the system. Therefore, as a vessel diameter decreases, the mean blood velocity will increase (Fig. 14.2). Elevated flow velocities correlate with the severity of vascular stenosis, and can be detected by the change in the frequency shift.

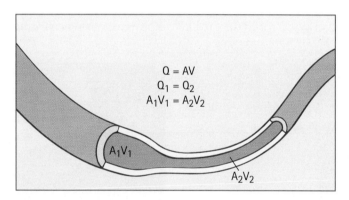

$$Q = AV$$
$$Q_1 = Q_2$$
$$A_1V_1 = A_2V_2$$

FIGURE 14.2 → According to the Bernoulli principle, flow (Q) through the larger cross-sectional area in the tube is equal to the flow in the constricted area. Since Q1=Q2, and the flow is equal to the cross-sectional area times the velocity, when the area is reduced in the constricted portion of the tube, the velocity will be increased proportionately.

The Doppler data can be represented in a number of different forms. A common method, known as spectral analysis, displays Doppler shift frequencies on the vertical axis, and time in the horizontal plane. As expected, the spectral analysis of hemodynamically significant stenosis shows increased Doppler shift frequencies, which are most pronounced in systole. In addition, spectral broadening that represents a wider range of frequencies may be detected, indicating the presence of turbulent flow. Detectable changes in the Doppler indices do not occur until the cross-sectional area of the arterial lumen is reduced by approximately 50%.

B-MODE ULTRASONOGRAPHY

Real time B-mode carotid ultrasonography can visualize the vessel wall and the characteristics of most atherosclerotic plaques (Fig. 14.3). Although it has been reported that cerebral angiography is better for assessing the dimension of the residual lumen, B-mode imaging more sensitively and specifically determines the characteristics of the arterial wall. When compared to specimens obtained at carotid endarterectomy, angiography has a sensitivity of 73% and a specificity of 62% in detecting ulcerated lesions; B-mode has respective sensitivities of 89% and 93%, and specificities of 87% and 84% in detecting plaque ulceration and intraplaque hemorrhage. The ability of B-mode to determine the severity of common carotid bifurcation stenosis has also been compared to arteriography. B-mode has an approximate sensitivity of 85% in detecting lesions that reduce the arterial lumen by up to 39%. It also has a sensitivity of 72% for 40%–69% stenosis, 55% for 70%–99% stenosis, and 51% for total occlusion. These findings suggest that B-mode ultrasonography can image vessels with mild to moderate degrees of reduction in luminal diameter. Technical limitations include the inability to reliably show plaques of low echogenicity ("soft plaques"), and to visualize intraluminal thrombi, which have an acoustic impedance that resembles blood. In addition, plaque calcification can cause ultrasonic shadowing, which may obscure the image. Because of these limitations, B-mode is usually utilized in conjunction with other noninvasive tests such as Doppler sonography and oculoplethysmography.

DOPPLER SONOGRAPHY

The severity of carotid stenosis can be estimated with the use of Doppler ultrasonography. Increased peak systolic and diastolic frequencies, as well as spectral broadening are the criteria for determining a vascular lesion's severity. These findings reflect intraluminal hemodynamic changes, but are not affected by mildly or moderately stenotic lesions, which may serve as a potential source for emboli. As a result, Doppler sonography can evaluate plaques that cause greater than 50%

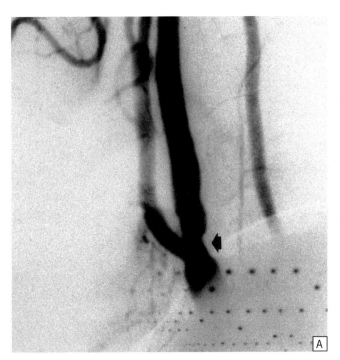
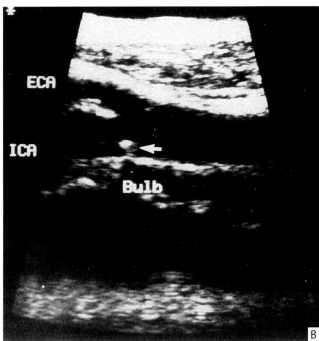

FIGURE 14.3 → Angiographic (**A**) and ultrasound (**B**) studies of the common carotid bifurcation show evidence of mild-to-moderate atherosclerotic plaque (arrows). (Courtesy of Dr. Charles Hyde)

luminal stenosis with an approximate sensitivity of 83% and a specificity of 90%, but is inaccurate in assessing arteries with lesser degrees of stenosis. Other limitations in this technique include poor discrimination between severe stenoses and complete arterial occlusions. Incorrect identification of arteries may occur, as this technique does not provide direct imaging of the vessel under study. In the past, Doppler sonography was used almost exclusively to detect stenotic lesions, but recent reports suggest that in patients with atrial fibrillation (AF), or in those undergoing cardiac surgery, it may be able to detect emboli moving through the carotid artery. The experience with emboli detection however, is limited, and the clinical significance of these findings remains unclear.

DUPLEX IMAGING

The combination of high resolution real time B-mode imaging with Doppler spectral analysis is a most accurate noninvasive method for evaluating carotid occlusive disease and has largely replaced other noninvasive ultrasound imaging modalities. Duplex scanning (DS) directly images carotid arteries by B-mode high resolution ultrasound, providing information on flow velocity in a small sample volume along the ultrasound beam by the Doppler technique. As a result, both plaque morphology and the severity of the hemodynamic changes can be assessed (Fig. 14.4). DS has

been extensively used to evaluate the cervical carotid arteries in patients with ischemic cerebrovascular disease (Fig. 14.5). Several large multicenter trials have compared DS to conventional contrast angiography and to pathologic specimens obtained at carotid endarterectomy. In one study, DS detected arteriographically-determined stenotic lesions causing greater than 75% reduction in a cross-sectional area, with a sensitivity of 87%, a specificity of 91%, and an accuracy of 90%. Other investigators have reported an accuracy of 95%.

Vertebral artery (VA) flow has also been evaluated with the duplex technique, as the course of the VAs from the subclavian artery origin into the transverse foramina can be insonated. Subclavian steal and flow characteristics in stenotic VAs can be studied, but DS is only 80% accurate when compared to angiography in determining VA characteristics.

The main shortcomings of DS include its inability to detect lesions located either proximal or distal to the common carotid bifurcation. These areas include the aortic arch and the carotid siphon. Other limitations concern the tendency to overestimate the severity of stenotic lesions when compared to angiography, and unreliability in discriminating between severe stenosis and occlusion. Hypoechoic lesions, such as intraluminal thrombi and calcified plaques, may also affect the overall accuracy of the results.

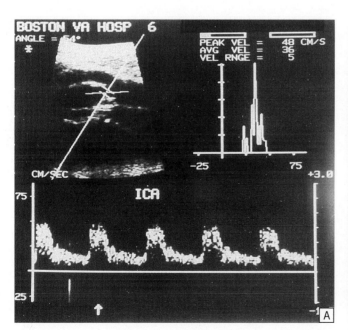
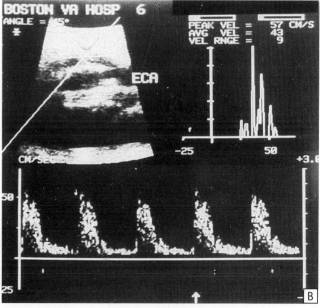

FIGURE 14.4 → A, The Duplex study shows evidence of mild to moderate atherosclerotic plaque in the distal common and proximal internal carotid arteries (ICAs), without significant Doppler shift. **B**, A normal study of the external carotid artery (ECA). (Courtesy of Dr. Charles Hyde)

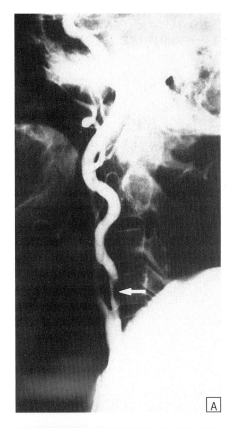

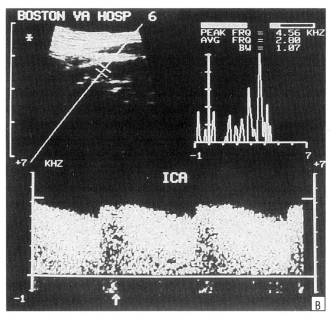

FIGURE 14.5 → Carotid angiography and duplex imaging of the common carotid artery (CCA) bifurcation. **A**, Evidence of severe proximal ICA stenosis is seen (arrow). **B**, The duplex study shows Doppler findings consistant with severe stenosis; these include increased peak systolic and diastolic frequencies and spectral broadening. (Courtesy of Dr. Charles Hyde)

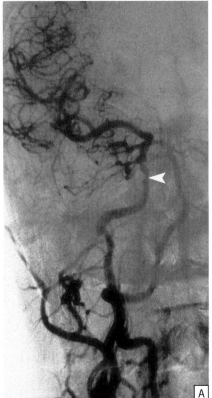

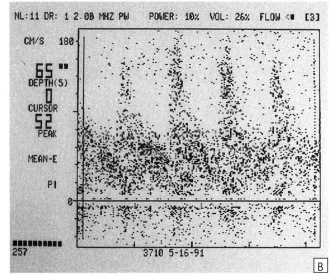

FIGURE 14.6 → **A**, This angiogram shows evidence of carotid siphon stenosis (arrow). **B**, Transcranial Doppler ultrasonography using the transorbital window reveals increased flow velocities in the carotid siphon. (Peak systolic flow velocity = 180 cm/sec)

The strength of DS lies in its ability to accurately detect extracranial disease noninvasively. It effectively screens both asymptomatic and symptomatic patients, and monitors disease progression in individuals with known carotid plaques. DS is most effective for evaluating the carotid-ophthalmic and intracranial arterial circulations when used in conjunction with other noninvasive diagnostic procedures such as transcranial Doppler ultrasound or oculoplethysmography.

COLOR FLOW IMAGING

The addition of velocity-coded color flow (CF) on the gray scale B-mode image provides the opportunity to image abnormal flow patterns directly on the video monitor while studying arterial structures. Blood flow is color coded according to the direction of flow. Blood flowing toward the transducer is coded red, while flow in the opposite direction is blue. Flow velocity is indicated by brightness. A white hue represents the highest velocities, while absence of flow is noted by lack of color. The direction of blood flow can be ascertained in the carotid as well as in the VAs, with measurements sampled along the flow stream and analyzed by viewing the frequency shift spectrum. CF can evaluate both the heart and the peripheral vascular system. It can also assess the intracranial vessels of neonates and aneurysmal flow patterns in adults.

CF studies of the common carotid bifurcation have shown that flow reversal along the posterior wall of normal arteries occurs mainly in systole and occupies approximately one third of the vascular lumen. The absence of this phenomenon may be abnormal. In patients with atherosclerotic carotid arteries, CF has been especially useful in evaluating tortuous vessels and in detecting slow flow, as well as high velocity jets, in areas of severe stenosis. This characteristic has made it possible to image highly stenotic lesions that allow the passage of only a trickle of blood. As a result, CF is more accurate than duplex imaging in identifying complete occlusions. CF is said to have a 97% sensitivity in detecting these lesions, and an accuracy of 94% in detecting lesions causing more than 50% stenosis of the carotid lumen. Its accuracy, however, is unsatisfactory for lesser degrees of stenosis. In addition, CF tends to overestimate the severity of stenotic lesions. CF is a relatively new method that promises to add to the noninvasive evaluation of carotid artery disease by improving diagnostic accuracy and increasing understanding of complex hemodynamic flow patterns.

TRANSCRANIAL DOPPLER SONOGRAPHY

Transcranial Doppler sonography (TCD), which was first introduced to clinical use in 1982 by Aaslid and his colleagues, has since been extensively utilized to evaluate patients with subarachnoid hemorrhage and ischemic cerebrovascular disease. Many reports de-scribe the use of this technology to monitor cerebral blood flow during carotid endarterectomy and cardiac surgery, and to assess the effects of therapeutic procedures on arteriovenous malformations. TCD can also help in the clinical diagnosis of brain death.

TCD is based on the same physical principles as ultrasound equipment utilized in carotid and cardiac imaging, but a lower frequency probe (2 MHz) is required to allow insonation through the cranium. Three transcranial windows are used to insonate intracranial arteries: 1) the transtemporal window insonates the supraclinoid internal carotid artery (ICA), the main stem of the middle cerebral artery (MCA), the A1 segment of the anterior cerebral artery (ACA), and the P1 segment of the posterior cerebral artery (PCA). It should be noted that in approximately 5% to 15% of individuals, recordings through the transtemporal window cannot be obtained; 2) the transorbital window is utilized to insonate portions of the ICA siphon and the ophthalmic artery; 3) a suboccipital approach through the foramen magnum can assess flow through the distal VA and proximal basilar artery (BA). A number of variables, including age, arterial partial CO_2 pressure (which has secondary effects on vasomotor tone), hematocrit, and various other pathologic processes can affect the hemodynamic indices that can be measured with TCD.

Ischemic Cerebrovascular Disease

Although TCD can detect emboli moving in the MCA, at present it is most commonly used to detect the hemodynamic effects of large arterial lesions.

Intracranial arterial lesions. TCD can detect structural abnormalities, including dolichoectatic and stenotic changes of the intracranial basal arteries. ICA siphon (Fig. 14.6) and MCA main trunk (Fig. 14.7) severe stenoses have been associated with 5% to 10% of carotid distribution cerebral infarcts. These lesions are beyond the area of insonation of duplex scanners. TCD permits detection of these lesions with an approximate sensitivity of 80%, specificity of 98%, and accuracy of 92%. Stenotic segments of the proximal ACAs and PCAs are detected less accurately, possibly because of anatomic variations at the circle of Willis. Hemodynamically significant stenoses of the intracranial VAs and of the proximal to mid portion of the basilar artery (BA) can be detected with an accuracy of approximately 80%. In some patients with acute cerebral infarction, TCD can help detect an MCA occlusion and subsequent "natural" recanalization. In the future, this ability may prove highly useful to monitor the effects of thrombolytic agents on symptomatic occluded arteries.

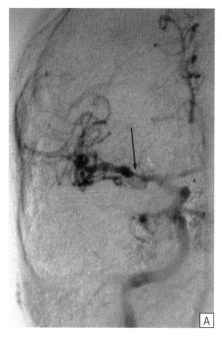

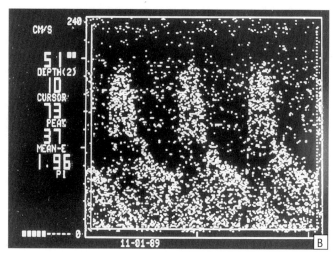

FIGURE 14.7 → **A**, Evidence of middle cerebral artery (MCA) stenosis (arrow) is seen on this angiogram. **B**, The transcranial Doppler ultrasound using the transtemporal window indicates the presence of an increased flow velocity in the MCA. Peak systolic flow velocity = 200 cm/sec.

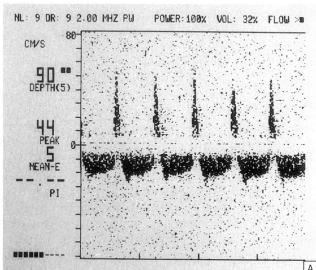

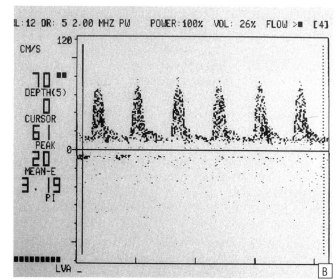

FIGURE 14.8 → On the transcranial Doppler ultrasound image using the suboccipital window, there is evidence of subclavian steal. **A**, The flow through the basilar artery (BA) is retrograde in diastole as well as in most of systole. **B**, The left vertebral artery (VA) also shows evidence of retrograde flow on the side of the subclavian stenosis. **C**, Flow in the right VA is antegrade.

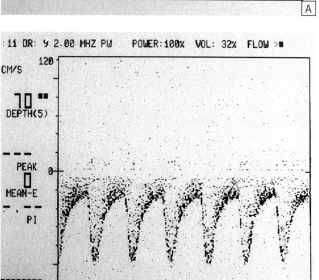

Extracranial arterial lesions. In approximately 50% of patients with hemodynamically significant cervical ICA stenosis, TCD can detect a decrease in flow velocity in the ipsilateral MCA. In such patients, collateral flow with a reversal in the usual direction of blood flow in the anterior communicating artery can be detected with approximately 70% sensitivity, 75% specificity, and 73% accuracy. In some patients, reversal of flow in the ipsilateral ophthalmic artery may occur as well. Subclavian artery stenosis, resulting in steal syndromes, can also be assessed with TCD. Findings include retrograde flow in the vertebrobasilar system (Fig. 14.8).

In summary, TCD can help detect the hemodynamic effects of intracranial and cervical arterial stenoses. In the setting of extracranial carotid stenosis, TCD is best combined with duplex scanning of the common carotid bifurcation.

Aneurysmal Subarachnoid Hemorrhage

The significant causes of morbidity and mortality in patients who survive aneurysmal subarachnoid hemorrhage include recurrent hemorrhage and arterial vasospasm. The latter is usually delayed by 3 or 4 days following the initial hemorrhage, reaches a maximum by days 5 to 10, frequently resolving after day 12. It can be detected angiographically in 30% to 70% of patients, but only 20% to 30% will develop symptoms of cerebral ischemia and infarction.

Although cerebral angiography remains the method of choice to demonstrate vasospasm, it is associated with significant morbidity and cannot be repeated often because of radiation exposure. TCD has been widely used to evaluate vasospasm, and presents an alternative method for monitoring patients with subarachnoid hemorrhage. Because it is noninvasive and can be performed at the bedside, serial studies can be obtained to monitor the effects of therapy. In some patients with vasospasm, TCD also has the advantage of detecting blood flow velocity changes before the clinical signs of cerebral ischemia develop.

Some degree of arterial spasm can be demonstrated by angiography at mean flow velocities of 120 cm/sec, but is seldom associated with symptoms of cerebral ischemia. Although a flow velocity threshold for cerebral ischemia has not been established, mean velocities ranging between 140 and 200 cm/sec have been used to initiate specific therapy against vasospasm. Depending on the selection criteria used, TCD is 60% to 80% sensitive and 98% to 100% specific in detecting MCA vasospasm. It is less accurate in assessing spasm of the ACA. Since there are limitations in the sensitivity of TCD in detecting arterial spasm, a negative study may require further evaluation with conventional angiography.

Arteriovenous Malformations

TCD can reliably detect and follow up intracranial arteriovascular vascular malformations (AVMs). Although many AVMs are diagnosed by brain CT, MRI, and MRA, these techniques cannot demonstrate the physiologic circulatory disturbances in vascular malformations. TCD can be helpful in the initial noninvasive diagnosis of these lesions. Significant findings on TCD include increased flow velocities and low pulsatility indexes, which are a measure of the resistance in the vascular beds of the arterial shunting system (Fig. 14.9). Feeding arteries, steal phenomena, and abnormal patterns of collateralization can also be detected.

Therapeutic modalities currently include surgical resection, embolization, and proton beam radiation. TCD can quantitate hemodynamic indexes in both feeding and nonfeeding arteries prior to and following treatment.

Intraoperative Monitoring

TCD has been used intraoperatively to monitor cerebral blood flow during carotid endarterectomy and, more recently, in cardiac surgery. A decrease in the MCA flow velocity has been shown to precede electroencephalographic changes during cross-clamping. Recent reports indicate that TCD can also detect cerebral emboli by noting changes in the visual Doppler spectrum, and by specific auditory signals. This ability can provide important information during cardiac and carotid surgical procedures, when there is the potential for embolic material to be dislodged into the cerebral circulation.

In summary, TCD uniquely provides physiologic information about flow characteristics of intracranial arteries. It is noninvasive and can be repeated to monitor changes reflecting disease progression or the response to therapy. At present, it is most useful in managing patients with subarachnoid hemorrhage and ischemic cerebrovascular disease. The detection of cerebral emboli seems to present a significant advance in noninvasive monitoring, but the data remain limited. The main limitations of TCD relate to the uncertainty in positively identifying individual vessels when congenital or acquired anatomic variations in the intracranial vasculature are present. TCD is most valuable when used in conjunction with other noninvasive and neuroimaging studies.

OCULOPLETHYSMOGRAPHY

Measurements of retinal artery pressure have been obtained with ophthalmodynamometers since 1917, but are no longer used to assess disease in the carotid distribution. Present day oculoplethysmographs assess blood flow characteristics in the ophthalmic artery (the first major branch of the ICA) with pressure measurements that have been found to approximate that of the

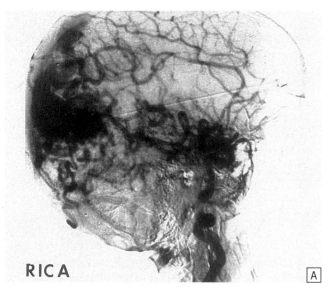

RICA

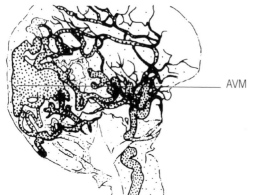

AVM

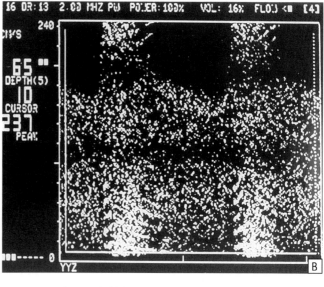

FIGURE 14.9 → **A,** This right carotid angiogram shows a large arteriovenous malformation (AVM). **B,** The transcranial Doppler image shows evidence of increased peak systolic and end diastolic flow velocities in the ICA.

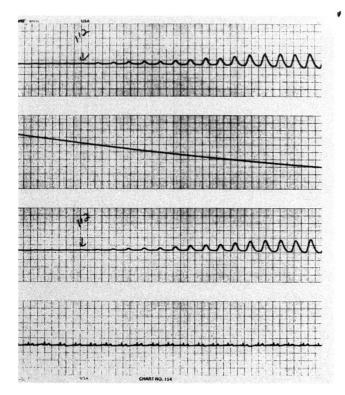

FIGURE 14.10 → Normal oculoplethysmography (OPG) study. (Courtesy of Dr Willard C. Johnson)

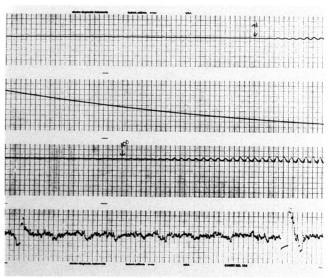

FIGURE 14.11 → The OPG image indicates a delay in the arrival time of the ophthalmic artery pulse, a finding that is consistent with a hemodynamically significant ipsilateral carotid stenosis. The ophthalmic artery pressure on the left (top) is 71 mm Hg while that on the right (bottom) is 100 mm Hg. The difference is significant. (Courtesy of Dr. Willard C. Johnson)

internal carotid siphon. Several instruments that use slightly different techniques are currently available. With the OPG-Gee instrument, an eyecup is placed on the sclera of each eye, while a pressure vacuum of 300 to 500 mm Hg is applied under the cups. The vacuum is then gradually degraded while the first ocular pulse is recorded from each eye. This method determines the ophthalmic artery systolic pressure (Fig. 14.10). In patients with severe carotid artery stenoses, the pressure in the ipsilateral eye drops when compared to the pressure in the contralateral carotid artery or to the ipsilateral brachial artery (Fig. 14.11).

OPG-Gee can detect only "hemodynamically significant" lesions that decrease ophthalmic artery pressure. Such lesions are associated with an approximately 70% reduction of the carotid artery cross-sectional area. It is for this reason that OPG is thought to better estimate the degree of hemodynamically significant carotid stenosis than angiography. OPG can also suggest the presence of lesions located both distal (e.g. carotid siphon) and proximal (e.g. innominate artery) to the common carotid bifurcation, which are out of the range of duplex instruments. OPG can confirm vessel patency following carotid endarterectomy, as duplex imaging cannot be performed at the operative site during the immediate postsurgical period. When compared to conventional contrast angiography, OPG has a sensitivity of approximately 80% to 90%, a specificity of 85% to 95%, and an accuracy of 85% to 92% in detecting hemodynamically significant carotid artery stenoses.

A significant limitation with OPG remains its inability to differentiate between severely stenotic and occluded carotid arteries. Bilateral carotid lesions are also a frequent source of error. Contraindications to the use of OPG include elevated intraocular pressure as seen in glaucoma, retinal detachment, and recent ocular surgery. For these reasons, approximately 15% of patients referred to carotid noninvasive laboratories are not suitable for OPG testing.

Duplex technology is a more accurate method than OPG for evaluating carotid bifurcation disease. The combined use of both technologies further improves diagnostic accuracy by providing hemodynamic data from a more extensive segment of the cerebral arterial tree.

ECHOCARDIOGRAPHY AND CARDIAC IMAGING

A cardiac source of cerebral embolism is the suspected etiology of approximately 15% to 20% of ischemic cerebral infarctions. For this reason, evaluation of the heart is an integral part of the diagnostic assessment of many stroke patients. Cardiac imaging techniques currently in use include transthoracic echocardiography (TTE) and transesophageal echocardiography (TEE), ultrafast CT, MRI, and indium-111 labeled platelet scintography. Long-term Holter monitoring, although helpful in detecting cardiac arrythmias, is not as frequently utilized to evaluate stroke patients because cardiac rhythm disorders, with the exception of atrial fibrillation (AF), are infrequently associated with focal neurologic disorders.

"Echocardiography" refers to the combined use of four ultrasonic diagnostic modalities to evaluate the heart: M-mode, 2-dimensional (2D) and Doppler echocardiography, as well as color flow imaging. "Contrast" echocardiography, obtained after intravenous injection of air micro-bubbles, can also assist in identifying patent foramina and other septal defects. Not all of the preceding modalities are used during each study. The combined 2D and Doppler examination are standard for stroke patients. The basis of high resolution ultrasound imaging, and the principles of the Doppler shift have been reviewed in the introduction to this chapter.

A successful echocardiographic examination enables one to image valvular structure and function, assess left ventricular chamber size, wall motion, and ejection fraction, and search for the presence of mural thrombi or tumors. Echocardiographic imaging of the heart can be obtained through either the transthoracic or the transesophageal approach. These techniques are reviewed in the following paragraphs.

Transthoracic Echocardiography

With the exception of electrocardiography, TTE is the technique that is most often used in the cardiac evaluation of patients with cerebral ischemia. TTE provides images of the heart through windows located in the third, fourth, and fifth intercostal spaces along the left sternal border. When appropriate, the aortic arch can be imaged through the suprasternal window. Most studies concur that TTE is especially successful in the evaluation of cerebrovascular disorders in young patients with a history of heart disease. Other indications include evaluation when rheumatic heart disease, mitral valve prolapse, prosthetic valves, atrial tumor, or valvular vegetations are suspected. In these patients, TTE can be useful to monitor the effects of therapy. Contrast-TTE can detect patent foramen ovale in young stroke patients. High quality studies may be difficult to obtain in patients with chronic obstructive lung disease.

In spite of its frequent use, TTE has a less than 5% yield in detecting clinically significant cardiac lesions in patients with cerebrovascular disease who have no evidence of cardiac disease by history or physical examination. When clinical evidence of heart disease is present, the prevalence of cardiac lesions has been reported to vary between 10% and 25%. Even in the latter group, however, thrombi are rarely visualized; some of the reported structural abnormalities, such as left ventricular hypertrophy, have an unclear relationship to cerebral embolism. The left atrium and atrial appendage, which are common sites of thrombus formation in AF, are not well imaged on TTE because of their posterior location. Visualization of the ascending aorta and the interatrial septum is also limited. In addition, TTE does not permit reliable discrimination of thrombi from other structures. For these reasons, TTE remains a technique of limited utility for evaluating stroke patients.

Transesophageal Echocardiography
TEE requires the use of an ultrasound probe attached to a flexible modified endoscope, which is advanced in the esophagus to a position behind the heart. The cardiac structures that lie close to the esophagus can be imaged, including the posteriorly located left atrium, the left atrial appendage, the mitral valve, the atrial septum, and the ascending aorta. The transducer can also be advanced into the gastric fundus to assess the left ventricle. Unlike TTE, where the ribs and air-filled lungs interfere with imaging, the clarity of the images and the anatomic resolution in TEE are much improved. TEE, however, is an invasive procedure and has been associated with an approximately 1% risk for complications, which can include cardiac arrhythmias, aspiration, and esophageal injury. It can be performed at the bedside, and takes approximately 20 minutes.

Most studies comparing the use of TTE and TEE suggest that the latter is a more sensitive method to detect sources of cerebral emboli. In one recent study, potential cardiac sources for embolism were identified by TTE in 14% and by TEE in 42% of patients with clinical symptoms of cerebrovascular disease. Several reports indicate that in 30% to 40% of

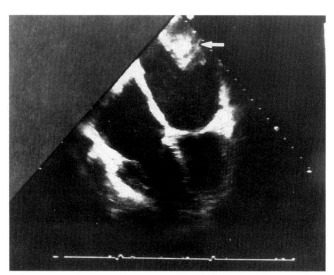 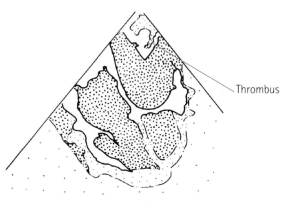

FIGURE 14.12 → Transesophageal echo (TEE) shows a large thrombus in the left atrium. (Courtesy of Dr. Mara T. Slawsky)

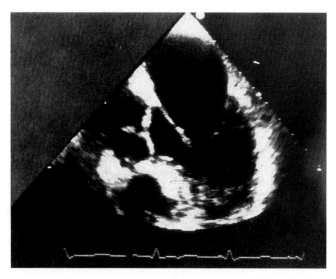 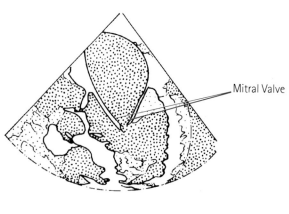

FIGURE 14.13 → Prolapse of the mitral valve into the left atrium is seen in this TEE. (Courtesy of Dr. Mara T. Slawsky)

stroke patients with negative TTE studies, TEE shows significant cardiac lesions, including thrombi in the left atrium and atrial appendage (Fig. 14.12), patent foramen ovale, myxomatous mitral valve degeneration, prolapse of the mitral valve (Fig. 14.13), septal aneurysm, and valvular vegetations. As with TTE, TEE has its highest yield in patients with clinically suspected cardiac lesions.

Although TEE remains qualitative and has limitations in evaluating patients with prosthetic or calcified cardiac valves, it has been proposed as the method of choice for detecting cardiac sources of embolism in patients with stroke syndromes. At present, however, experience with this technology remains limited. Further studies are needed to fully assess its shortcomings in patients with cerebrovascular disease.

MAGNETIC RESONANCE ANGIOGRAPHY

MRA is based on the same physical principles as MRI. In MRI, a radiofrequency pulse in the form of electromagnetic energy is delivered in a specifically timed sequence to protons in a magnetic field of interest. As the radiofrequency pulse is applied, protons become excited; they first absorb energy, then release it as they return to equilibrium. The energy is received as a radiofrequency signal, which in turn depends on the proton density of the tissue under study. Specific time sequences of the emitted pulse are utilized to best visualize both normal anatomy and abnormal pathology. The physical characteristics of various tissues determine their appearance on different scanning sequences. Blood flowing through the vasculature produces a signal void as the returning signals from the moving protons (hydrogen nuclei in water) are not recorded. Although MRI may indicate the presence of visible flow voids in normal vasculature and the absence of such in cases of vascular stenosis, it does not permit optimal imaging of vascular pathology.

MRA uses two techniques to visualize arterial and venous structures. These are known as "time of flight" and "phase contrast" imaging. The time of flight method can detect rapidly flowing blood as it is visualized in each anatomic slice under study. Inflowing intravascular blood, which was not initially exposed to the radiofrequency pulse, has a brighter signal than the stationary, adjacent tissues. The phase contrast method exposes all tissues to a radiofrequency pulse sequence and subtracts the signal from stationary tissues, leaving a visible signal from the flowing blood. The two methods are complementary. Time of flight can reduce the loss of signal from phase dispersion seen in images obtained by phase contrast techniques, hence limiting the artifactual reduction in arterial diameter. Phase contrast imaging has the advantage of detecting slower blood flow and the potential to measure blood flow.

MRA can visualize the cervical and intracranial cerebral vasculature, including the circle of Willis, the first and second order branches of the ACA, MCA, and PCA, as well as the vertebrobasilar system. It has been used to evaluate extracranial and intracranial arterial stenotic lesions, arteriovenous malformations, intracranial aneurysms, and tumors. Recent research also suggests that it may be applied to study intracranial collateral flow.

In patients with cerebral ischemia and infarction, MRA has been valuable in assessing the degree of stenosis at the common carotid bifurcation (Fig. 14.14). Stenotic lesions or occlusions of intracranial arteries such as the M1 segment of the MCA, the VA, and the BA have been visualized (Fig. 14.15). Results regarding the reliability of the technique have varied among

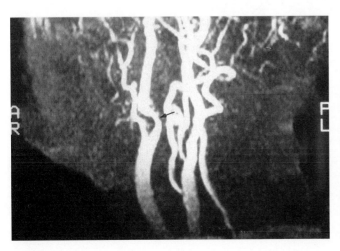

FIGURE 14.14 → MRA image of the extracranial anterior circulation shows a mild to moderate stenosis of the right ICA (arrow).

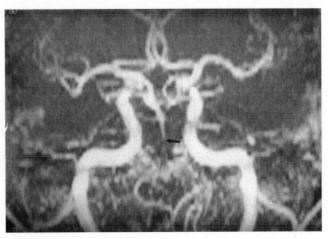

FIGURE 14.15 → The MRA image shows evidence of a probable BA occlusion (arrow).

centers. The sensitivity and specificity of MRA when compared to angiography in detecting common carotid bifurcation lesions causing more than 70% luminal stenosis varies between 86%–100% and 90%–92%, respectively. MRA can also visualize the feeding arteries and draining veins of AVMs (Fig. 14.16). Aneurysms as small as 3 mm can be identified as they arise from the circle of Willis (Fig. 14.17). In one study, 17 of 19 angiographically demonstrated aneurysms were detected by a combination of MRI and MRA. Patients with a familial history of cerebral aneurysms or with polycystic kidney disease can be noninvasively evaluated with MRA. Intracranial venous structures can also be assessed (Fig. 14.18).

Although MRA can detect stenotic lesions, it tends to overestimate the degree of stenosis. This may reflect the low signal recorded from blood flowing more slowly near the vessel wall, causing the vessel diameter to appear smaller than it would on cerebral angiography. MRA can also underestimate occlusions that may instead be interpreted as severe stenoses. In addition, MRA may not be able to provide optimal visualization of the carotid siphon. For this reason, until experience proves otherwise, MRA should only be considered a screening modality for extracranial carotid disease. Cerebral angiography is still a necessary study prior to carotid endarterectomy in most patients. MRA may also fail to detect aneurysms and dolichoectatic vessels with slow flow as well as aneurysms that are less than 3 or 4 mm. This shortcoming may be overcome with technical improvements.

The experience with MRA is still relatively limited. Its main advantage over angiography is its noninvasive capability. It does not require the use of contrast media, catheterization of vessels, nor does it deliver ionizing radiation. Computerized reconstructions allow the images to be projected in various anatomic planes in two or three dimensions, thus providing specific details of complex vascular relationships. It should also be noted that by performing the usual MRI sequences to visualize brain parenchyma in conjunction with MRA, the evaluation of cerebral infarction can be more complete. MRA is expected to evolve in the forthcoming years. With the introduction of newer techniques and contrast media, it will be increasingly used in the evaluation of patients with cerebrovascular disease.

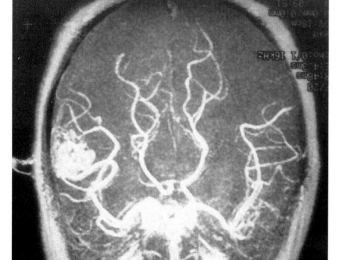

FIGURE 14.16 → MRA image reveals a large AVM.

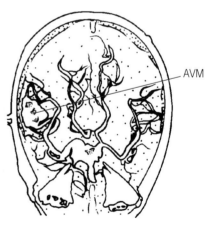

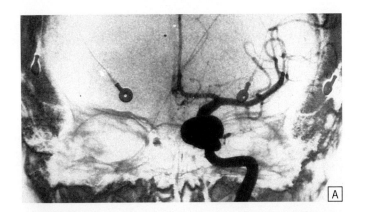

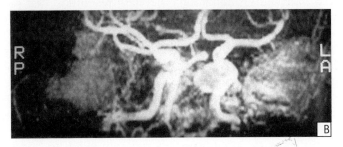

FIGURE 14.17 → **A**, Angiogram shows a large aneurysm in the cavernous portion of the ICA (black area). **B**, MRA image in the same patient.

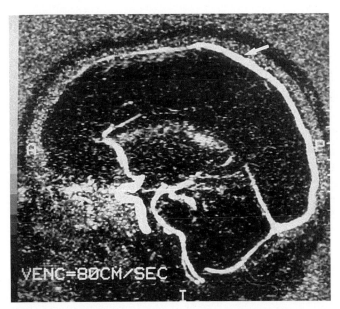

FIGURE 14.18 → The MRA image shows arterial and venous structures including the superior sagittal sinus (arrow).

CLINICAL APPLICATIONS

An explosive increase in the number of diagnostic tests available to evaluate patients with cerebrovascular disease has taken place over the last 20 years, resulting in an improved understanding of the pathophysiology of stroke and its treatment. Some of the technologies described earlier in this chapter have similar imaging capabilities. Questions often asked by the clinician concern test selection in a given clinical setting. In general, the selection of a test should depend on an individual patient's clinical presentation, using data derived from a thorough examination and clinical evaluation. A sound understanding of the advantages and limitations of each specific technology, as well as the availability and cost of the diagnostic test, must be considered. Some of the pros and cons of different testing modalities are presented below, based on the clinical presentation of stroke patients. Definitive recommendations for test selection cannot be made at the present time, however, as there are only a few studies comparing the accuracies of these tests. In addition, some technologies, such as TCD and MRA, are still evolving and have been in clinical use for relatively brief periods of time. As new technological developments are introduced and further experience is acquired, the selection criteria for these tests will likely be clarified.

In patients presenting with symptoms of *cerebral ischemia in the carotid territory*, the cervical carotid artery should be imaged. Duplex (or color flow) imaging and MRA are probably of comparable accuracy in assessing the severity of common carotid bifurcation stenosis. Duplex has the advantage of having been in use for a relatively long period of time, of being widely available, and of costing considerably less than MRA. It can also be performed at the bedside and in some agitated patients. In the clinical context of acute stroke, the combined use of brain CT and duplex imaging may have an additional advantage, as CT can assess hemorrhagic lesions with acceptable accuracy. MRA may be more accurate in detecting carotid dissection and can provide simultaneous images of the brain parenchyma. However, both MRA and duplex imaging can lead to errors in diagnosis when estimating the degree of luminal stenosis. Neither can accurately distinguish between severe stenosis and occlusion. For these reasons, cerebral angiography is still recommended prior to carotid endarterectomy for most patients. The therapeutic implication of asymptomatic, severe carotid stenosis is unclear, but is presently under investigation.

If the common carotid artery bifurcation is normal on MRA or duplex imaging, the distal carotid tree must be evaluated, since both techniques can miss carotid siphon stenosis and duplex imaging does not permit detection of lesions that are located more distally in the arterial tree. MRA can detect intracranial stenoses, but there are currently no data assessing its accuracy in detecting these lesions. The experience with TCD is considerably more extensive, and published data regarding its accuracy are available. TCD also permits evaluation of the carotid siphon. Although both tests can be used for screening, angiography is still required for a definitive diagnosis if anticoagulation is considered in this setting.

In patients with *lacunar infarcts* in whom small-vessel disease is suspected, MRI can provide the detailed resolution that permits identification of these lesions. Patients with lacunes should be evaluated in a similar manner to those with cortical infarcts. When *disease in the vertebrobasilar territory* is suspected, both TCD and MRA can provide an assesment of arterial lesions. MRI has the advantage of providing images of the posterior fossa, an area not well visualized on brain CT. Again, the use of MRA has been limited to date in this setting; conventional angiography is recommended to confirm findings on noninvasive tests when long-term anticoagulation is considered.

Transthoracic echocardiography is known to be of limited utility when evaluating stroke patients. Several studies indicate that TEE has a higher yield in detecting *cardiac lesions* of clinical significance in this population. TEE is more expensive and more prone to complication than TTE, but its advantages probably outweigh these considerations. As TEE replaces TTE, it is likely that a larger proportion of stroke patients will be found to have cardiac sources of cerebral embolism. Echocardiography remains most useful when evaluating individuals with clinically suspected cardiac lesions and young stroke patients.

In patients presenting with symptoms of *intracerebral hemorrhage,* brain CT remains the method of choice for early evaluation. Follow-up MRI or CT studies may be necessary when further bleeding or hydrocephalus is suspected. Angiography is indicated in some patients to rule out AVMs or aneurysms.

In the setting of suspected *subarachnoid hemorrhage,* brain CT should be performed immediately, and should be followed with a lumbar puncture if the CT does not show evidence of subarachnoid blood. Angiography is currently the definitive procedure to diagnose the presence of cerebral aneurysms or AVMs. TCD can monitor vasospasm and the effects of treatment in these patients. MRA is the screening method of choice for asymptomatic patients at high risk for aneurysms, including individuals with polycystic kidney disease, and those with a family history of intracranial aneurysms. In those with a suspected AVM, MRA can also be used as a screening technique.

REFERENCES

Abu Rahma AF, Diethrich EB. Comparison of various oculoplethysmography modalities. *J Vasc Surg.* 1985; 2:288–291.

Blasberg DJ. Duplex sonography for carotid artery disease: an accurate technique. *AJNR.* 1982; 3;609–614.

Comerota AJ, Cranley JJ, Cook SE. Real-time B-mode carotid imaging in diagnosis of cerebrovascular disease. *Surgery,* 1981; 89:718–729.

Mattle HP, Kent KC, Edelman RR, et al. Evaluation of the extracranial carotid arteries: correlation of magnetic resonance angiography, duplex ultrasonography, and conventional angiography. *J Vasc Surg.* 1990; 13:838–845.

Newell DW, Aaslid R (eds). *Transcranial Doppler.* New York: Raven Press, 1992.

O'Donnell TF, Erdoes L, Mackey WC, et al. Correlation of B-mode ultrasound imaging and arteriography with pathologic findings at carotid endarterectomy. *Arch Surg.* 1985; 120:443–449.

Pearson AC, Labovitz AJ, Tatineni S, et al. Superiority of transesophageal echocardiography in detecting cardiac source of embolism in patients with cerebral ischemia of uncertain etiology. *J Am Coll Cardiol.* 1991; 17:66–72.

Pop G, Sutherland GR, Koudstaal PJ, et al. Transesophageal echocardiography in the detection of intracardiac embolic sources in patients with transient ischemic attacks. *Stroke.* 1990; 21:560–565.

Ross JS, Masaryk TJ, Modic MT, et al. Magnetic resonance angiography of the extracranial carotid arteries and intracranial vessels: a review. *Neurology.* 1989; 39:1369–1376.

Sumner DS. Use of color-flow imaging technique in carotid artery disease. *Surg Clin North Am.* 1990; 70:201–211.

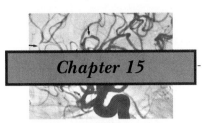

Chapter 15

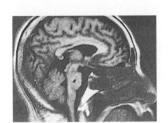

JAMES LINGLEY

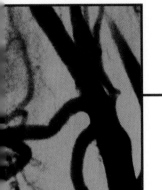

Neuroradiology of Stroke

IMAGING ISCHEMIC or hemorrhagic stroke requires multiple modalities, including noninvasive studies such as ultrasound and magnetic resonance imaging (MRI), in addition to the more invasive and sometimes therapeutic techniques of angiography. Ultrasound has already been discussed in Chapter 14. Therefore, this chapter will concentrate on computed tomography (CT), MRI, magnetic resonance angiography (MRA), and conventional angiography, as well as their applications to particular clinical presentations. "Stroke" syndromes will be divided into patients presenting with ischemic symptoms and those with hemorrhagic events. The clinical findings associated with these subtypes are discussed in Chapter 2.

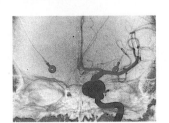

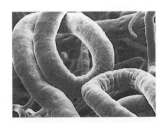

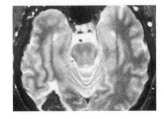

ISCHEMIC STROKE

COMPUTED TOMOGRAPHY

CT is often the first neuroradiologic test used when the patient presents with symptoms suggesting ischemic infarction or hemorrhage. The classical CT findings of an ischemic infarct are those of a low density region corresponding to a vascular territory (Fig. 15.1). The earliest time of detection varies somewhat, depending on the size of the infarct and its location. Supratentorial infarcts are more easily seen than posterior fossa infarcts, due to the absence of beam-hardening artifacts above the petrous bones. Larger infarcts are more readily and rapidly apparent than small insults. Six hours is usually the earliest that changes can be detected on CT in patients with a large middle cerebral artery infarct (Fig. 15.2). Occasionally, a hyperintense thrombus may be demonstrated on CT (Fig. 15.3).

As the infarct ages, its density on CT decreases, eventually becoming equal to water density. At this time there may be evidence of adjacent, local ventricular dilatation (Fig. 15.4). Lacunar infarcts or small brainstem infarcts may be difficult to appreciate acutely on CT because of their often small size and slight contrast difference with adjacent brain tissue. However, these infarcts do evolve toward water density on CT, thus becoming more readily apparent (Fig. 15.5).

Infarcts enhance on CT as early as one week after onset, although the peak time for contrast enhancement is around two weeks. Generally, the

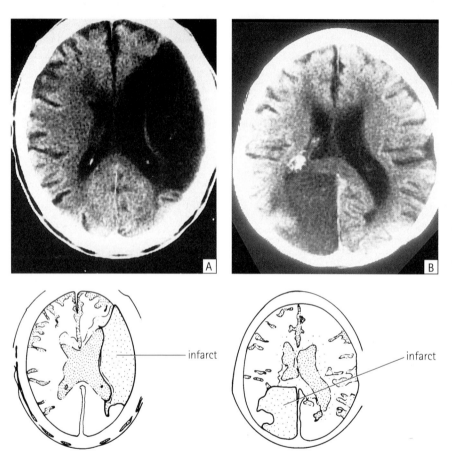

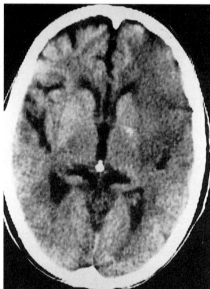

FIGURE 15.1 → **A,** Noncontrast CT demonstrates a large, low-density infarct bounded by the expected vascular territory of the left middle cerebral artery (MCA). The lesion has all the characteristics of an old infarct, including ipsilateral dilatation of the adjacent lateral ventricle. This infarct occurred six months previously. **B,** Posterior cerebral infarct. Axial unenhanced CT scan was obtained 24 hours after onset of symptoms. Low density of infarct corresponds to vascular territory of the posterior cerebral artery (PCA).

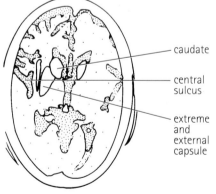

FIGURE 15.2 → Axial unenhanced CT. Note the large area of diminished density in much of the left hemisphere in the territory of the MCA. There is loss of grey/white matter contrast and compression of the central sulcus secondary to acute edema. Right side is normal.

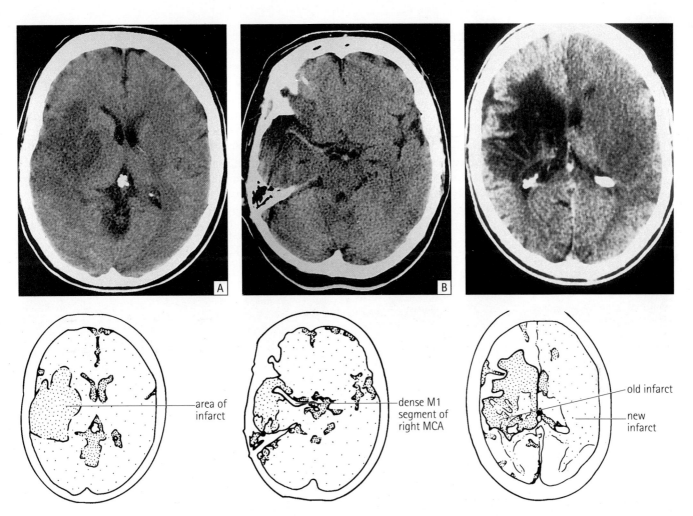

FIGURE 15.3 → Right MCA Infarct. **A,** Noncontrast CT shows a large, low-density lesion in the vascular territory of the right MCA. **B,** This infarct is secondary to thrombosis, with high-density clot in the right MCA noted on noncontrast CT.

FIGURE 15.4 → Unenhanced axial CT shows bilateral infarcts in territories of the right MCA and the left internal carotid artery (ICA). The right-sided infarct is 6 months old and shows expected findings of cerebrospinal fluid (CSF) density in addition to right lateral ventricular dilatation. The acute, left-sided infarct is hypointense due to edema.

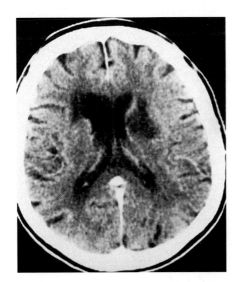

FIGURE 15.5 → Bilateral lacunar infarcts are noted. The larger infarct is hypointense, but not yet of water density. Clinical history suggested that the larger infarct was 3 days old.

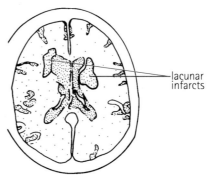

use of intravenous contrast is not helpful acutely and may be confusing if only a contrast-enhanced scan is obtained. (The CT scan may render an infarct isointense, causing it to be missed.)

MAGNETIC RESONANCE IMAGING

A discussion on the neuroradiology of stroke would be incomplete without mentioning the emerging techniques that are related to nuclear magnetic resonance. MRI has been well established for several years. As it has become more widely available, it has supplanted CT imaging in many instances. MRI generally will detect infarcts sooner than CT because of its greater contrast sensitivity.

MRI's contrast sensitivity allows earlier diagnosis of smaller, lacunar infarcts. Infarcts will show enhancement after injection of gadolinium on MRI, although the experience with contrast enhancement is not yet as extensive as with CT. There appear to be three types of MRI contrast enhancement. *Cortical blood vessels* in the territory of occlusion often enhance. Except for diffusion imaging, this is the earliest sign of an infarct on MRI. It can be seen almost immediately—certainly within two hours. *Deep infarcts, infarcts in watershed zones,* and *areas of ischemia without infarction* may enhance as early as two or three days. *Major cortical infarcts* enhance in a pattern similar to CT, namely beginning at 7 to 10 days (Fig. 15.6). The

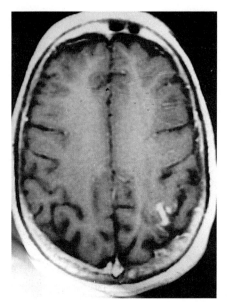

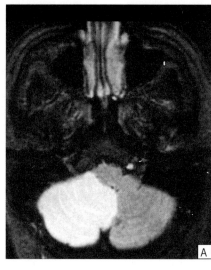

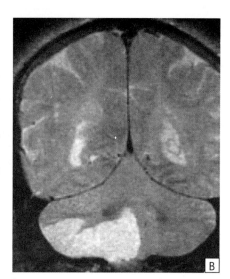

FIGURE 15.6 → Enhancing infarct. Axial T1 MRI after gadolinium. On the same scan before enhancement there was no signal brightening. A T2-weighted scan showed a typical infarct. The gadolinium-enhanced scan shows gyral enhancement; the scan was performed 9 days after the acute event.

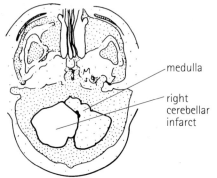

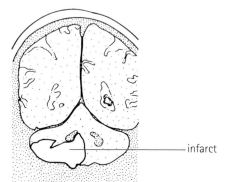

FIGURE 15.7 → **A,** Axial T2-weighted MRI. Increased signal intensity is very sharply demarcated from the normal left cerebellum and medulla. The anatomy corresponds to the territory of the right posterior inferior cerebellar artery (PICA). **B,** Coronal T2-weighted MRI shows similar findings. The patient presented with a lateral medullary syndrome.

various mechanisms for the different types of enhancement can be found in the references.

MRI can also demonstrate changes of cerebral infarction sooner than CT can. With the development of vasogenic edema, an infarct will be hyperintense on T2-weighted MRI scans. While abnormal T2-weighted scans have been reported as early as 2 hours after the development of symptoms, most patients do not develop obviously abnormal T2-weighted scans until 8 to 18 hours after the infarct. Since the dense bones at the base of the skull cause no artifact, MRI is much more sensitive than CT for evaluating posterior fossa infarcts (Fig. 15.7). With time, the hyperintensity of T2-weighted scans

becomes more obvious and equal to that of cerebrospinal fluid (CSF). T1-weighted images show hypointensity. Both T1 and T2 scans eventually demonstrate the local ventricular dilatation seen on CT (Fig. 15.8).

The acute changes of infarction shown on MRI are those of increased signal intensity on T2-weighted images reflecting increased water content—probably vasogenic edema. Even MRI, however, is not sensitive to changes produced by cerebral infarction until 2 to 6 hours after the event. Newer techniques that are still in the experimental stage, such as diffusion or perfusion imaging and MRI spectroscopy, have the potential to demonstrate physiologic and

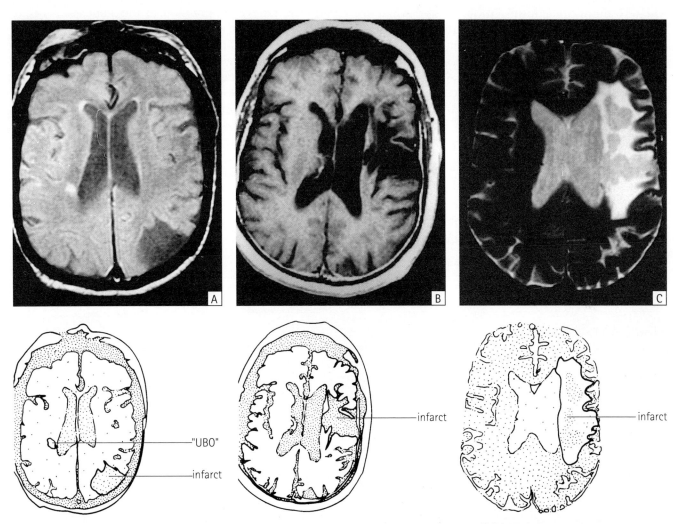

FIGURE 15.8 → **A,** Axial proton density (TR 2000, TE30) MRI. There is a triangular, CSF density lesion on the left at the junction of the left middle and posterior cerebral vascular territories. Note the typical wedge shape of an infarct; the lesion had signal characteristics of CSF on all pulse sequences. Note also the nonspecific hyperintense lesion adjacent to the right lateral ventricle. Lesions near the ventricles in deep white matter are seen increasingly with age and are also associated with hypertension and diabetes. Pathologically, they may represent areas of perivascular

gliosis or small white-matter infarcts, and have been referred to as "UBOs" (unidentified bright objects). **B,** Left frontoparietal infarct. Axial MRI, T1-weighted scan shows a vestige of an old infarct; low density (equivalent to CSF) is seen in the left frontoparietal operculum and adjacent deep white matter. **C,** Axial MRI, T2-weighted scan shows expected high signal intensity (even higher than CSF) secondary to increased water content and gliosis in the old infarct.

anatomic changes within minutes of the ischemic event. Figure 15.9 shows an experimental animal study in which diffusion imaging studies demonstrated the area of diminished flow and ischemia within 30 minutes of carotid ligation. These techniques are not yet clinically useful, but hold great promise. The reader is referred to the reference on recent advances in MRI imaging for more detailed information.

In view of MRI's ability to detect smaller infarcts and posterior fossa infarcts better and earlier than CT, MRI would appear to be the procedure of choice were it equally available and within the same price range. Generally, those conditions do not exist. Also, some patients are too unstable, cannot be adequately monitored during MRI, or have some contraindication to MRI such as a cardiac pacemaker. From a practical point of view, an emergency CT exam answers the usual clinical question as to whether the patient has an infarct or hemorrhage. Since CT can accurately detect acute hemorrhages and is probably better than MRI in detecting subarachnoid hemorrhage (SAH), a negative CT effectively excludes an intracranial hemorrhage (IH) and, in the appropriate clininical setting, strongly suggests an infarct.

MAGNETIC RESONANCE ANGIOGRAPHY

MRA is available in many established MRI sites and is currently used to clinically evaluate patients at risk for cerebrovascular disease. It already has been shown to be at least as sensitive and accurate as ultrasound. It can also provide noninvasive images of the brain vasculature that cannot be obtained with ultrasound or other techniques. For a more exhaustive discussion of the signal characteristics of flow and MRA, see Chapter 14.

VASCULAR IMAGING

In many patients, the etiology of an ischemic stroke is arterial atherosclerosis and its variable manifestations (Fig. 15.10). Symptoms may be the result of stenotic, occlusive, or ulcerative atherosclerotic plaques. The symptoms are determined by a large number of factors, including the adequacy of intracranial collaterals and the rate of progression of the stenosis or occlusion. Patients may be asymptomatic or present with symptoms of TIA, RIND, or completed infarct. Patients with ulcerated atherosclerotic plaques may present with amaurosis fugax (Figs. 15.11, 15.12). Regardless of the particular clinical presentation, after the appropriate initial noninvasive workup, angiography remains the diagnostic procedure of choice when operative intervention is to be considered. The purpose of angiography is diagnostic when the presenting symptoms are confusing and not clearly related to primary vascular disease. Arch and selective carotid angiography supply diagnostic confirmation and preoperative roadmapping for patients with clear-cut

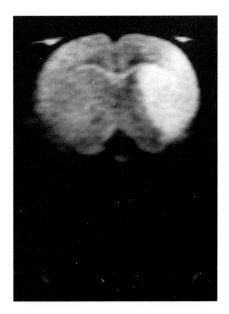

FIGURE 15.9 → Diffusion MRI in a rat model, 30 minutes after carotid occlusion. Area of infarct is hyperintense.

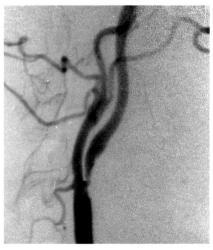

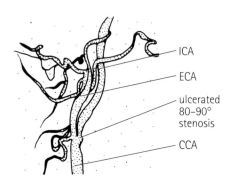

FIGURE 15.10 → Carotid stenosis. Lateral view of left common carotid digital arteriogram. There is a high grade, 80–90% stenosis at the origin of the left internal cartoid artery (ICA). The severity of this lesion could be appreciated only on the lateral projection. (CCA=common carotid artery)

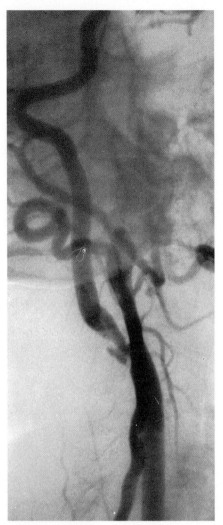

FIGURE 15.11 → Ulcerated carotid stenosis. In this oblique view of an arch aortogram, a large collection of contrast projects into the atheromatous plaque at the origin of the right ICA. (VA=vertebral artery)

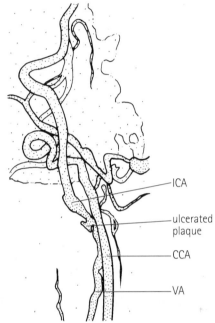

ICA

ulcerated plaque

CCA

VA

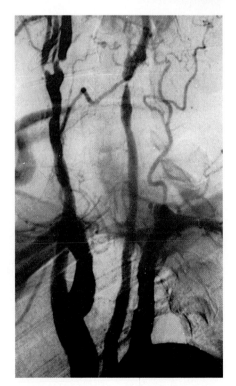

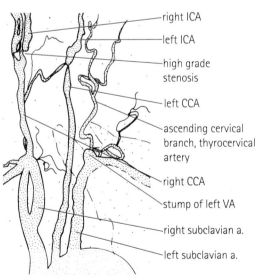

right ICA

left ICA

high grade stenosis

left CCA

ascending cervical branch, thyrocervical artery

right CCA

stump of left VA

right subclavian a.

left subclavian a.

FIGURE 15.12 → Multiple vascular lesions. Arch aortogram, left anterior oblique (LAO) projection, shows diffuse vascular disease, including occlusion of both VAs and very high grade stenoses of both proximal ICAs. Multiple views (not shown) confirmed the vertebral occlusions, with the distal VAs filling from thyrocervical collaterals.

symptoms whose noninvasive studies strongly suggest a significant carotid stenosis. Duplex ultrasound is currently the modality of choice as a noninvasive screening procedure, but in the near future, MRA will probably supplement both ultrasound and invasive angiography in many, if not most, patients.

The advent of intraarterial digital arteriography has provided complete studies of the arch, carotid, and vertebral arteries (VAs) with much smaller amounts of contrast (typically about 90–100cc of dilute contrast—less than the usual dose used for an intravenous pyelogram). The study can be obtained with smaller catheters, yet yield a more complete examination when compared to previous examinations that used full strength contrast and standard film screen combinations. Although angiography is invasive, its rate of serious complication (stroke, major hemorrhage) is less than 1%. A complete evaluation includes views of the aortic arch to identify the origins of the great vessels and an examination of both carotid arteries, including visualization of the intracranial vasculature. In patients with posterior fossa symptoms or subclavian steal syndrome, injections of contrast to the subclavian arteries may be necessary. Selective vertebral catheterization for atherosclerotic disease is usually unnecessary. The importance of a complete angiographic evaluation is shown in Figures 15.13 and 15.14. Cervical carotid examination alone would have missed the significant carotid siphon lesion exhibited in Figure 15.13. Similarly, the significant carotid siphon lesion in Figure 15.14 would have been missed if the intracranial vessels had not be evaluated; the result would have been an inappropriate carotid endarterectomy. The surgical management of both these patients was significantly altered by a complete radiographic evaluation.

At least two views of the carotid bifurcation are necessary to exclude asymmetric plaques and to

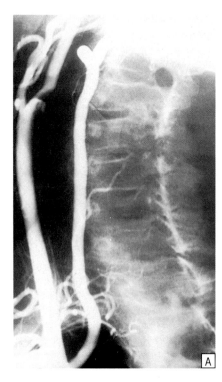

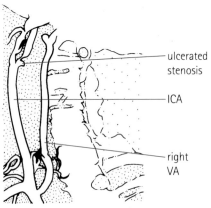

ulcerated stenosis

ICA

right VA

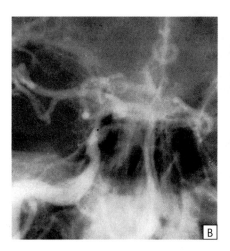

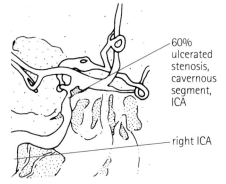

60% ulcerated stenosis, cavernous segment, ICA

right ICA

FIGURE 15.13 → Serial carotid stenoses. **A,** Right brachial arteriogram (LAO projection) demonstrates a highly significant ulcerated stenosis of the proximal ICA in a patient presenting with right hemispheric transient ischemic attacks (TIAs). **B,** Right brachial arteriogram, anteroposterior (AP) intracranial study shows a second significant carotid stenosis.

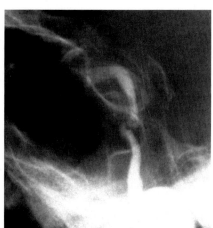

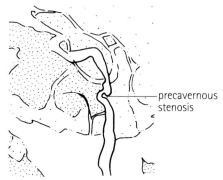

precavernous stenosis

FIGURE 15.14 → Cavernous carotid stenosis. Lateral view, left carotid arteriogram demonstrates a high grade stenosis of the ICA in its precavernous portion. The cervical portion of the ICA (not shown) was normal.

demonstrate subtle ulcerations. In general, a 50% or greater linear stenosis of the carotid artery is considered significant—a 50% linear stenosis is equivalent to a 75% reduction in cross-sectional diameter. Other angiographic factors of importance are the length of the lesion, the presence or absence of ulceration, and the presence of other stenoses. Atheromatous ulcerations may be subtle or large, and require high resolution angiography with multiple views.

While atherosclerosis is responsible for the large majority of patients with ischemic symptoms, angiography occasionally reveals some surprises (Fig. 15.15). Dissection of the carotid artery can occur following cervical trauma, but often is spontaneous, usually in the young to middle age groups, and may be bilateral. It is sometimes associated with fibromuscular dysplasia (Fig. 15.16). The dissection usually ends at the point where the carotid artery enters into the skull base, although it can extend intracranially. The lesions, which can be treated with anticoagulation therapy, often regress with very little residual angiographic deformity. The angiographic finding is typically a long, tapered ICA that begins to narrow at or above the corner carotid bifurcation. The luminal narrowing extends to the base of the skull, sometimes continuing to the carotid siphon. In view of occasional vertebral involvement, complete cerebrovascular angiogrphy is recommended.

Atherosclerotic or posttraumatic aneurysms may be a source of emboli. A palpable mass may be clinically obvious; the role of angiography is to demonstrate the aneurysm's proximal and distal extent, the anatomy of the carotid artery distal to the aneurysm, and the status of the remaining cerebral vessels prior to definitive treatment. Ischemic symptoms may also arise from tumor encasement of the

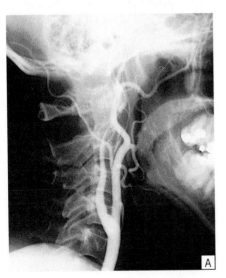
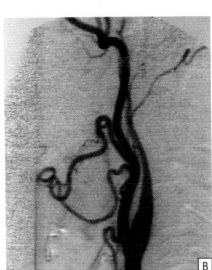
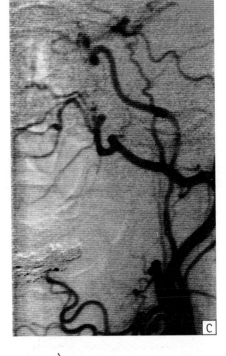
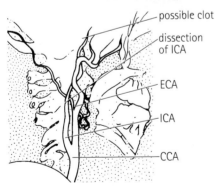
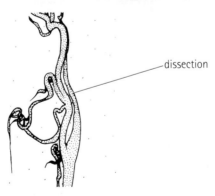

FIGURE 15.15 → Carotid dissection. A, Lateral view of left common carotid arteriogram. The origin of the ICA is normal; tapered narrowing begins at the level of C-3 and progresses to virtual occlusion at the level of the odontoid, with probable clot just above this level. Later films showed a normal ICA above the base of the skull. B, Left carotid arteriogram, lateral view (different patient). The ICA tapers above the carotid bulb. C, Left carotid arteriogram, LAO view (same patient as B). The carotid is narrowed in its cervical portion and resumes a more normal caliber as it enters the skull base. Additional views showed totally normal intracranial circulation. (ECA=external carotid artery)

cervical portion of the common carotid artery (CCA) or ICA, typically in patients with malignancies of the upper airway, mouth, and pharynx. The major risk to these patients, however, is hemorrhage.

The intracranial vascular causes of ischemic strokes include atherosclerosis, vasculitis, meningitis, tumor encasement, emboli, intracranial arteriovenous malformations with steal phenomenon, subclavian steal, moyamoya, and venous occlusive disease. Diagnostic angiography may suggest vasculitis when the typical changes of irregular luminal walls or beading with alternating areas of ectasia and stenosis, or even occlusion, are seen (Fig. 15.17). From a strictly angiographic point of view, the changes of the vas-

culitis may sometimes be difficult to distinguish from intracranial atherosclerotic disease, although the clinical presentations are usually much different. Bacterial or fungal meningitis may be associated with arterial narrowing, particularly in the arteries of the basal cisterns after fungal or tuberculous meningitis (Fig. 15.18). Moyamoya ("puff of smoke") syndrome derives its name from the hazy appearance of numerous, small, collateral lenticulostriate arteries (Fig. 15.19). Both ICAs may be occluded in their supraclinoid portion. The posterior circulation may also be involved. Patients may present with either ischemic symptoms or SAH, presumably from one of the multiple, tortuous, basal collaterals.

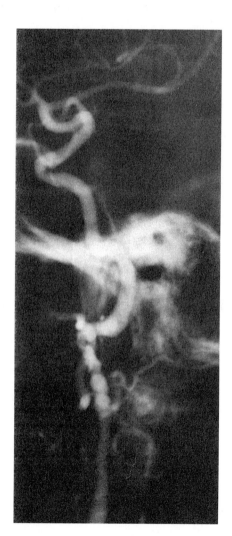

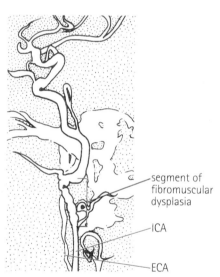

FIGURE 15.16 → Fibromuscular dysplasia. Lateral view, right carotid arteriogram shows typical "string of beads" appearance. Patient also had similar changes in both renal arteries. There was no dissection in this patient.

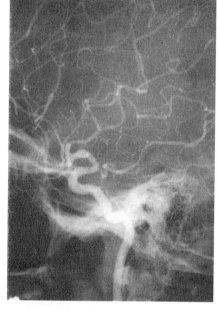

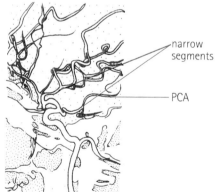

FIGURE 15.17 → Lupus vasculitis. In this lateral view, right ICA arteriogram, careful inspection reveals multiple areas of cortical arterial narrowing in the anterior MCAs and PCAs. There also are some areas of ectasia; similar changes were noted on the left. The patient was known to have lupus and also had multiple small cerebral infarcts.

Intracranial embolic disease is not often studied angiographically. The angiographic finding is an abrupt occlusion of an intracranial vessel or vessels by a small intraluminal filling defect (Fig. 15.20). Often, however, the angiogram is done days later, after the embolus has lysed and the specific occluding lesion is not demonstrated angiographically.

"Steal" phenomenon describes a clinical syndrome of ischemic symptoms produced by redirection of flow from normal brain tissue to any area of increased demand. In the central nervous system, this situation occurs most frequently in relation to the sub-

clavian steal syndrome, where blood flow is diverted in a retrograde manner down the vertebral artery (VA) ipsilateral to a proximal subclavian stenosis, providing collateral circulation to the ipsilateral arm. This is easily demonstrated angiographically. Interestingly, patients with subclavian stenosis have been treated with balloon angioplasty without the complications of emboli to the posterior fossa and with good clinical result. A "steal" syndrome may also occur in areas in the brain that are adjacent to an arteriovenous malformation (AVM), but the clinical findings are usually dominated by the AVM's symptoms.

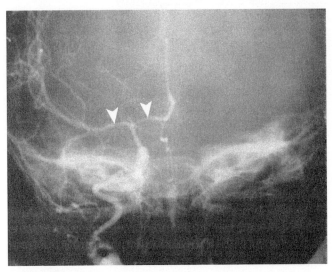

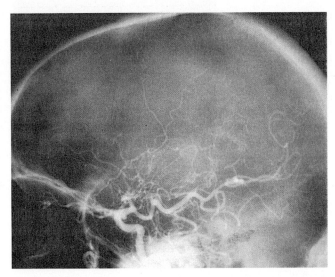

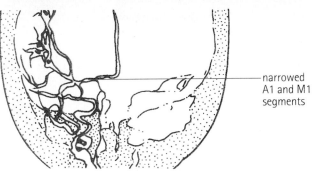

narrowed A1 and M1 segments

middle meningeal artery

"moyamoya" blush basal ganglia aa. collaterals

intact PCA

OA

ICA

FIGURE 15.18 → Tuberculous meningitis. AP view left carotid arteriogram shows narrowed A1 and M1 segments at the anterior and middle cerebral arteries (arrows). Child had proven tuberculous meningitis. (Courtesy of Dr. Milton Weiner, Worcester, Massachusetts)

FIGURE 15.19→ Moyamoya. Left carotid arteriogram, lateral view, shows the ICA is occluded. Numerous lenticuloctriate collaterals are exhibited clearly, in part due to the absence of overlying middle cerebral vessels on this early phase film. The right ICA study showed similar findings. Patient presented with a subarachnoid hemorrhage (SAH) and had a prior history of symptoms that resembled TIAs. (OA=ophthalmic artery)

STROKE SUBTYPES AND IMAGING TECHNIQUES

INTRACEREBRAL HEMORRHAGE

CT and MRI

The most common causes of IH are preexistent hypertension, intracranial aneurysms, arteriovenous malformations (AVMs), infarctions (both venous and embolic) and amyloid angiography. Tumors (especially metastatic melanoma, lung, and hypernephroma), vas-culitides, and moyamoya are less common causes. In all cases, CT without contrast remains the first important diagnostic step after the initial clinical evaluation. MRI is certainly capable of detecting intraparenchymal hemorrhage, but is less accurate in the detection of SAH and is generally less available than CT.

Hypertensive hemorrhages occur most frequently in the basal ganglia, less commonly in the temporal lobe, pons, and cerebellar hemispheres (Fig. 15.21). On CT, there is high density from the acute hemorrhage, with variable mass effect on the

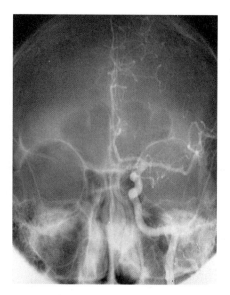

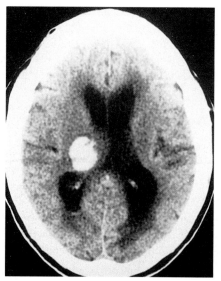

FIGURE 15.21 → Hypertensive bleed in the right thalamus is seen on an axial unenhanced CT.

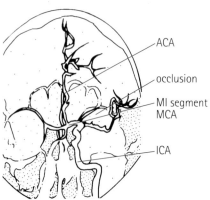

ACA

occlusion

MI segment MCA

ICA

FIGURE 15.20 → Embolic occlusion of the right MCA branch. The posterior division of the right MCA in this carotid arteriogram, AP view, is abruptly occluded. An actual intraluminal thrombus is not seen, but the lack of atherosclerotic change elsewhere (on this film and on all other series) makes an embolic etiology very likely. The patient had mitral valve disease and atrial fibrillation.

third ventricle and ipsilateral lateral ventricle. Hemorrhages involving the thalamus often rupture into the ventricular system. CT shows blood in the third or lateral ventricle (Fig. 15.22). Within a few days, the density of the hematoma decreases. Follow-up scanning will eventually show a water density lesion in the area of the resorbed hemorrhage. The MRI findings of IH are complex and depend on the hematoma's age and size (Fig. 15.23). Briefly, the signal changes of IH are indicated in Figure 15.24 and summarized in Figure 15.25. Changes in signal inten-

sity reflect biochemical events that occur with the evolution of the hematoma and help to pinpoint its age. While CT remains the most important initial imaging modality, MRI can be very helpful in the follow-up examination of hemorrhage patients who have had an event of uncertain etiology sometime previously. In general, MRI will detect parenchymal hemorrhage with greater sensitivity and for a much longer period of time than will CT. MRI is particularly sensitive for detecting small petechial hemorrhages that occur in infarcts. Generally, however, these tiny hemorrhages,

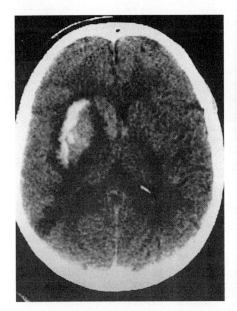

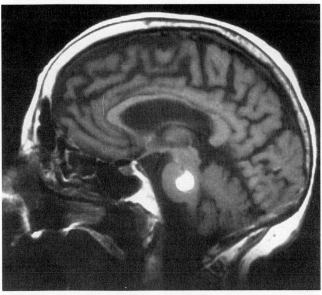

FIGURE 15.23 → Pontine hemorrhage. The hemorrhage in the middle of the pons is fairly acute, with increased signal intensity of acute blood on sagittal T1-weighted MRI scan. The patient was hypertensive.

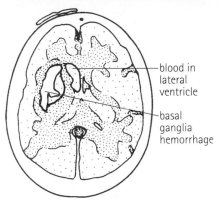

FIGURE 15.22 → Intraventricular rupture. Axial enhanced CT shows a hypertensive hemorrhage originating in the right globus pallidus, putamen, and caudate, with rupture into the right lateral ventricle. CT a few days later showed a blood/CSF level in both lateral ventricles.

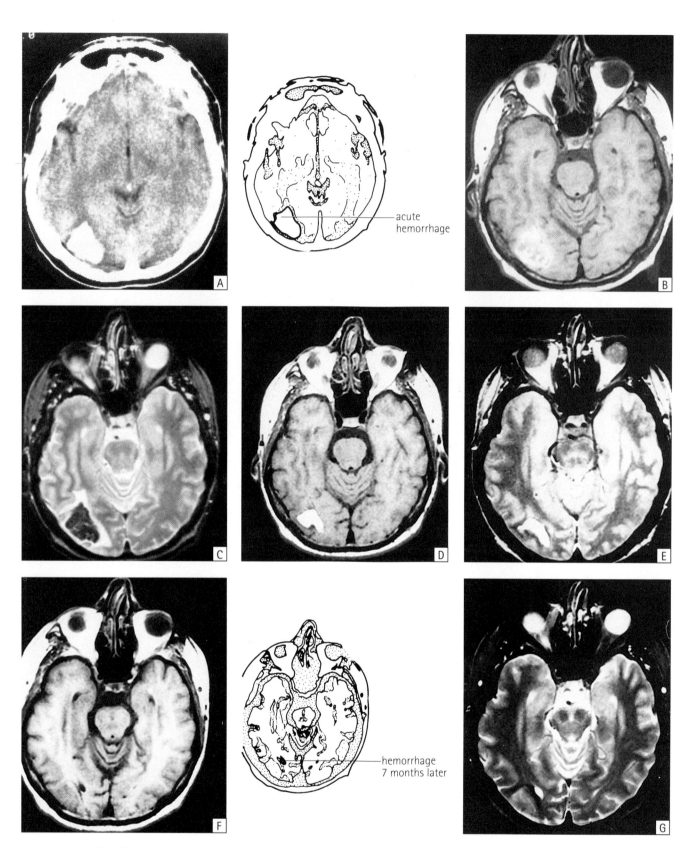

FIGURE 15.24 → Evolution of hemorrhage on MRI. Axial CT at time of ictus **(A)** shows high density acute hemorrhage on right. Axial MRI with T1- **(B)** and T2-weighting **(C)** at same level as CT, 3 days later. Bright on T1, dark on T2 with some hyperintense surrounding edema, these findings correspond to an acute intracerebral hemorrhage (IH). MRI with T1- **(D)** and T2-weighting **(E)** 4 weeks later. Hyperintensity on both T1 and T2 are consistent with subacute to chronic bleed. Edema has resolved and the lesion is smaller. MRI 7 months later, T1- **(F)** and T2-weighted **(G)** at same level. Lesion is much smaller, with a low signal on T1. Increased signal on T2 may simply represent fluid in a small area of necrosis.

seen in both embolic and thrombotic infarcts, are not of any clinical significance. Large hemorrhagic infarcts may develop within embolic infarcts or in patients with large thrombotic infarcts, particularly after anticoagulation. Such larger acute hemorrhagic infarcts are equally well demonstrated by CT or MRI (Figs. 15.26, 15.27).

Venous infarcts are typically hemorrhagic, with the area of hemorrhage usually occurring near the cortical medullary junction. Hemorrhagic changes

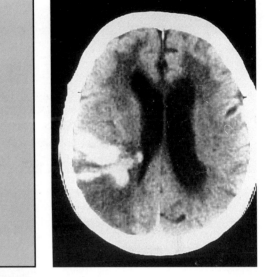

FIGURE 15.25 → EVOLUTION OF SIGNAL CHANGES OF BLOOD ON SPIN-ECHO HIGH FIELD STRENGTH MRI

	T1-WEIGHTED	T2-WEIGHTED
Acute (1–3 days)	Hypo- to isointense	Hypointense
Subacute (3–14 days)	Hyperintense	Hypo- to becoming hyperintense
Chronic (greater than 1 month)	Hyperintense, becoming hypointense	Become markedly hypointense from the periphery

Intensity of signal is in relation to brain parenchyma.

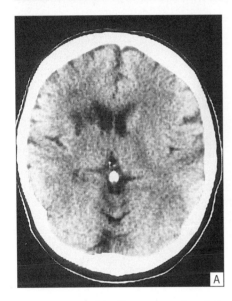

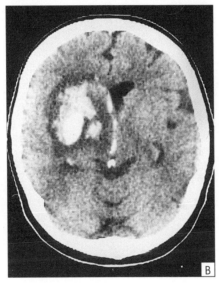

FIGURE 15.26 → Hemorrhage into infarct. **A,** An area of diminished density within the head of the caudate nucleus, adjacent white matter, as well as the anterior putamen and globus pallidus can be seen on this initial unenhanced CT. **B,** Unenhanced CT 9 days later. The patient deteriorated after anticoagulation. High-density, acute blood is is shown outlining the infarct.

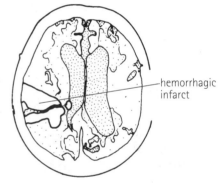

hemorrhagic infarct

FIGURE 15.27 → Hemorrhagic infarct. Axial CT at the level of the lateral ventricles exhibits high-density blood from an acute hemorrhage, which is noted primarily in the cortex of the right parietal lobe. Other sections showed blood in the vascular territory of the posterior division of the right MCA. The infarct was secondary to embolus from the left ventricle following myocardial infarction.

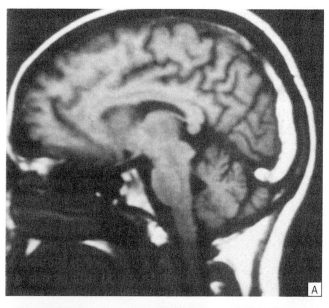

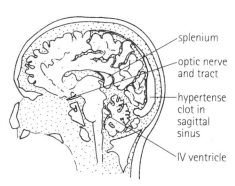

splenium

optic nerve
and tract

hypertense
clot in
sagittal
sinus

IV ventricle

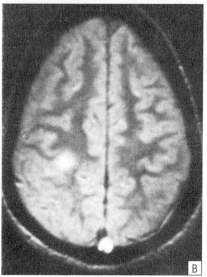

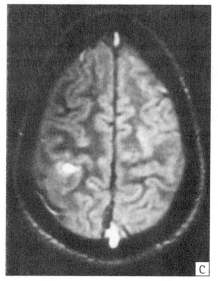

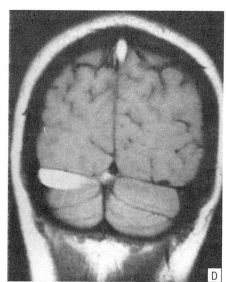

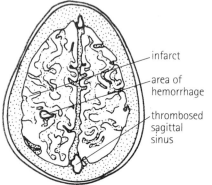

infarct

area of
hemorrhage

thrombosed
sagittal
sinus

FIGURE 15.28 → Sagittal sinus
thrombosis. **A,** Hyperintense signal on
sagittal T1 MRI is noted from the thrombus within the superior sagittal sinus.
Normally, the sagittal sinus has low signal on this sequence due to blood flow.
B,C: Axial proton density MRI demonstrates the cortical infarction (secondary
to venous thrombosis) with hypertense
signal due to blood within the infarct.
D, Coronal T1 MRI. The thrombosus
(hyperintense) extends into the lateral
sinus. Other images showed extension
into the jugular vein.

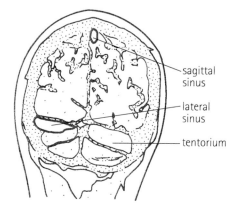

sagittal
sinus

lateral
sinus

tentorium

can be detected by MRI (Fig. 15.28), which has the additional advantage of being able to directly demonstrate the thrombosis of a cortical vein and possibly other dural sinus thromboses. In fact, a patient with venous infarct is probably best studied with MRI and MRA, as these technologies are quite sensitive in evaluating the presence or absence of venous flow. Diagnosing cortical vein thrombosis may be quite difficult angiographically and may sometimes be presumed only by the absence of filling of the cortical veins (Fig. 15.29).

ANEURYSMS

CT, MRI, and MRA

Patients with symptomatic intracranial aneurysms usually present with SAH, although occasionally the presenting symptom is secondary to mass effect, as in a posterior communicating artery aneurysm leading to a third nerve palsy. CT without contrast is highly reliable for diagnosing SAH and is probably as accurate as lumbar puncture (Fig. 15.30). On CT, the CSF space is obscured by high density or isodense blood. Sometimes a focal collection indicates the exact site of the bleed. It is very important that the patient suspected of SAH be scanned without intravenous contrast; the detection of subarachnoid blood may be very difficult after contrast enhancement. CT may also demonstrate the aneurysm itself but, in general, angiography is required for diagnosis and for preparing surgical or endovascular therapy. Special MRI and MRA techniques may be able to detect aneurysms as small as 2 or 3 mm, but their reliability has not been fully tested. MRA's usefulness in replacing conventional

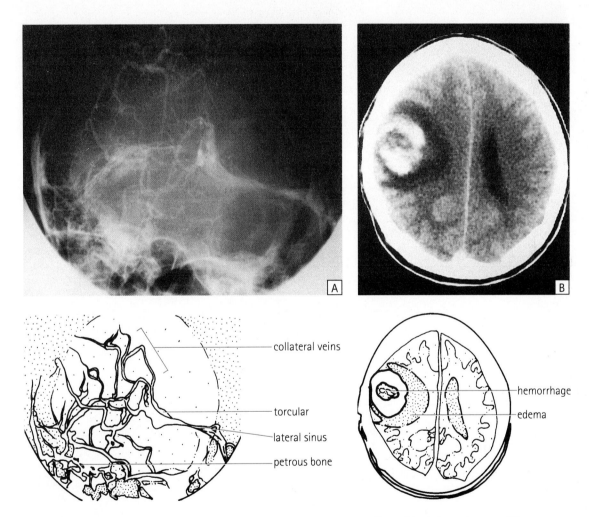

FIGURE 15.29 → Sagittal sinus thrombosis with venous infarct. **A,** The sagittal sinus does not fill. Numerous small-to-medium-sized cortical veins act as collaterals to the lateral dural sinus on this oblique, axial projection carotid arteriogram, venous phase. **B,** Axial unenhanced CT shows central high-density blood with surrounding edema, representing the venous infarct secondary to sagittal sinus thrombosis.

angiography awaits more experience, confidence, and some further technical improvements (Figs. 15.31, 15.32). In the near future, MRA will probably supplant conventional angiography in the diagnosis and preoperative treatment planning for patients with intracranial aneurysms. MRA is used as a screening procedure in high risk patients, in patients for whom angiographic evaluation could not be completed, and as a diagnostic tool in patients with SAH who may undergo further invasive or surgical procedures.

Angiography

Conventional angiography, properly performed, can reliably show an aneurysm (Fig. 15.33). Complete evaluation of the intracranial vessels requires selective carotid and vertebral studies with views in multiple

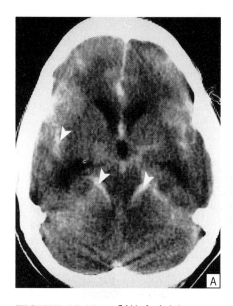 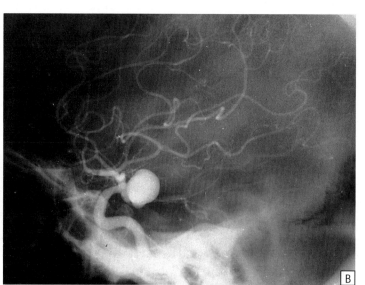

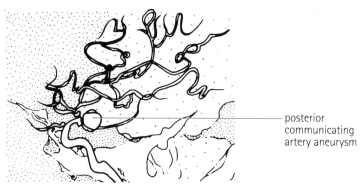

FIGURE 15.30 → SAH. **A,** Axial unenhanced CT demonstrates high-density blood throughout the subarachnoid spaces (arrows). **B,** Left carotid aneurysm as seen on internal carotid arteriogram. (An aneurysm this large would have been easily identified on MRA.)

posterior communicating artery aneurysm

projections. Angiography should demonstrate the anatomy of the aneurysm, including the presence of a neck, the relation of the parent vessel to the aneurysm, the presence or absence of spasm, and/or mass effect (Figs. 15.34, 15.35). Twenty-five percent of patients with SAH and aneurysm will have more than one aneurysm, so a complete evaluation of the intracranial vasculature is necessary. In patients with multiple aneurysms, the largest aneurysm is usually the site of aneurysm rupture, although other features such as irregularity and local spasm can help identify the responsible aneurysm (see Fig. 15.35).

While neurosurgery has traditionally been the treatment of choice for aneurysms, selected cases may be referred for endovascular therapy. Detachable balloons, coils, or other occluding material are then

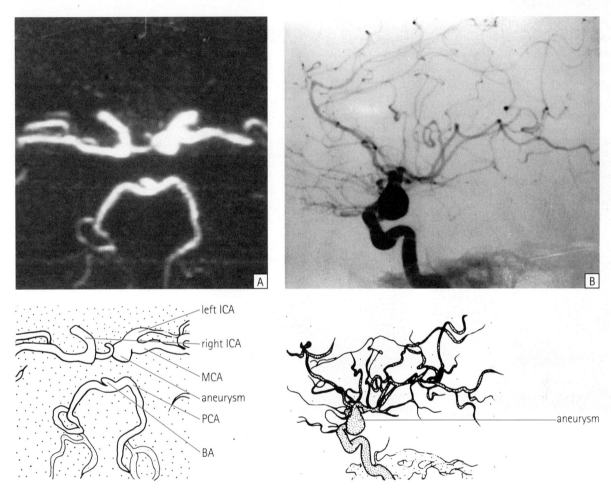

FIGURE 15.31 → Posterior communicating aneurysm. **A,** Axial projection MRA shows an abnormal flow signal, which projects from the distal left ICA at the origin of the posterior communicating artery. (The BA is projected end-on; other view showed no basilar aneurysm.) **B,** Left carotid arteriogram, lateral view, confirms the MRA findings.

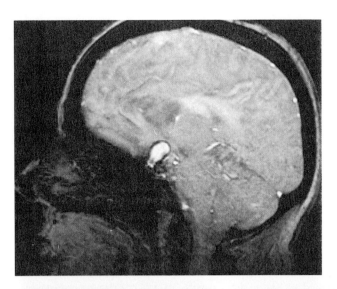

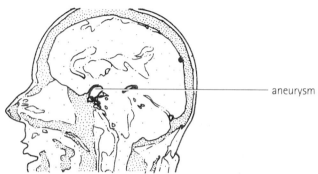

FIGURE 15.32 → Sagittal gradient-recalled MRI. In this sequence (GRASS), flowing blood appears bright (note small cortical veins). The patent aneurysm of the ICA is therefore outlined. In spin-echo pulse sequence for MRI, flowing blood usually appears dark.

aneurysm

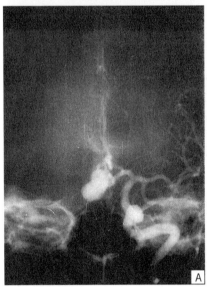

A

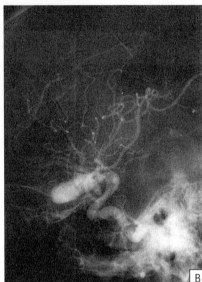

B

FIGURE 15.33 → Anterior communicating artery aneurysm. The left internal carotid arteriogram shows a large bilobed aneurysm. **A,** AP view. **B,** Lateral view.

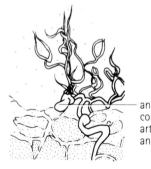

anterior communicating artery aneurysm

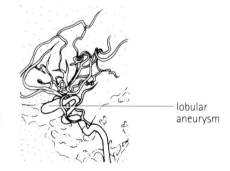

lobular aneurysm

used to occlude the aneurysm. Endovascular therapy is generally performed on patients who are ineligible for intracranial surgery, for whom surgery was unsuccessful, or for whom the preoperative angiogram suggests an aneurysm that is inaccessible to surgical approach.

ARTERIOVENOUS MALFORMATIONS

CT, MRI, and MRA

Arteriovenous malformations may announce their presence by SAH, but the initial symptoms, particularly in the younger population, may be seizures or may be related to mass effect. Rarely, patients present with ischemic symptoms secondary to steal phenomenon from the arterial venous shunting. In most patients with hemorrhage, CT is the first diagnostic procedure; it will show either SAH or intracranial hematoma. The dilated draining veins and feeding arteries, which may be seen even on C− scans, become obvious on C+ scans (Fig. 15.36). MRI and MRA are much more likely to be used diagnostically than CT in evaluating an AVM because of their sensitivity to flow (Fig. 15.37). Whatever the imaging modality, its purpose is to identify the AVM, its location, its relation to other critical structures, as well as

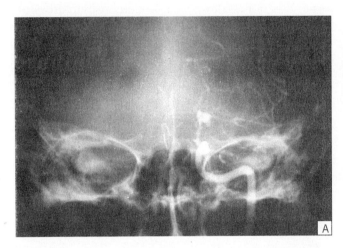

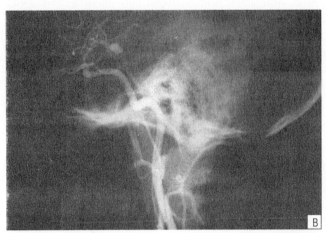

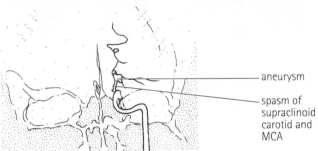

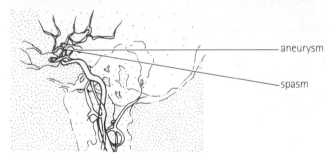

FIGURE 15.34 → Internal carotid aneurysm. A left internal carotid arteriogram demonstrates an irregular aneurysm with marked spasm of the adjacent supraclinoid carotid as well as the A1 and M1 segments. A, AP view. B, Lateral view.

the location and size of the feeding and draining blood vessels. Whether MRA will completely replace conventional diagnostic angiography is not clear at this time. Currently, conventional angiography is still required to provide the necessary preoperative details for neurosurgical or endovascular treatment.

AMYLOID ANGIOPATHY

CT and MRI

Intraparenchymal cortical hemorrhages in the middle-aged and older population are often caused by amyloid angiopathy. The CT (or MR) findings are those of a largely cortical hematoma, often in the parietal lobe. These superficial hemorrhages can occur in any lobe but spare white matter, deep gray matter, and the brainstem. Contrast scans show no contrast enhancement. The diagnosis is often presumptive if hypertension, tumor enhancement, or abnormal blood vessels are absent. MRI shows the changes of hemorrhage and

will also show no enhancement with gadolinium, nor any abnormal vascular supply. In general, patients with this type of hemorrhage are better evaluated with MRI because it can rule out any other lesions, date the abnormality, and evaluate for the presence or absence of abnormal blood vessels.

HEMORRHAGE INTO TUMORS

CT and MRI

Metastatic or primary intracranial tumors may present as IH. Usually, these patients have a known primary lesion, and the presence of other metastatic lesions on imaging studies of the brain or elsewhere is diagnostic. It is not at all unusual to demonstrate areas of hemorrhage within a malignant glioma (Fig. 15.38), but the clinical findings are commonly dominated by the tumor's effects. Only rarely do tumors initially present as hemorrhagic stroke. Metastatic lesions, however, are more apt to announce themselves by

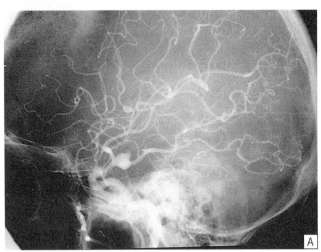

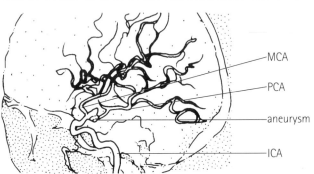

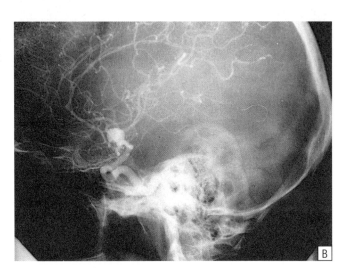

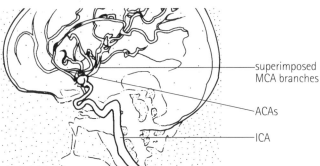

FIGURE 15.35 → Multiple aneurysms. **A,** Right carotid arteriogram, lateral view, shows a 1-cm lobular aneurysm arising from the distal ICA at the origin of the posterior communicating artery. The irregularity suggests that this aneurysm bled. The patient presented with SAH. **B,** In this left carotid arteriogram,

lateral view, a round, 1-cm aneurysm arises from the anterior communicating artery (AP view showed midline position of aneurysm). Note that both ACAs fill from the left carotid injection, a frequent normal finding.

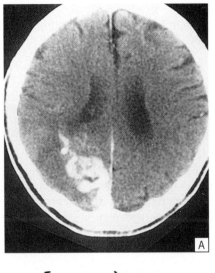

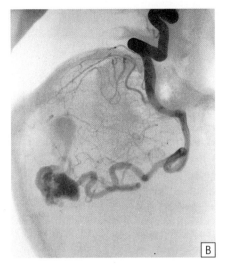

FIGURE 15.36 → AVM figure. **A,** Contrast-enhanced CT shows high density of AVM and enlarged draining vein to sagittal sinus close to the torcular. **B,** Corresponding left vertebral arteriogram. The PCA is markedly enlarged secondary to increased flow within the AVM.

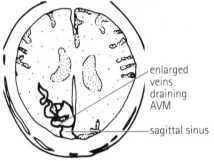

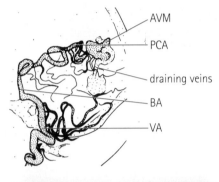

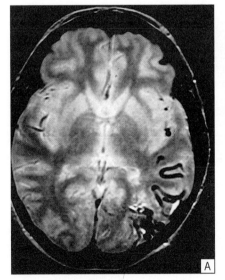

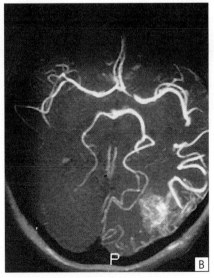

FIGURE 15.37 → AVM. **A,** Axial MRI, proton density (spin echo). **B,** Axial projection MRA (gradient echo). Both sequences demonstrate the enlarged feeding arteries and tortuous veins. Signal characteristics of flowing blood can be altered by the type of protocol. In general, spin-echo techniques show flowing blood as black. Gradient echo techniques, if properly selected, show flowing blood as bright.

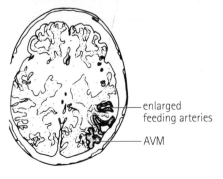

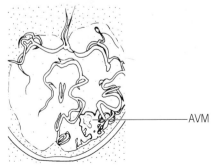

virtue of hemorrhage (Fig. 15.39). Metastatic melanoma, lung tumor, and hypernephroma are the lesions that most commonly cause intracranial bleeding. On CT, the findings are those of a dense lesion, which is often found at the cortical medullary junction but can also occur in the basal ganglia or posterior fossa. On MRI, the lesion will sometimes appear as areas of hyperintensity on T1 images and, depending on the age, hypo- or hyperintense on T2-weighting. The hyperintensity on MRI and the increased density of CT may obscure the underlying tumor, making it difficult to determine whether there is any abnormal enhancement after gadolinium (MRI) or iodinated (CT) contrast. In a few cases, it may be necessary to obtain follow-up scans in several weeks to evaluate the presence or absence of metastatic disease after the obscuring signal characteristics of the acute/subacute hemorrhage have resolved.

CONCLUSION

This chapter has highlighted the imaging findings in patients presenting with ischemic or hemorrhagic strokes. Neuroradiology is entering an exciting period where imaging of neurologic diseases will encompass both anatomic and physiologic information. The early studies on spectroscopy, diffusion, and perfusion imaging promise great advances in the understanding of stoke, its early diagnosis, and treatment.

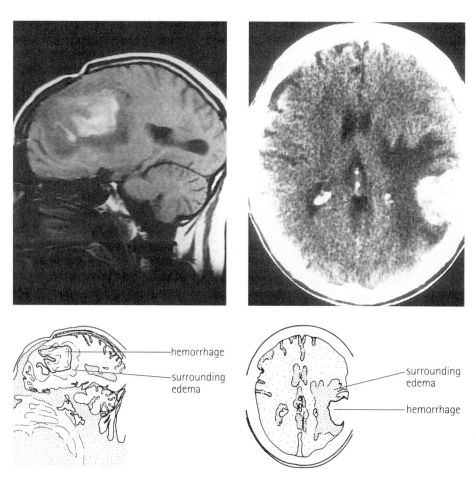

FIGURE 15.38 → Hemorrhage in frontal glioma. Hyperintensity on sagittal T1-weighted MRIs can be seen with blood, acutely and subacutely. Low-signal intensity on T1 scans is consistent with increased water content, as in surrounding edema. The patient had a known high-grade glioma and had abrupt clinical deterioration two days before this scan.

FIGURE 15.39 → Hemorrhagic metastasis. Unenhanced CT shows high-density hemorrhage in left parietal region with extensive surrounding vasogenis edema. Area of hemorrhage is not homogenous and the pattern of edema is suspicious. The patient had oat cell carcinoma.

REFERENCES

Baker LL, Kucharczyk J, Sevick RJ, et al. Recent advances in MR imaging/spectroscopy of cerebral ischemia. *Am J Roentgenol.* 1991; 156:1133-1143.

Bryan RN. Imaging of acute stroke. *Radiology.* 1990; 177:615–616.

Bryan RN, Whitlow WD, Levy LM. Cerebral infarction and ischemic disease. In: Atlas SW (ed). *Magnetic Resonance Imaging of the Brain and Spine.* New York: Raven Press. 1991; pp 411–438.

Edelman RR, Mattle HP, Atkinson DJ, Hoogewoud HM. MR angiography. *Am J Roentgenol.* 1990; 159:937–946.

Elster AD. MR contrast enhancement in brainstem and deep cerebral infarction. *Am J Roentgenol.* 1992; 158:173–178.

Haughton VM. Vascular diseases. In: Williams AL, Haughton VM (eds). *Cranial Computed Tomography.* New York: C.V. Mosby. 1985; 88–147.

Houser OW, Mokri B, Sundt TM, et al. Spontaneous cervical cephalic dissection and its residuum: angiographic spectrum. *ANJR.* 1984; 5:27–34.

Motarjeme A, Keifer JW, Zuska AJ, Nabawi P. Percutaneous transluminal angioplasty for treatment of subclavian steal. *Radiology.* 1985; 155:611–613.

Thulbern KR, Atlas SW. Intracranial hemorrhage. In: Atlas SW (ed). *Magnetic Resonance Imaging of the Brain and Spine.* New York: Raven Press. 1991; pp 175–222.

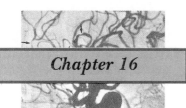

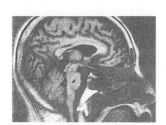

Chapter 16

MARC FISHER

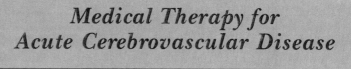

Medical Therapy for Acute Cerebrovascular Disease

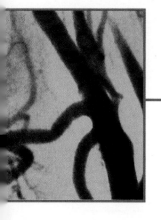

ISCHEMIC STROKE PREVENTION

The prolonged decline of ischemic stroke incidence, which may now be leveling off, can be related to many developments, including the identification of risk factors. Much of the reduction in incidence is, in fact, directly related to ameliorating risk (Fig. 16.1). Therapy for risk factors such as hypertension, cigarette smoking, hyperlipidemia, certain cardiac disorders, and prior transient ischemic attack (TIA) helps reduce subsequent stroke incidence. Lowering elevated blood pressure with various pharmacologic mechanisms, for instance, will minimize the subsequent stroke risk and related mortality. The cessation of cigarette smoking also reduces risk. Elevated levels of total and LDL cholesterol appear to be independent stroke risk factors, but although reducing them lowers cardiovascular disease incidence and mortality, no such relationship with ischemic stroke has been proven. As previously outlined, a variety of cardiac disorders and TIA are also associated with an increased risk for ischemic stroke. The identification of at-risk patients has generated intervention trials with platelet inhibitors and anticoagulants, which have demonstrated significant reductions in subsequent stroke risk.

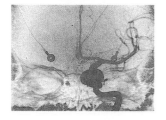

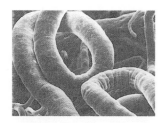

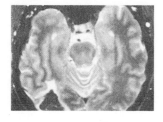

Many trials have evaluated the effects of aspirin on stroke incidence in patients who have had a TIA or minor stroke (Fig. 16.2). The consensus is that aspirin reduces stroke risk by approximately 25% to 30% over a wide dose range (40–1200 mg/d). Lower doses appear to be associated with fewer side effects, especially in the gastrointestinal system. Aspirin, therefore, can be recommended as a prevention for patients with TIA or minor stroke if they are not candidates for carotid endarterectomy. The dose remains unsettled, but 325 mg/d is standard. Aspirin prophylaxis has also been studied in patients with atrial fibrillation (AF), to reduce the risk of first stroke. Conflicting results have been reported, but 325 mg/d may be effective. Another medication with platelet inhibitory effects, ticlopidine, also reduces subsequent stroke risk in TIA and stroke patients. Ticlopidine seems to be more effective than aspirin, but cost and side effects such as leukopenia and gastrointestinal disturbances may limit use. Dipyridamole has not been shown to be effective in stroke prevention.

Intravenous and oral anticoagulants have been evaluated in many clinical conditions associated with an increased stroke risk. They have not been

FIGURE 16.1 → RISK FACTORS FOR STROKE: TREATMENT EFFECTIVE OR POSSIBLY EFFECTIVE

- Hypertension
- Cigarette smoking
- Cardiac source: AF, valvular disease
- Prior TIA or stroke
- Hyperlipidemia
- Excessive alcohol consumption

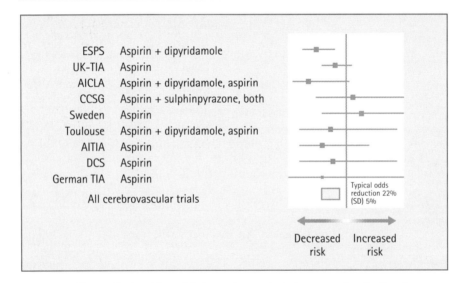

FIGURE 16.2 → Trials with aspirin have demonstrated an overall reduction in subsequent stroke risk of 22%. (Adapted with permission, from Norris JW, Hachinski VC, 1991)

proven to be effective therapies for reducing stroke risk after TIA or minor stroke from atherothrombotic causes. This deficiency may in part be related to inadequate therapeutic trials. Anticoagulants are empirically used in TIA patients who continue to have episodes despite aspirin therapy or who initially present with multiple events. Oral anticoagulation reduces primary stroke risk in patients with AF and can be recommended for all such patients who do not have a contraindication (Fig. 16.3). There is no definitive proof of efficacy for oral anticoagulants to prevent secondary stroke in AF patients, but ongoing studies will provide an answer shortly. Anticoagulants may also reduce the high risk of stroke in patients who have suffered an anterior wall, transmural myocardial infarction. Patients with mechanical prosthetic cardiac valves are also at high risk for stroke; long-term oral anticoagulation is often recommended. Oral anticoagulation may also be indicated for a variety of other cardiac conditions associated with an enhanced stroke risk.

Intravenous (IV) anticoagulation with heparin is used by some clinicians acutely after atherothrombotic stroke onset (Fig. 16.4), especially if the neuro-

FIGURE 16.3 → EFFECTS OF ORAL ANTICOAGULANTS ON ATRIAL FIBRILLATION

	DANISH TRIAL	AMERICAN TRIAL	BOSTON TRIAL	AGGREGATE
PLACEBO GROUP				
Patient years	413	244	435	1092
Number of strokes	19	17	13	49
Percent strokes				
per year	4.6	7.0	3.0	4.5
TREATMENT GROUP				
Treatment years	105	168	369	642
Strokes	1	2	2	5
Percent strokes				
per year	1.0	1.2	0.5	0.8

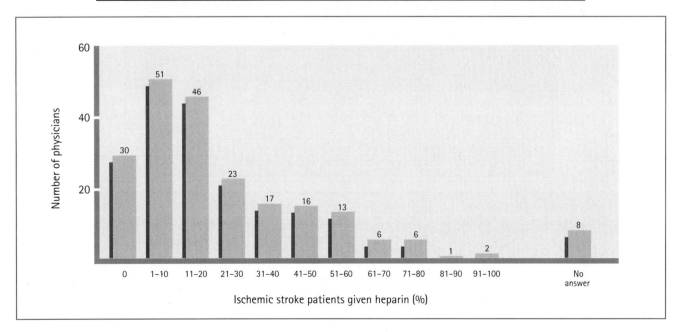

FIGURE 16.4 → Despite the lack of proven efficacy, heparin is frequently used in ischemic stroke patients. (Reproduced with permission of Edgell Communications, Inc.)

logic deficits are incomplete. The value of heparin in this setting remains uncertain. Patients with cardioembolic stroke frequently receive IV heparin for 5 to 7 days before oral anticoagulation is initiated to reduce the early risk of stroke recurrence. This practice may be unnecessary if the early risk approximates 3% to 5% over the first two weeks after stroke onset, as compared to previous estimates of 10% to 12%. Heparin therapy is also widely employed for patients with progressing or evolving stroke, but proof of efficacy is unavailable. Fibrinolytic therapy may be more appropriate for progressing stroke patients; its efficacy and safety, however, require clinical investigation.

ACUTE STROKE THERAPY

STANDARD INTERVENTION
Much of the decline in acute ischemic stroke mortality can be ascribed to improved medical and nursing management, as no specific therapy for the ischemic neurologic injury exists. The evaluation and treatment of acute ischemic stroke patients probably can be performed most easily and effectively in a dedicated stroke care unit (SCU), headed by an expertly trained management team of physicians, nurses, rehabilitation specialists, and social workers. The establishment of SCUs will become more vital as acute stroke care evolves to rapid intervention within hours of onset. Stroke care should eventually emulate the standards presently employed for acute myocardial infarction in coronary care units.

A variety of general medical and nursing interventions are available for acute ischemic stroke patients (Fig. 16.5). Cardiovascular and respiratory support may be necessary in some patients. Blood pressure must be closely followed, but typically will decline to an acceptable range within hours after admission. Because autoregulation is impaired in ischemic cerebral tissue, unacceptably high blood pressure must be lowered carefully. A precipitous drop in blood pressure further compromises cerebral blood, and could lead to an extension of the ischemic penumbra to infarction. Intravenous fluids, which are necessary for many stroke patients during the first several days, should be kept on the low side of bodily requirements (1500–2000 mL/d). Fluid overloading might exacerbate cerebral edema. Glucose and electrolytes should be followed; if imbalances are detected, appropriate adjustments should be made. Excessive glucose levels have been associated with a poorer prognosis in animal stroke models, presumably related to enhanced lactate production. The role of elevated glucose in human stroke prognosis is less certain, but it may be wise to gently lower glucose levels that are above 200–250 mg during the acute phase of ischemic stroke.

Infections frequently complicate acute ischemic stroke. A fever above 38°C should not be ascribed to tissue destruction. Aspiration pneumonia, urinary tract infection, and septicemia are the most commonly encountered infections. Early oral feeding should not be attempted unless the patient can swallow easily.

FIGURE 16.5 → SUPPORTIVE AND GENERAL MEDICAL THERAPIES FOR ACUTE ISCHEMIC STROKE

- Blood pressure evaluation and treatment
- Cardiovascular and respiratory support
- Fluid management
- Prevention and treatment of infections
- Deep vein thrombosis prophylaxis
- Rehabilitative services

FIGURE 16.6 → EFFECTS OF DEXAMETHASONE IN ACUTE STROKE

STUDY	PATIENTS	STROKE TYPE	DEXAMETHASONE DOSE	OUTCOME
Dyken	36	Infarct	?–21 days	Worse
Patton	31	Infarct & hemorrhage	200 mg–17 days	Improved
Bauer	54	Infarct	120 mg–10 days	No effect
Norris	53	Infarct	140 mg–14 days	Worse
Norris & Hachinski	113	Infarct	480 mg–12 days	No effect
Poungvarin	93	Hemorrhage	30 mg–9 days	No effect

Instrumentation should be avoided—except when absolutely necessary—because in-dwelling urinary catheters and intravenous access lines can lead to infectious complications.

Immobilized acute stroke patients may develop deep vein thrombosis and pulmonary emboli. Early mobilization, range of motion exercises, and compression stockings are suggested. Subcutaneous heparin should be considered for patients who are likely to remain immobile for more than a few days. Rehabilitative services such as physical, occupational, and speech therapies can help appropriate patients; a rehabilitation evaluation should be performed as soon as possible. Social service evaluation for discharge planning is another important aspect of comprehensive stroke care.

CEREBRAL EDEMA

The most common neurologic cause of early mortality in acute ischemic stroke occurs secondary to massive cerebral edema, leading to herniation syndromes. Edema develops by both cytotoxic and vasogenic mechanisms, exhibiting its maximal clinical effects 48 to 72 hours after stroke onset. Effective therapy to prevent or ameliorate the consequences of cerebral edema does not yet exist. Corticosteroids, primarily dexamethasone, have been widely evaluated with conflicting results (Fig. 16.6). Elevation of glucose levels by corticosteroids might actually worsen the outcome. Newer corticosteroid derivatives without glucocorticoid effects are now being developed, and these drugs might be valuable in the future. Although osmotic diuretic agents (e.g., mannitol and glycerol) are not generally believed to be effective for ischemic cerebral edema, they may be helpful in desperate situations, especially if a surgical decompressive procedure is being considered for the near future. Hyperventilation of intubated patients may also be of limited value. Occasionally, younger patients with massive cerebral edema will benefit from a bone flap that allows external decompression. An effective safe therapy for ischemic edema remains an essential but elusive component in early stroke therapy.

POTENTIAL MEDICAL THERAPIES FOR ISCHEMIC STROKE

ENHANCED BLOOD FLOW

Quickly and safely restoring blood flow to an ischemic region might help to preserve uninfarcted tissue. Thrombolytic therapy for acute myocardial infarction has successfully reduced acute mortality in association with reperfusion of initially occluded vessels. Both exogenous, non–clot-specific thrombolytic agents such as streptokinase and urokinase, and relatively clot-specific agents such as tissue plasminogen activator (TPA) are effective. A major concern with thrombolytics is their potential for hemorrhagic side effects (Fig. 16.7), but no significant difference in cerebral hemorrhage development exists between clot-specific and nonspecific drugs when they are used for myocardial infarction.

Restoring flow to occluded cerebral vessels is an enticing goal that remains unattained despite many attempts. Early endeavors with streptokinase and urokinase were associated with substantial hemorrhagic complications and little evidence of clinical improvement. The development of clot-specific thrombolytic drugs has revived interest in thrombolytic therapy. Clot-specific thrombolytic therapy theoretically has less risk for local cerebral hemorrhagic complications than nonspecific thrombolytic therapy, because it avoids a systemic lytic state (Fig. 16.8). Intravenous infusion of TPA in animal experiments demonstrated that intracranial arteries can be rapidly

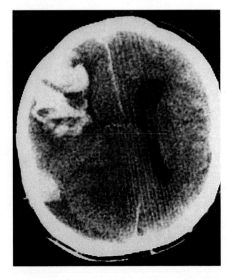

FIGURE 16.7 → CT documentation of an acute, extensive intracerebral and subdural hematoma in a patient who received TPA and heparin for the treatment of an acute myocardial infarction.

reperfused with no increased risk for intracerebral hemorrhage (Fig. 16.9). A reduction of infarct size and improved neurologic outcome has also been documented in animals that received TPA after stroke onset. Preliminary human trials with TPA include a dose-escalation safety trial that demonstrated a 4% hemorrhagic rate in 74 patients. Another study evaluated safety and angiographic efficacy in 94 patients. Parenchymatous hemorrhage was observed in 9.6% of patients, and partial or complete reperfusion was demonstrated in 35% of previously occluded arteries. The therapy was most effective in patients with distal middle cerebral artery occlusion, but was ineffective in proximal carotid artery occlusion. A Japanese study observed a 66% recanalization rate with TPA in cardioembolic stroke. Hemorrhagic complications were common, but typically not clinically significant. Efficacy trials of TPA for acute ischemic stroke are underway; a preliminary result suggests that it can produce significant clinical improvement. Thrombolytic therapy is undergoing a rapid evolution. Newer approaches, such as combined therapy with TPA and an exogenous thrombolytic drug, or more clot-specific TPA molecules, may prove to have a better therapeutic index than current therapy.

Lowering the hematocrit reduces serum viscosity, thereby increasing cerebral blood flow. A hematocrit in the range of 30% to 33% appears to maximize flow without compromising the blood's oxygen-carrying capacity (Fig. 16.10). A normal hematocrit can be reduced to this range by either isovolemic or hypervolemic hemodilution. The clinical trials that have been performed have not documented clinical benefits, in part because of delayed time to treatment. In one study, hypervolemic hemodilution was associated with a greater than 50% improvement rate, but also with an unacceptably high incidence of fatal cerebral edema. This observation suggests that further study of hypervolemic hemodilution may be appropriate in patients with a low risk for developing cerebral edema.

CYTOPROTECTIVE THERAPY

Protecting cells against ischemic injury's biochemical and metabolic consequences reduces infarct size, preserves tissue, and improves clinical outcome. The most widely studied cytoprotective therapies are voltage-regulated calcium channel antagonists, NMDA calcium channel inhibitors, free radical inhibitors, and gangliosides. The mechanism of action

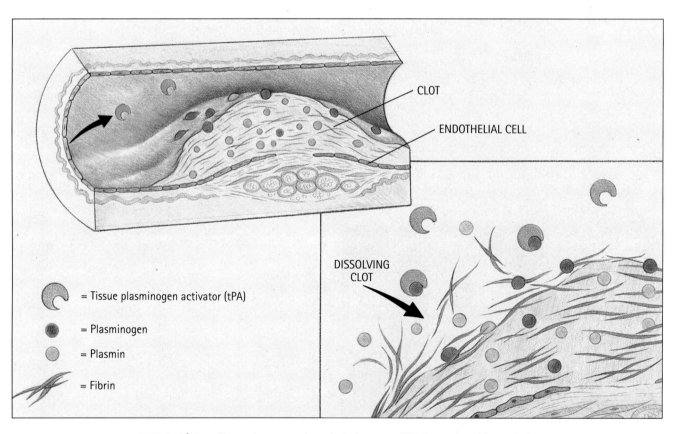

FIGURE 16.8 → The endogenous thrombolytic agent, TPA, is produced by endothelial cells and converts plasminogen to plasmin, promoting rapid arterial clot lysis.

of each cytoprotective drug group is different and synergistic effects are possible.

Voltage-Regulated Calcium Channel Antagonists
As discussed in Chapter 2, the entry of Ca^{++} into ischemic cells via voltage-regulated and receptor-mediated Ca^{++} channels may cause irreversible injury. Calcium channel antagonists of the dihydropyridine group (e.g., nimodipine, nicardipine, and isradipine), which have been most frequently evaluated in experimental and clinical ischemic stroke, have several potentially beneficial effects (Fig. 16.11).

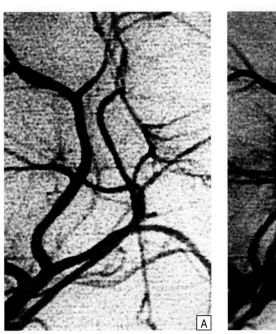
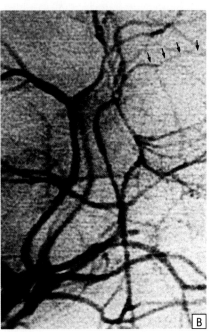

FIGURE 16.9 → **A,** Intravenous TPA reperfused occluded middle cerebral artery branches in a rabbit embolic stroke model. **B,** Flow return is documented (arrows).

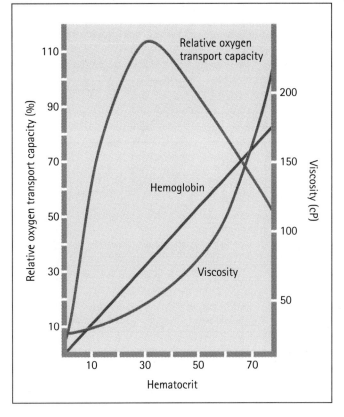

FIGURE 16.10 →
The relationship between blood oxygen carrying capacity, viscosity, hematocrit and hemoglobin suggests that a hematocrit of 30% to 33% may be best for providing maximal flow and tissue oxygenation. (Reproduced, with permission, from Wood JH, 1981.)

They inhibit the passage of Ca^{++} through the slow L channel but do not affect other Ca^{++} channels. They are also vasodilators of both peripheral and cerebral vessels. Vasodilation of cerebral vessels can enhance blood flow, but can also cause systemic hypotension, which could reduce cerebral perfusion. Flow may be increased by inhibiting red blood cell deformability. None of the current voltage-mediated calcium channel antagonists affect only the cerebral blood vessels. Other potential side effects include cardiac rhythm disturbances, gastrointestinal upset, dizziness, muscle cramping, and peripheral edema.

Studies of voltage-regulated calcium channel antagonists in stroke models have yielded mixed results, especially when given after the onset of ischemia. In humans, nimodipine has been the most widely evaluated drug (Fig. 16.12). An early study demonstrated that initiating oral nimodipine within 24 hours of stroke onset reduced mortality (9% vs. 20%) and improved clinical outcome. Four other oral nimodipine trials have reported conflicting results. Subgroup analysis suggests that patients who are ran-domized early (12 h from onset) or have moderate neurologic deficits may benefit, but there is no conclusive data. Nicardipine, given intravenously within 12 hours from stroke onset, has been preliminarily evaluated without a control group. Unfortunately, no studies of patients treated within 6 hours of stroke onset are available. At this time it is uncertain if voltage-regulated calcium antagonists are effective treatment for acute ischemic stroke; their use cannot be recommended.

NMDA Channel Antagonists

The NMDA channel seems to be an important mediator of calcium influx related to ischemic injury. Activation of the glycine or polyamine receptors of the NMDA receptor complex potentiates glutamate binding to a membrane receptor site, thus energizing the NMDA channel. Several receptor sites are associated with the ion channel itself, and activation of the magnesium, zinc, or channel antagonist (PCP) sites inhibits Ca^{++} influx. Under ischemic conditions, large quantities of glutamate are released that activate the NMDA channel, potentiating irreversible cellular

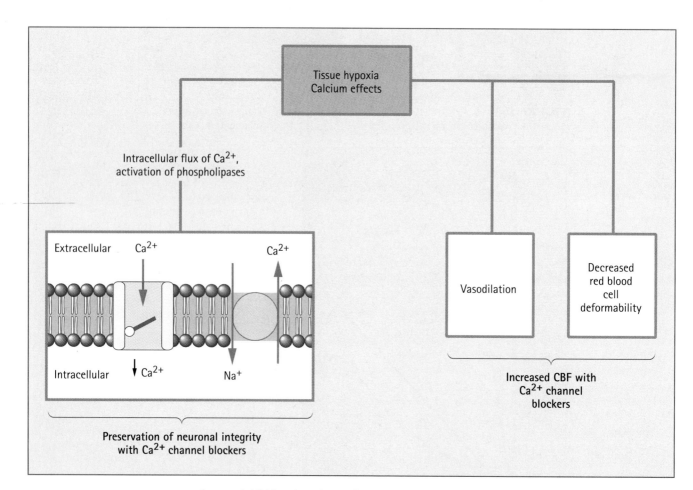

FIGURE 16.11 → Inhibiting the release of calcium during brain tissue ischemia has a variety of potentially beneficial effects.

injury. The complicated structure of the NMDA receptor-channel complex suggests that a variety of inhibitory approaches are possible (Fig. 16.13).

NMDA receptor-channel inhibitors can be divided into two major groups: those that competitively inhibit the glutamate, glycine, or polyamine sites, and noncompetitive inhibitors that bind to the PCP site within the ion channel. Specific competitive inhibitors of the glutamate, glycine, and polyamine sites have been developed, but most do not satisfac-torily cross the blood-brain barrier. Several of these drugs have substantially reduced infarct size in animal stroke models when given up to 3 hours after onset of ischemia. However, side effects such as respiratory suppression, hypotension, memory impairment, and behavior disturbances have been observed. Noncompetitive antagonists such as MK-801 have also been evaluated in animal models. Dramatic reductions of infarct size have been obtained with treatment beginning up to 2 hours after stroke onset (Fig. 16.14). Side effects were

FIGURE 16.12 → CLINICAL TRIALS OF VOLTAGE-MEDIATED CALCIUM ANTAGONISTS IN FOCAL ISCHEMIA

STUDY	DRUG AND DOSE	# PATIENTS AND TIME TO TREATMENT	FOCAL ISCHEMIA OUTCOME
Gelmers et al.	Nimodipine 30 mg p.o. QID x 4 weeks	180 patients 24 h	Significant and in deaths and clinical improvement/secure patients
Hornig et al.	Nimodipine 120 mg qd p.o. X 3 weeks	365 patients 48 h	No treatment effect
Trust study group	Nimodipine 120 mg qd p.o. X 3 weeks	1,215 patients 48 h	No treatment effect
Martinez-Villa et al.	Nimodipine 120 mg qd p.o. X 4 weeks	164 patients 48 h	No treatment effect
Mohr et al.	Nimodipine 20, 40, or 80mg q8h X 3 weeks	1,064 patients 48 h	Overall no effect, but patients receiving 20, 40mg dose in less than 12 h had improved outcome

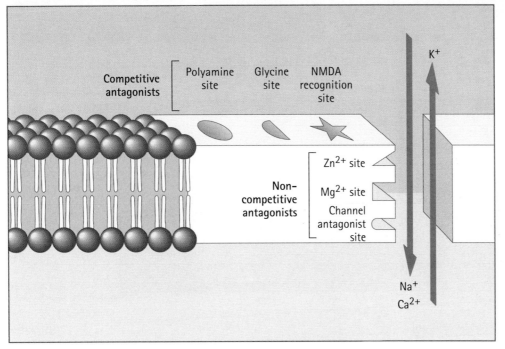

FIGURE 16.13 → Competitive and noncompetitive antagonists of the NMDA channel have been developed to impede calcium influx through this important site.

similar to those observed with competitive NMDA antagonists, but an additional problem is apparent neurotoxicity. Vacuolization of cortical neurons has been seen, which lessens with delayed observation or prolonged treatment. Stroke therapy will probably be administered only briefly. Some side effects should be short-lived, while other long-term effects can be avoided. Safety trials with several competitive and noncompetitive antagonists are in progress. If they are positive, efficacy trials in human stroke should quickly follow. We can also anticipate combination therapy with an NMDA channel antagonist and voltage channel antagonist to synergistically reduce Ca^{++} influx via these two channels.

Free Radical Inhibitors

Oxygen free radicals, which contain an unpaired electron in the outer ring, are highly toxic molecules produced via the mitochondrial electron transport chain, the interaction of NADH and NADPH, the activity of xanthine oxidase, or arachidonic acid metabolism. The primary oxygen free radicals include superoxide, as well as the hydroxyl radical and its associated molecule, hydrogen peroxide. Oxygen free radicals are not generated in completely ischemic regions, but in partially perfused or reperfused tissue. They can mediate tissue injury by oxidizing lipids, proteins, nucleic acids, glycosaminoglycans, and by other mechanisms (Fig. 16.15). Polymorphonuclear leukocytes, which are recruited early to ischemic regions, produce large quantities of oxygen free radicals and may be an important source of tissue injury. Normally, the brain contains intrinsic protective mechanisms such as superoxide dismutase (SOD), glutathione peroxidase, and catalase to neutralize oxygen free radicals. Unfortunately, these antioxidant resources are limited and easily overwhelmed.

Ischemic injury is currently being treated with naturally occurring enzymes and synthetic antioxidants, especially after reperfusion. SOD does not cross the blood-brain barrier easily, but can be entrapped within liposomes or attached to carrier molecules such as

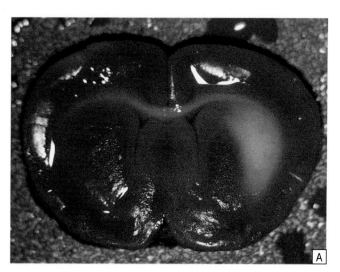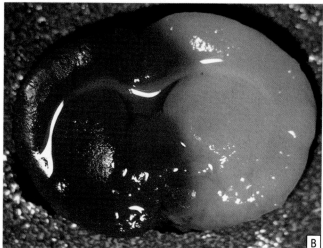

FIGURE 16.14 → The light area represents infarcted tissue on TTC staining. The animal that received the noncompetitive NMDA antagonist, MK-801 (A), has a much smaller lesion than the control animal (B).

FIGURE 16.15 → CELLULAR INJURY MEDIATED BY OXYGEN FREE RADICALS

- Lipid membranes oxidized
- Damage to proteins, nucleic acids, and glycosaminoglycans
- Membrane permeability increased
- Release of intracellular calcium
- Mitrochondria destroyed
- Cytoskeletal disruption

polyethylene glycol. Complexed SOD reduces infarct size in animal stroke models. Synthetic antioxidants such as the 21-aminosteroids derived from methyl-prednisolone, scavenge oxygen free radicals and lipid peroxyl radicals, as well as inhibit production by polymorphonuclear leukocytes (Fig. 16.16). The 21-aminosteroids preserve ischemic neurons and reduce infarct size in animal stroke models. Another antioxidant, OPC-14117, has similar effects (Fig. 16.17). Safety trials with these drugs are underway in humans, and efficacy trials for stroke outcome are planned. Antioxidants may perform best when combined with thrombolytic therapy or other initial cytoprotective agents.

Gangliosides and Other Interventions

The gangliosides are naturally occurring sphingolipids that may alleviate central and peripheral nervous system injury. Their neuronal protective abilities appear to ameliorate the effects of intracellular Ca++ overload secondary to NMDA channel activation. The gangliosides enhance dissociation of protein kinase C

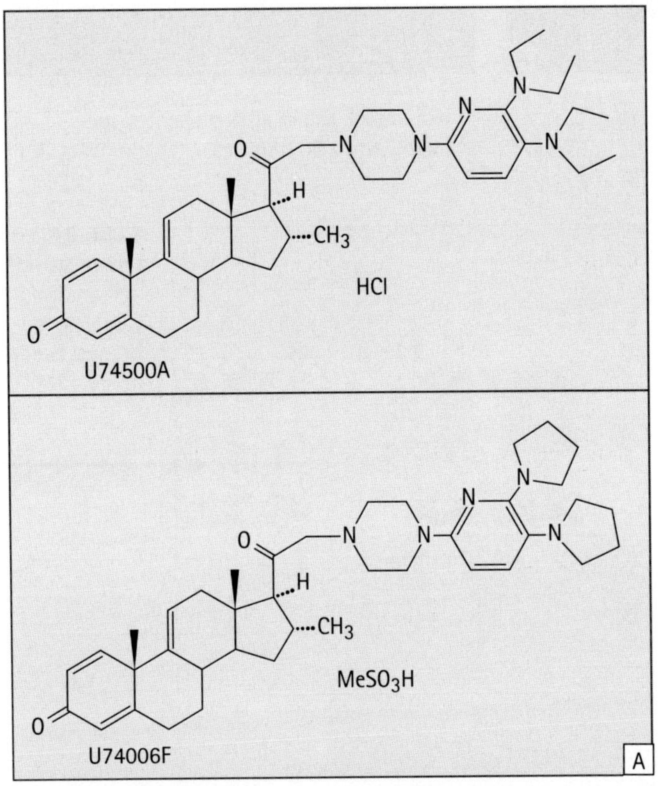

FIGURE 16.16 → A, The structures of two 21-aminosteroids, derived from methylprednisolone. **B,** The 21-aminosteroid, U74500A, markedly inhibits oxygen free radical production by stimulated human polymorphonuclear leukocytes and monocytes.

FIGURE 16.16B → EFFECT OF U74500A ON LEUKOCYTE HYDROGEN PEROXIDE GENERATION AND CHEMILUMINESCENCE

U74500A (µM)	HYDROGEN PEROXIDE POLYMORPHONUCLEAR LEUKOCYTES (NMOL/106 CELLS/30 M)	MONOCYTES (COUNTS/103 CELLS/5 MIN)
0	24.1 ± 2.4	25.4 ± 3.4
1	19.9 ± 3.2	20.5 ± 4.8
5	6.7 ± 1.9	0.3 ± 0.2
10	1.6 ± 1.1	0
	CHEMILUMINESCENCE	
0	89 ± 19	461 ± 204
100	171 ± 103	108 ± 81

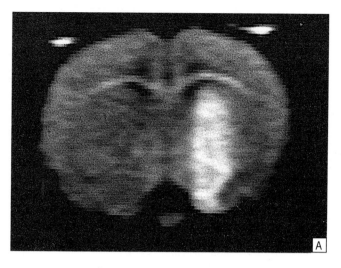 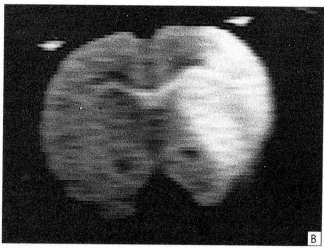

FIGURE 16.17 → Another free radical inhibitor, OPC 14117, reduces the extent of ischemic lesions denoted by the lightish area (A) as compared to animals receiving placebo (B) in a rat stroke model. The images presented are diffusion weighted MRI scans obtained 30 minutes after the onset of ischemia.

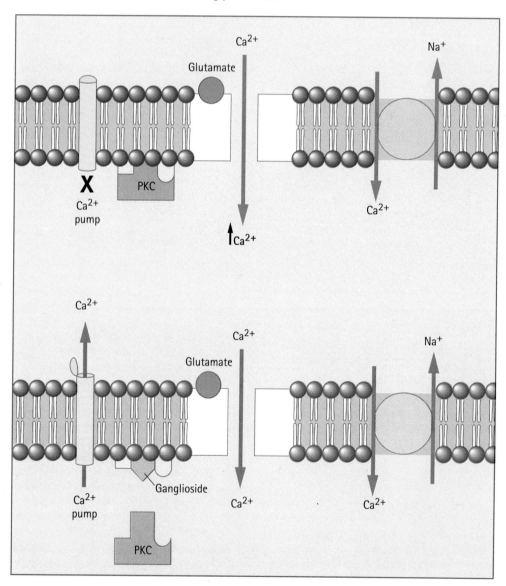

FIGURE 16.18 → Glutamate enhances intracellular calcium accumulation and protein Kinase C interaction with cell membranes. Gangliosides appear to ameliorate these developments.

from cell membranes, helping to prevent overload of cytosolic Ca++ caused by Ca++ channel activation (Fig.16.18). In vitro studies with gangliosides demonstrated a protective effect on glutamate mediated injury. A beneficial effect of GM-l was observed in a cat stroke model. Human trials have been conducted with delayed treatment that began up to 12 hours after stroke onset, but no sustained benefit was obtained. The results of an important trial with enrollment in less than 4 hours after stroke onset are pending. Other purportedly cytoprotective therapies that have been evaluated in experimental and clinical stroke include naloxone (an opioid receptor antagonist), propentofylline (a xanthine derivative), and inhibitors of polymorphonuclear leukocyte adhesion and activation. The data on these drugs are preliminary; these approaches are less likely to be beneficial than those previously outlined.

MEDICAL TREATMENT OF PRIMARY INTRACEREBRAL AND SUBARACHNOID HEMORRHAGE

PRIMARY INTRACEREBRAL HEMORRHAGE
The prognosis of medium to large primary intracerebral hemorrhage (PIH) is dismal, and it is unclear if any intervention can alter the outcome. Several supportive medical therapies may be helpful in selected patients (Fig.16.19). Many PIH patients have respiratory compromise and require supplemental oxygenation or artificial ventilation. Acute elevation of blood pressure or exacerbation of underlying hypertension is common and requires intervention if the blood pressure remains elevated for more than a few hours. An appropriate goal is to lower the blood pressure to preictal levels, if they are known, because sustained high blood pressure can enhance cerebral perfusion and cerebral edema. Beta-blockers and diuretics given intravenously with careful monitoring are the

drugs of choice. Calcium channel blockers, nipride, and hydralazine should be avoided; their vasodilatory effects can lead to greater amounts of cerebral edema. The treatment of cerebral edema and elevated intracranial pressure (ICP) PIHremains problematic. Hyperventilating intubated patients may help for short time periods. Osmotic diuretics such as low-dose mannitol, sorbitol, and glycerol may be effective for several days in selected patients and should be tried. Corticosteroids, especially dexamethasone, were frequently used in PIH patients, with conflicting results. A recent study demonstrated a worse outcome with dexamethasone. Its use is not recommended. For paralyzed patients, range of motion exercises is recommended. Compression stockings and pneumatic boots should be considered to prevent deep vein thrombosis, but subcutaneous heparin probably should be avoided.

SUBARACHNOID HEMORRHAGE
Medical management of subarachnoid hemorrhage (SAH) patients (Fig. 16.20) should be undertaken in most cases in an intensive care unit or SCU. These settings provide close nursing observation and the capability to easily perform cardiac and other physiologic monitoring. The SAH patient should be kept in a dark quiet room with few visitors. Mild sedation is recommended—a short-acting benzodiazepine can be used. Alternatively, 30 to 60 mg phenobarbital every 6 hours can work as a sedative and provide prophylactic protection against seizures. Although there is no convincing evidence that seizures alter the course in SAH patients, avoiding them is prudent. Analgesics will be necessary in most patients to control headache. Meperidine and codeine are the standard medications. Straining at stool or with urination should be prevented with a high fiber diet and stool softener. SAH patients may develop hyponatremia secondary to inappropriate antidiuretic hormone secretion or central salt-wasting. Fluids should be

---

FIGURE 16.19 → SUPPORTIVE MEDICAL THERAPY FOR PRIMARY INTRACEREBRAL HEMORRHAGE

- Reduce severe high blood pressure
- Maintain respiratory and cardiovascular status
- Attempt to reduce elevated intracranial pressure: hyperventilation, osmotic diuretics
- Prevent pulmonary emboli and sepsis

FIGURE 16.20 → MEDICAL THERAPY FOR SUBARACHNOID HEMORRHAGE

- Quiet and restful nursing environment
- Mild–moderate sedation
- Appropriate analgesia
- Stool softeners, urinary catheter (selected patients)
- Careful fluid management and blood pressure control to avoid and treat cerebral vasospasm
- Electrolyte management

restricted when inappropriate antidiuretic hormone secretion occurs and normal saline, packed red cells, or colloids should be considered for central wasting. Therapy may be necessary if cardiac arrhythmias or hypertension develop. A large variety of ECG changes occur in SAH patients; ß-blockers such as propranolol may be useful. A systolic blood pressure above 170 mm/hg should be carefully lowered, as vasospasm may develop if the blood pressure drops precipitously.

Rebleeding and vasospasm are two SAH complications that may be medically treated. Rebleeding most often occurs during the first week after the initial SAH. Bed rest and hypotension apparently do not prevent this problem. Antifibrinolytic drugs such as epsilon-aminocaproic acid and tranexamic acid have been used with conflicting results. Antifibrinolytic drugs are of uncertain value to the prevention of rebleeding, but may be used for a few days if surgery is delayed. Cerebral vasospasm causing cerebral ischemia typically develops 3 to 10 days after SAH and is directly related to the amount of blood in the subarachnoid space on admission. A variety of approaches to prevent or treat vasospasm have been tried (Fig. 16.21). Nimodipine appears to reduce the development of delayed cerebral ischemia after SAH, although it may not reduce vasospasm. Other calcium channel blockers such as nicardipine have been found to inhibit spasm and may improve outcome. Once vasospasm and ischemia occur, therapy is difficult. Volume expansion and blood pressure elevation under careful monitoring may be helpful in some cases.

FIGURE 16.21 → TREATMENT FOR CEREBRAL VASOSPASM

PREVENTION
- Surgical or thrombolytic removal of clot
- Pharmacologic: anti-inflammatories, antioxidants, calcium antagonists (nicardipine)

REVERSAL OF SPASM
- Hypervolemic, hypertensive hemodilution
- Mechanical therapy: angioplasty
- Pharmacologic (?): nitroglycerin, papaverine, calcitonin-peptide

PREVENT ISCHEMIC EFFECTS
- Avoid hypovolemia
- Calcium antagonists (nimodipine)

REFERENCES

Antiplatelet Trialist's Collaboration. Secondary prevention of vascular disease by prolonged antiplatelet treatment. *Br Med J.* 1988; 296:320–331.

Asplund K. Hemodilution in acute stroke. *Cerebrovasc Dis.* 1991; 1 (Suppl 1):129–138.

Braughler JM, Hall ED, Jacobson EJ, et al. The 21-aminosteroids: potent inhibitors of lipid peroxidation for the treatment of central nervous system trauma and ischemia. *Drugs Fut.* 1989; 14:143–152.

Choi DW. Methods for antagonizing glutamate neurotoxicity. *Cerebrovasc Brain Metab Rev.* 1990; 2:105–147.

Del Zoppo GJ, Poeck K, Pessin MS, et al. Recombinant tissue plasminogen activator in acute thrombotic and embolic stroke. *Ann Neurol.* (In press)

Dyken ML. Stroke risk factors. In: Norris JW, Hachinski VC, eds. *Prevention of Stroke.* New York: Springer-Verlag. 1991; 83–102.

Favarson M, Maneu H, Vicini S, et al. Prevention of excitatory amino acid-induced neurotoxicity by natural and semisynthetic sphingoglyoclipids. In: Guidotti A, ed. *Neurotoxicity of Excitatory Amino Acids.* New York: Raven Press. 1990; 243–258.

Findlay JM, Macdonald RL, Weis BKA. Current concepts pathophysiology and management of cerebral vasospasm following aneurysmal subarachnoid hemorrhage. *Cerebrovasc Brain Metab Rev.* 1991; 3:336–361.

Fisher M. Clinical pharmacology of cerebral ischemia. *Cerebrovasc Dis.* 1991; 1 (Suppl l): 112–119.

Grotta JC. Clinical aspects of the use of calcium antagonists in cerebrovascular disease. *Clin Neuropharm.* 1991; 17:373–390.

Kase CS, Fisher M, Babikian VL, Moher JP. Cerebrovascular disease. In: Rosenberg RN. *Comprehensive Neurology.* New York: Raven Press. 1991; 97–156.

Marsh EE, Adams HP, Biller J, et al. Use of antithrombotic drugs in the treatment of acute ischemic stroke. *Neurology.* 1989; 39:1631–1637.

Norris JW, Hachinski VC. *Prevention of Stroke.* New York: Springer Verlag. 1991; 122.

Poungvarin N, Bhoopat W, Viriyave Jakul A, et al. Effects of dexamethasone in primary intracerebral hemorrhage. *N Engl J Med.* 1987; 316:1229-1233.

Schmidley JW. Free radicals in central nervous system ischemia. *Stroke.* 1990; 21:1081–1090.

Sherman DG, Dyken ML, Fisher M, et al. Antithrombotic therapy and cerebral embolism. *Chest.* 1989; 95:140s–155s

Wood JH. *Cerebral Blood Flow.* New York: McGraw-Hill Book Co. 1981.

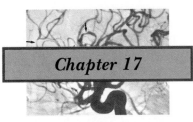

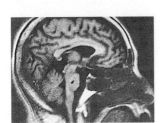

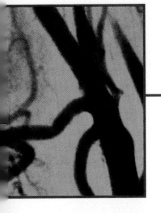

Chapter 17

MASSIMO S. FIANDACA

Surgical Therapy for Cerebral Ischemia

SURGICAL THERAPY for cerebral ischemia dates back at least 40 years. During these four decades, many technical contributions and innovations have been made in the surgical approaches toward lesions responsible for ischemic strokes. Thanks to the clinical/pathologic studies of Fisher and others, surgical approaches to various stroke syndromes can be tailored to address individual abnormalities of the cerebrovascular system. Along with these highly-specialized procedures came the development of cerebrovascular medicine, which unites neurology, radiology, medicine, pathology, and surgery into one discipline. Physicians in these areas continue to strive to better understand the pathogenesis of cerebrovascular disease so that new information can be used in logical, relatively safe methods of treatment, and ultimately, in the prevention of brain ischemia.

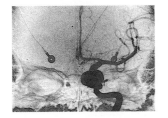

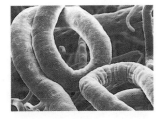

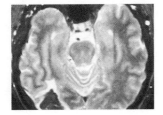

Investigators in cerebrovascular medicine are currently attempting to determine whether the most commonly performed surgical procedures for the treatment of cerebral ischemia are actually better able to prevent stroke than medical therapy. The negative results of multicenter randomized clinical trials have deemed the extracranial-intracranial (EC-IC) bypass procedures ineffective, and therefore they should not be utilized, except in rare instances. While carotid endarterectomy for symptomatic extracranial carotid high-grade stenosis (70–99%) proved more effective than the best medical therapy, studies assessing this operation's role in patients with asymptomatic lesions or in symptomatic patients with nonhemodynamically significant (<70% stenosis) lesions have not yet delivered a verdict.

Many more clinical trials in the future will evaluate medical and surgical therapies for cerebral ischemia. In this chapter some of the more common surgical procedures for treating the various pathologies that lead to clinical cerebral ischemia will be highlighted, emphasizing the current indications for the procedure and in most cases the surgical technique is briefly described and depicted. References to other sections of this book dealing more specifically with nonsurgical aspects of treatment will be noted.

EXTRACRANIAL CAROTID ARTERY SURGERY

ATHEROSCLEROTIC DISEASE

By far, the surgical pathology most responsible for cerebral ischemia worldwide occurs at the carotid bifurcation and is secondary to atheromatous changes in the vessel walls. These changes result in vessel stenosis, ulceration with artery to distal artery embolization, and eventually occlusion. The results of the recent NASCET study have shown that carotid endarterectomy is better than the best available medical therapy in patients who have symptoms of cerebral ischemia with high-grade (70–99%) internal carotid stenosis. This is only true, however, if the surgical team has a low operative morbidity and mortality (risk of major stroke or death <2.5%).

Surgical candidates are primarily selected based on their general medical condition, especially cardiac and pulmonary status, which indicates their tolerance for general anesthesia. In some cases, due either to the surgeon's preference or to the patient's unstable condition, carotid endarterectomy can be performed using local anesthesia and mild intravenous sedation. Currently, most cerebrovascular physicians agree that a patient with significant symptomatic atherosclerotic cerebrovascular disease (>70% stenosis of the ipsilateral internal carotid artery [ICA]) who can tolerate anesthesia from the cardiovascular and pulmonary perspective, is a candidate

for carotid endarterectomy. Special situations obviously occur. The following are some particularly common clinical examples and their recommended surgical therapies.

In a unilaterally symptomatic patient with bilateral high-grade carotid stenosis, operation on the more stenotic of the two vessels, even if it is on the asymptomatic side, is recommended, followed within a week by surgery on the other side. In the case of bilateral symptoms and bilateral high-grade stenoses, the tightest lesion should be operated on first. Trials are currently evaluating the surgical efficacy of best medical therapy versus carotid endarterectomy in cases of moderate (30–69%) stenoses in symptomatic and asymptomatic patients. This objective information should be available soon, to indicate the possible role of surgery and help guide us in managing these additional problematic cases.

Shallow ulcerations, unless associated with a significantly stenotic atherosclerotic lesion, are thought to carry a fairly low risk of future stroke. Deep ulcers, however, especially if irregular and associated with dye-pooling on delayed angiographic films, have in some series been associated with significantly increased risk of stroke, prompting them to be operated on repeatedly. It remains to be seen whether these lesion subgroups have a natural history that is significantly different from nonulcerated plaques in patients who have low- and moderate-grade stenoses.

Carotid artery occlusion remains a condition primarily treated by medical therapy at this time, unless it is associated with acute thrombosis or a significantly stenotic contralateral ICA. In the former, embolectomy and endarterectomy are quite effective in reestablishing the patency of the carotid artery, while in the latter, carotid endarterectomy on the contralateral side may ameliorate the symptoms and signs of cerebral ischemia.

Specific Surgical Techniques and Considerations
Carotid endarterectomy as a surgical technique has evolved over the years due to the experience and innovations of the surgeons who perform it. The procedure is not extremely difficult, but it must be carried out with extreme precision and meticulous technique to prevent associated morbidity and mortality. Attention to detail begins in the patient selection, since operative results partly depend on the patient's preclinical status and risk factors (see previous chapters). To obtain excellent results, compulsive attention to detail is maintained in the operating room and postoperatively.

Intraoperatively, most carotid endarterectomies are performed with the patient under general anesthesia. However, local anesthesia and mild intravenous sedatives alone are sometimes successful.

Having the patient awake during the procedure allows the surgeon to monitor neurologic function, including speech. The surgeon and anesthesiologist could be alerted to transient ischemic episodes by a change in intraoperative neurologic status, which is extremely sensitive to such occurrences, allowing prompt treatment. Besides the surgeon's preference, endarterectomies under local anesthesia should be considered in the occasionally hemodynamically unstable patient or in other situations where general anesthesia may be too risky. Bupivicaine and xylocaine are the standard agents used to obtain local anesthesia for carotid endarterectomy. The planned incision site along the anterior border of the sternocleidomastoid muscle edge is infiltrated with either one or both of these local anesthetics, avoiding direct injection into the external jugular vein. Deeper injections are carried out under direct vision during the operative dissection to prevent direct injection into vital deep structures, such as the carotid artery and internal jugular vein. Additional local anesthetic injections can be given during the procedure to keep the patient relatively pain-free. Intravenous anxiolytics can assist in keeping the patient as comfortable and relaxed as possible. Relative contraindications to performing endarterectomies under local anesthesia include extreme patient anxiety or uncooperativeness, a high ICA bifurcation, and the potential need for EEG burst-suppression with barbiturates.

Most endarterectomy cases are performed under general anesthesia with the patient supine, and begin with the induction of anesthesia with intravenous barbiturates. In many medical centers and community hospitals it has become routine to monitor EEG from both hemispheres before, during, and after the procedure. Scalp electrodes are placed and baseline preanesthesia recordings are carried out. Particular attention is paid to differences between the right and left sides, since the development of EEG asymmetry may indicate an ischemic event. The patient is hydrated prior to induction with nonglucose-containing crystalloid and/or colloid to prevent the hypotension associated with barbiturates. Pneumatic boots are placed to prevent venous pooling in the lower extremities. Orotracheal intubation follows, with the maintenance of anesthesia usually consisting of inhalational isoflurane/nitrous oxide/oxygen. Baseline EEG is obtained following induction so that it can be compared to that occurring during the procedure. Some EEG units give a compressed spectral array that can quickly appraise the surgeon and anesthesiologist of changes in amplitude and frequency of the EEG burst pattern. Others prefer 16-channel recording units. After securing the endotracheal tube without compromising the superior exposure in the neck, the patient's head is gently rotated contralateral to the operative site and a small roll is placed between the patient's scapulae to induce slight neck extension.

After injecting local anesthetic into the skin and subcutaneous tissues along the anterior border of the sternocleidomastoid muscle, an incision is made through the platysma (Fig. 17.1). A plane of dissection is developed beneath the platysma so that it can be closed at the end of the case without significant adherence to the underlying tissues. The fascia

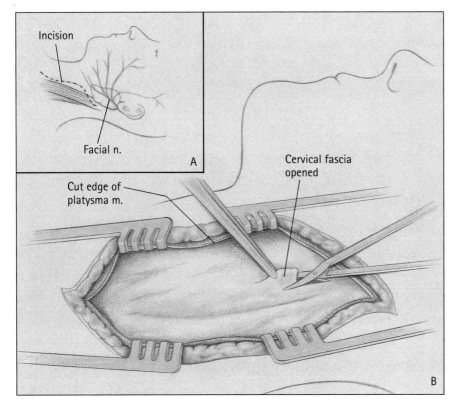

Incision

Facial n.

A

Cut edge of platysma m.

Cervical fascia opened

B

FIGURE 17.1 → **A,** Curvilinear skin incision (dashed line) used for most carotid approaches. **B,** After cutting through the platysma, the deep fascia connecting the medial edge of the sternocleidomastoid to the strap muscles is cut. (Adapted with permission from Sundt TM Jr, 1987)

connecting the medial border of the sternocleidomastoid to the medial strap muscles is then sharply incised in the direction of the skin incision. Using blunt dissection, a plane is then developed between the sternocleidomastoid muscle laterally and the strap muscles medially, exposing the internal jugular vein and carotid sheath. At this point, blunt self-retaining retractors are placed to assist in the deeper dissection. In most cases, the omohyoid muscle and descendens hypoglossi are cut to improve the caudal and rostral exposure, respectively (Fig. 17.2A). The common facial vein is doubly ligated and cut, facilitating lateral retrac-

tion of the internal jugular vein. The ICA, common carotid artery (CCA), external carotid artery (ECA), internal jugular vein, and deep tissues should be further dissected, paying careful attention to the anatomic details and variability. Technical pitfalls encountered during this portion of the surgery include injury to the great vessels, the vagus, recurrent laryngeal, superior laryngeal, or hypoglossal nerves, as well as the trachea and esophagus. During this portion of the dissection, some surgeons inject the adventitia of the carotid bifurcation with xylocaine (Fig. 17.2B), thereby blocking the carotid sinus response with its associated bradycardia

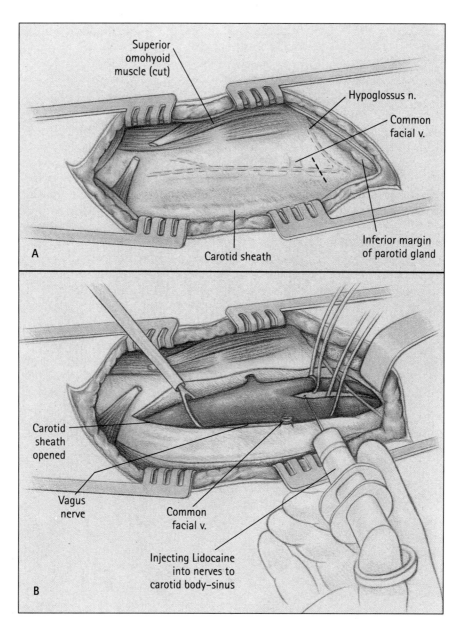

FIGURE 17.2 → **A,** Deeper dissection medial to the sternocleidomastoid reveals the carotid sheath. The omohyoid muscle and descendens hypoglossus nerve can be transected to improve inferior and superior exposure, respectively. **B,** Upon exposure of the carotid bifurcation, lidocaine may be injected in the adventitia of the carotid sinus to prevent reflex bradycardia and hypotension. (Adapted with permission from Sundt TM Jr, 1987)

and hypotension. By avoiding significant manipulation of the carotid bifurcation during the exposure, this response is prevented and atheromatous material associated with the plaque can be prevented from iatrogenically embolizing to the cerebral circulation.

Once the carotid bifurcation is dissected, vascular loops are placed around the CCA, ECA, and ICA to be used for occlusion during the endarterectomy. With careful attention paid to hemostasis of the wound, the patient is now given 5000 units of heparin intravenously. The anesthesiologist is asked to prepare to raise the blood pressure after carotid clamping with volume or inotropic agents, to maintain a systolic of at least 150 to 170 mm Hg. After allowing the heparin to circulate for approximately 5 minutes, a small aneurysm clip or double loop of 0-silk suture is placed around the superior thyroid artery to occlude it from the proximal ECA (Fig. 17.3). By this point, a decision should have been made about what type of cerebral protection to use during the actual endarterectomy.

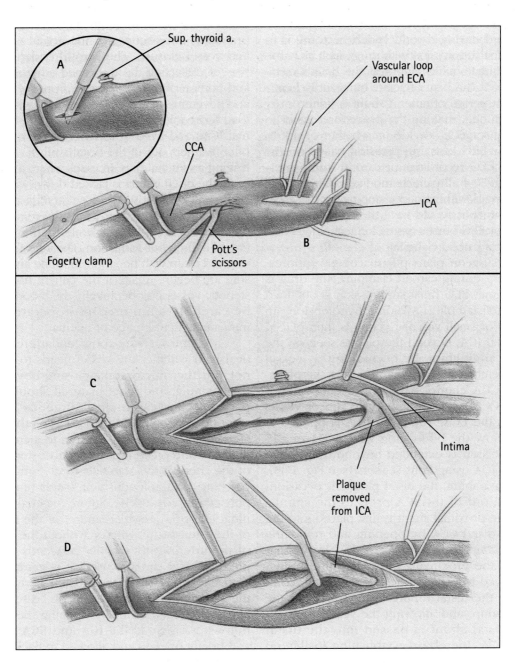

FIGURE 17.3 → A, An incision is made in the distal common carotid artery (CCA) with a #11 blade, gaining access to the carotid lumen. **B,** The incision is extended from the CCA into the internal carotid artery (ICA) using Potts scissors. **C,** The atherosclerotic media and intima are dissected free from the remaining vessel wall with a blunt dissector. **D,** The plaque extending up the ICA is allowed to "feather out." The entire plaque is then removed from the vessel lumen. (Adapted with permission from Sundt TM Jr, 1987)

bral ischemia in cases of carotid occlusion, tandem carotid lesions, and some cases of carotid occlusion with contralateral stenosis. The most common procedure involved the microvascular connection of the superficial temporal artery (STA) to an ipsilateral cortical branch of the MCA (STA-MCA) (Fig. 17.5). Despite this procedure's technical success, an international multicenter randomized trial in the early 1980s failed to prove it more efficacious than best medical therapy. This procedure has since been relegated to use in cases of planned iatrogenic occlusion of the ICA flow in the treatment of large ICA aneurysms or certain skull-base tumors. Patency rates for these anastomoses was >90% in most surgeons' experiences, but

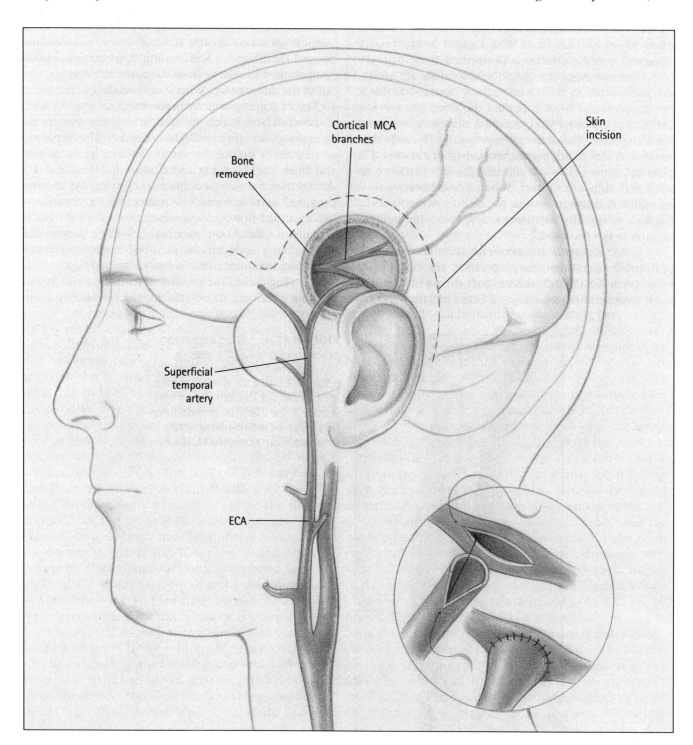

FIGURE 17.5 → The STA–MCA bypass operation takes a branch of the superficial temporal artery and anastomoses it with an intracranial branch of the MCA, to provide additional blood flow to the brain. (Adapted with permission from Sundt TM Jr, 1987)

Cerebrovascular Disorders

a drawback to using the STA to perfuse the hemisphere was the small caliber and amount of flow it could deliver. As the STA-MCA bypass matured, in most cases the vessel enlarged to handle more flow, but this took months and did not meet the acute needs of some patients. In an effort to develop a high flow anastomotic fistula to the hemisphere that could deliver enough blood flow to compensate for an acute carotid occlusion, autologous vein grafts connected proximally to either the ICA or ECA provided a readily available high flow vascular graft that was then anastomosed to the more proximal MCA (M1 or M2 segments). The microvascular anastomoses are performed with the operating microscope using 9-0 or 10-0 microvascular sutures on the MCA, which is temporarily occluded with temporary microvascular clips.

External carotid endarterectomy can be performed as an isolated procedure in the case of an ipsilateral ICA occlusion and badly stenotic ECA that on angiography reconstitutes the distal internal carotid via collaterals, or supplies the hemisphere directly via the ophthalmic artery. Transient ischemia under these circumstances may be related to the proximal obstruction to flow in this important collateral vessel. Surgical intervention is indicated when ongoing ischemic symptoms can be directly related to this proximal ECA stenosis or ulceration. Technically, the exposure and procedure is the same as for routine carotid endarterectomy surgery, except that the opening of the ECA is carried more distally. Since the proximal ICA is occluded, an extensive distal dissection of this vessel is unnecessary. Surgery for transient cerebral ischemia or stroke related to the *external carotid stump syndrome* usually requires angiographic evidence of ipsilateral ICA occlusion with a residual stump, and no other likely source of ipsilateral emboli other than the stump. Using an approach similar to that for endarterectomy, resection of the stump with vessel reconstruction can alleviate the patient's ischemic symptoms and prevent their recurrence (Fig. 17.6).

FIBROMUSCULAR DYSPLASIA

Symptomatic fibromuscular dysplasia (FMD) of the extracranial carotid artery is extremely rare. In most circumstances, angiographic FMD is an incidental angiographic finding in patients undergoing evaluation of cerebral ischemia or other cerebrovascular disorders. The most common pathologic entity, featuring small saccular dilations of the vessel alternating with rings of fibrous and muscular hyperplasia, is found in women during their fourth through sixth decades of life. FMD's natural history is not yet fully understood. Most symptomatic FMD patients have associated atherosclerotic disease of the extracranial carotid as well. With this in mind, the surgical indications for treating

fibromuscular dysplasia of the ICA are usually those associated with the atherosclerotic diasease. Rarely, a fibrous band will significantly restrict flow by itself or cause an intolerable bruit, thereby encouraging surgical intervention.

Direct surgical treatment of FMD is usually complicated by the disease's occurrence in the distal extracranial ICA, near the skull base. Direct surgical approaches to focal stenoses can be quite successful, with resection of the segment and reanastomosis of the vessel accompanied by patching. The surgical approach to expose the vessel is the same as for carotid endarterectomy, except that more distal exposure beneath the parotid gland and angle of the mandible may be necessary. Because the surgical exposures can be difficult, balloon angioplasty has been utilized effectively in some cases. The fragility of the vessels in this disease may lead to vessel rupture or dissection after percutaneous angioplasty procedures, resulting in the need for emergency surgery. Intraoperative dilation of the segment of FMD with Fogarty balloons or biliary duct dilators is a sound alternative, since most ruptures or dissections are treatable during the same procedure.

CAROTID DISSECTION

Traumatic and spontaneous dissections of the extracranial ICA have been clearly associated with cerebral ischemia. The dissection results from an intimal tear that allows blood to dissect the intima from the media, forming a false lumen or aneurysm that can significantly restrict distal blood flow. Additionally, thrombosis within the false lumen or true lumen can cause distal embolization and ischemia. Of the two types, traumatic dissections are more common clinically and are frequently associated with blunt neck trauma or forced head rotation. Most cases of spontaneous dissection have associated intrinsic vessel disease, such as FMD, which predispose the vessel wall to injury. In many cases of spontaneous dissection, however, there is also an associated history of minor trauma to the neck, such as seen in severe retching or coughing. Most cases can be managed medically with anticoagulation if there are ongoing transient neurologic deficits or a small fixed neurologic deficit associated with the dissection. In cases where medical therapy fails to prevent further ocular or cerebral ischemic events, or in cases of progressive neurologic deterioration associated with diminishing ipsilateral ICA flow, surgical intervention should be considered.

A symptomatic carotid dissection is technically exposed in the same manner as a carotid endarterectomy. In the area of the carotid dissection, the vessel usually looks larger in diameter than normal and the vessel wall is bluish, indicating the area of clot in the

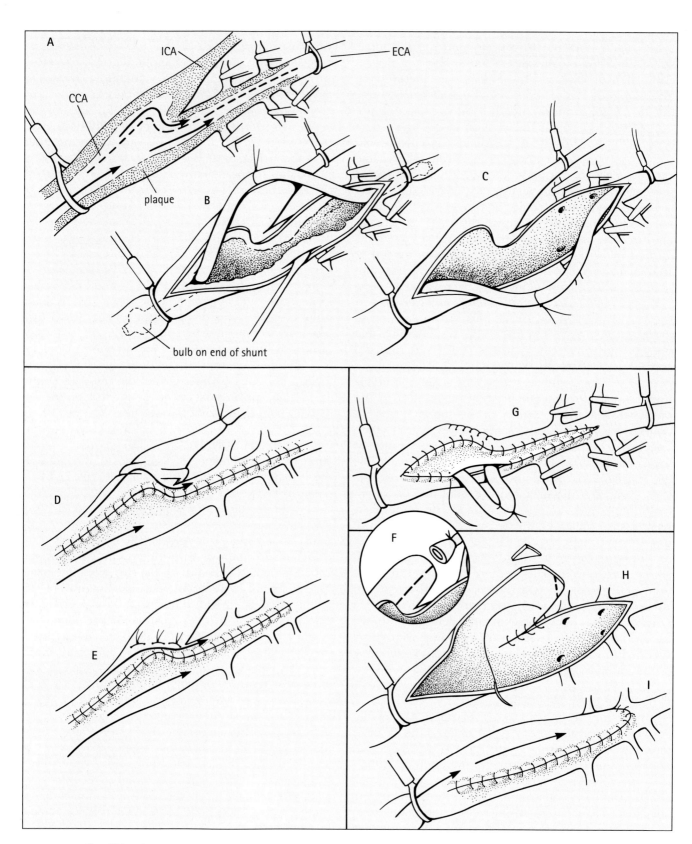

FIGURE 17.6 → ECA endarterectomy and stump angioplasty. **A,** ICA occlusion with proximal stump and ECA stenosis. Blood flow (arrows) shows thrombus forming an eddy in ICA stump. Incision for ECA endarterectomy (dashes) runs from distal CCA onto ECA, beyond proximal stenotic atherosclerotic plaque. ECA branches are temporarily occluded with aneurysm clips. **B,** After vessels are opened, intraluminal shunt maintains ipsilateral blood flow to the brain from CCA via ECA collaterals. **C,** ECA and proximal ICA stump endarterectomy with temporary shunt. **D,** After endarterectomy of proximal ICA stump, vessel may be plicated without disconnecting the distal ICA. **E,** Arteriotomy closed without a patch. **F,** Most other angioplasties disconnect proximal ICA stump from distal occluded ICA. **G,** Disconnected ICA stump can be oversewn while arteriotomy is closed, usually with a patch graft over a shunt. **H, I:** Proximal ICA stump—shaped into pedicle patch for closure of ECA arteriotomy—allows smooth flow of CCA blood into ECA. (Adapted with permission from Countee RG and Argila CR, 1989)

false lumen. Distal embolization must be prevented via the residually patent ICA by occluding its origin and minimally handling the wall of the vessel during the operative exposure to prevent possible rupture. As in treating an acute carotid occlusion, the vessel is opened just beyond the proximal clamp on the carotid bulb; backbleeding flushes any distal thrombus out of the vessel. The distal artery is then occluded for hemostasis and a carotid endarterectomy is performed, removing the dissected intima and clot in the false lumen. If the vessel is at all redundant and tortuous at the level of the dissection, an excision of the pathologic arterial segment is performed with either a primary reanastomosis of vessel or placement of a vein interposition graft. Since a shunt may not be technically feasible during the carotid occlusion, many of these patients require cerebral protection during clamping via EEG burst suppression, as previously noted.

EXTRACRANIAL VERTEBRAL ARTERY SURGERY

ATHEROSCLEROTIC DISEASE
Unlike symptomatic atherosclerotic disease in the carotid circulation most ischemic clinical symptoms related to the vertebrobasilar system are due to intracranial stenoses or occlusions. A very important subgroup of patients, however, have clinical symptoms related to extracranial vertebral artery (VA) disease. Unfortunate variations of anatomy, severe atherosclerosis, or both predispose most of these patients to develop vertebrobasilar ischemic symptoms or actual infarctions. Extracranial stenosis or occlusion of the VA commonly occurs at the vessel origin from the subclavian artery. In most symptomatic cases, the contralateral VA is either atretic or occluded, hypoplastic, or severely stenotic, making flow in the ipsilateral VA even more important to vertebrobasilar perfusion of the brain. Many of these patients also have extracranial carotid disease, complicating their clinical picture. In cases of combined symptomatic disease, the carotid disease should be treated either initially or at the same setting. After defining the pathologic anatomy angiographically, initial treatment for vertebrobasilar ischemia by most neurologists and internists has been with systemic anticoagulation. Although not supported to date by a randomized clinical trial, anticoagulation therapy usually stabilizes the patient and allows the ischemic symptoms to resolve. Patients should be considered for direct VA surgery if 1) signs and symptoms of vertebrobasilar ischemia persist despite surgically-treated symptomatic carotid atherosclerotic lesions and adequate anticoagulation; 2) they have not been devastated by stroke or associated medical conditions; 3) they have accessible atherosclerotic pathology. The mainstay of surgery is to create an uncompromised channel for blood flow to the hindbrain by direct surgical attack on the extracranial VA pathology. In rare cases, the extracranial pathology is not arterial. Instead, transient or permanent stenosis or occlusion of the extracranial VAs may be due to cervical spondylosis and associated abnormal spine movement. For the rare latter cases, decompression of the interosseous vertebral canal or cervical fusion may ameliorate extracranial VA blood flow.

Specific Surgical Techniques and Considerations
Vertebral-carotid transposition is a technically demanding procedure carried out in cases of symptomatic proximal atherosclerosis at the VA origin. Patients with transient ischemic attacks (TIAs) or minor strokes involving the vertebrobasilar system who have had their cerebral circulation fully evaluated and have recurrent clinical symptoms despite systemic anticoagulation should be considered for this procedure. The decision to utilize this operative technique rather than vertebral endarterectomy or other options is based upon the surgeon's preference and the patient's anatomy. In individuals where angiograms indicate that the anatomy may make exposure of the subclavian and vertebral origin difficult without a median sternotomy or thoracotomy, a transposition of the vessel should be considered and is the procedure of choice for symptomatic proximal VA disease. Experience with this approach has generally been good, although thorough objective evaluation of historical data is not available and neither is information from a multicenter randomized clinical trial.

The classic approach to the right VA origin is via a low transverse supraclavicular incision. Depending on the patient's anatomy and the surgeon's preference, the left VA origin can either be exposed in a similar manner, via a left thoracotomy or, occasionally, modified median sternotomy. In the former case, after the platysma has been incised transversely, 1 cm above the clavicle, the clavicular head of the sternocleidomastoid muscle is cut, leaving the sternal head of the muscle intact. The underlying fat and lymphoid tissue is dissected gently off the underlying anterior scalene muscle and the subclavian vein, inferiorly. The boundaries of the exposure feature the internal jugular vein medially, the omohyoid muscle passing in a transverse manner superiorly, the phrenic nerve passing down the lateral border of the anterior scalene, and the subclavian vein inferiorly. With careful attention to the phrenic nerve on either side, and also the thoracic duct passing toward the confluence of the subclavian vein and internal jugular vein on the left, the anterior scalene muscle is cut transversely near its origin on the first rib. The superior belly of this muscle is retracted cephalad, exposing the underlying subclavian artery and its proximal branches (VA, thyrocervical trunk, and internal mammary artery) (Fig. 17.7). The VA is then dissected from its origin to its insertion into the longus colli muscle and, in most cases, the foramen transversarium of the C-6 vertebral body. This distal dissection allows greater mobilization of the vessel for implantation of the proximal end into the CCA. Occasionally, sympathetic fibers crossing over the VA must be divided to obtain the necessary exposure. Patients need to be told preoperatively about the possibility of a Horner's syndrome ipsilateral to their surgery. Since many of these patients have precarious cerebrovascular hemodynamics, EEG burst suppression during the occlusion of the verterbral and anastomosis may be recommended for prevention of brain ischemia. The proximal VA is then doubly tied and transected distal to the sutures, occluding backflow from the VA with an aneurysm clip. The tip

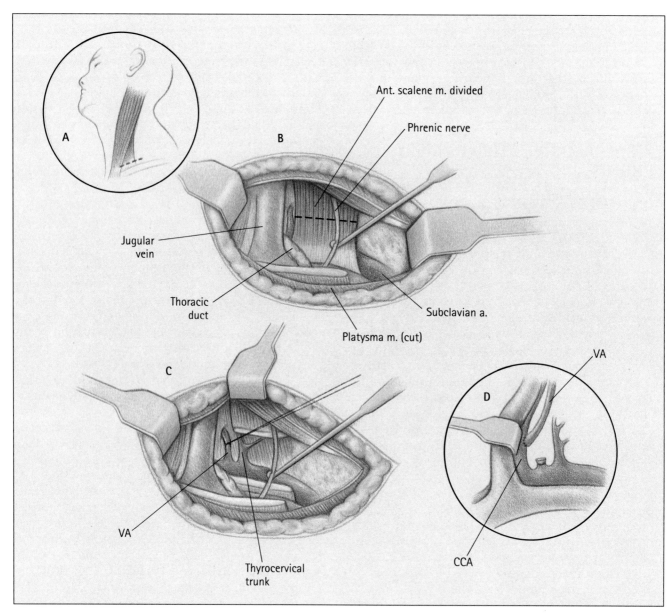

FIGURE 17.7 → Exposure for a vertebral-carotid transposition. **A,** The incision is placed low in the neck, 1 cm above the clavicle and at the lateral border of the sternocleidomastoid muscle. **B,** With the lateral sternocleidomastoid cut, the anterior scalene muscle is seen below fatty and lymphoid tissues. Attention must be paid to identifying the phrenic nerve (and the thoracic duct, on left-sided exposures). **C,** With division of the anterior scalene muscle, the proximal subclavian artery is identified along with its main branches. **D,** With the proximal vertebral artery (VA) ligated, the VA is mobilized, cut, and anastomosed with the CCA, thereby bypassing proximal vertebral or subclavian disease. (Adapted with permission from Sundt TM Jr, 1987)

of the VA, to be anastomosed to the CCA, is fish-mouthed, allowing an adequate orifice at the anastomotic site. The CCA is now exposed by dissecting the internal jugular vein superiorly and medially off the carotid sheath. Identifying the vagus nerve and recurrent laryngeal nerve (on the right) is essential in preventing injury to these structures. Once the CCA is exposed, it is either partially occluded at the planned site of anastomosis using a Wylie partial occlusion clamp, or proximally and distally occluded to allow the anastomosis to take place. A Goosen punch can make an arteriotomy in the CCA to accept the fish-mouthed proximal VA stump. The anastomosis is performed with 6-0 or 7-0 vascular suture.

Proximal vertebral endarterectomy is not as popular as vertebral-carotid transposition since surgeons usually find it technically more difficult. In the most common circumstance, the initial surgical approach is similar to that mentioned for the vertebral-carotid transposition. Once the origins of the subclavian artery and proximal branches are isolated and vascular loops are passed around the proximal and distal subclavian artery, the operative dissection is taken along the VA away from its origin, to obtain distal control of that vessel near the longus colli muscle. Just prior to clamping, some patients may be placed in EEG burst suppression for cerebral protection during the occlusion of the VA. The proximal and distal subclavian artery are then occluded by vascular clamps, while the thyrocervical trunk, internal mammary artery, and distal VA are occluded with aneurysm clips. The endarterectomy can be carried out through a longitudinal arteriotomy in the subclavian artery, since the VA may be too small to open directly. Another option is to incise from the subclavian artery into the VA, carry out the endarterectomy, then perform a patch angioplasty upon closing, again utilizing 6-0 or 7-0 suture.

The *subclavian steal phenomenon* results in brain ischemia due to pathology in the proximal subclavian artery, prior to the origin of the VA. By far, the most common pathologic entity causing this clinical syndrome is atherosclerotic disease, but congenital vessel abnormalities and trauma may also be responsible. Many patients are clinically asymptomatic, with the characteristic reversal of blood flow in the ipsilateral VA seen on angiography for other indications. Symptomatic patients have symptoms referable to vertebrobasilar or ipsilateral upper extremity ischemia, especially on excercising with the involved limb. Due to the proximal occlusion or severe stenosis of the subclavian, the ipsilateral arm is nourished by retrograde blood flow from the VA. In symptomatic cases, the diversion of this blood from the vertebrobasilar system to the upper extremity is enough to cause neurologic symptoms and signs. Surgical options with symptomatic subclavian steal phenomenon include reanastomosis of the subclavian distal to the occlusion (or stenosis) to the CCA, bypass grafting from CCA to subclavian, ligation of the VA, vertebral-carotid transposition, and subclavian thromboendarterectomy. Most surgeons treating this disorder for cerebral ischemia prefer the previously described vertebral-carotid transposition as a way of improving flow to the vertebrobasilar system.

FIBROMUSCLAR DYSPLASIA

FMD is rarely associated with the extracranial VA alone. It is usually found in patients who show evidence of FMD in the ICA. FMD in the VA most commonly occurs in the distal VA as it winds around the atlas and axis. In those rare symptomatic circumstances, many surgeons recommend treating the internal carotid FMD rather than the vertebral disease, even with primarily vertebrobasilar ischemic symptoms.

DISSECTIONS

Extracranial VA dissections are quite rare, being 25% to 33% less common than those occuring in the ICAs. Angiographically typified by a tapered eccentric stenosis, most extracranial vertebral dissections occur at the level of C-2 and usually involve a short vessel segment. As in carotid dissections, most cases are asymptomatic or resolve spontaneously, whether traumatic or spontaneous. Spontaneous cases are often associated with FMD. Surgical intervention is rarely indicated; most cases probably do not warrant any treatment at all. Like carotid dissections, however, ischemic symptoms have been treated successfully with anticoagulation. Rarely, surgical intervention with distal VA occlusion or trapping of the involved segment is carried out in cases refractory to systemic anticoagulation.

INTRACRANIAL CAROTID ARTERY SURGERY

Intracranial carotid artery disease responsible for cerebral ischemia is an uncommon, technically challenging entity. With advances in microsurgery, especially over the last 15 years, many more intracranial vascular procedures are carried out successfully for planned occlusion of the intracranial carotid artery, in association with tumors or vascular lesions, or occasionally for severe carotid siphon disease.

ATHEROSCLEROTIC DISEASE

The major area of intracranial atherosclerosis in the anterior circulation occurs in the carotid siphon region of the ICA, a difficult position to approach surgically. Not infrequently this focal region of vessel wall disease is coupled with extracranial carotid bifurcation disease, causing clinical symptoms. In these cases, the extracranial pathology is often more significant and should be treated with carotid endarterectomy. The residual siphon lesion is then treated medically with antiplatelet therapy, or occasionally, anticoagulation. In rare circumstances, however, the distal stenosis is the more significant of the two lesions or is the sole pathologic lesion of the ICA. If the proximal internal carotid stenosis is greater than 70%, a carotid endarterectomy should be performed despite the more significant distal lesion. With a residually significant siphon lesion, if medical therapy (antiplatelet drugs or anticoagulants) fails to relieve symptoms of cerebral ischemia, an EC-IC bypass or a petrous carotid-supraclinoid carotid bypass should be considered. Both of these therapeutic options, although not proven to be beneficial via randomized clinical trials, have been quite useful in reestablishing a high flow shunt of blood to the distal intracranial internal carotid and its branches.

Aneurysms of the cavernous carotid artery and distal ICA artery may develop in association with atherosclerotic vessel disease. Occasionally, thrombus formation within these large vessel outpouchings is responsible for distal embolization and resultant clinical ischemia. In most circumstances, these aneurysms do not cause ischemic problems, rather they present clinically with signs of mass effect or subarachnoid hemorrhage (SAH). If the particular aneurysm is not amenable to microsurgical clip ligation, as noted on surgical exploration, primary treatment options include interventional radiologic balloon occlusion of the aneurysm versus trapping of the aneurysm, either via percutaneous catheter techniques or surgically.

Specific Surgical Techniques and Considerations
Petrous carotid-supraclinoid carotid bypass was developed in 1986 by Dr. Fukushima to deal specifically with the need of a high-flow bypass when electively occluding the cavernous carotid artery. When treating intracavernous carotid disease, whether it is atherosclerosis, tumor, or aneurysm, this technique allows permanent occlusion of the ICA in the region of pathology while maintaining excellent blood flow to the hemisphere (Fig. 17.8).

Using a standard frontotemporal craniotomy on the lesion's side, the intradural internal carotid is dissected to its bifurcation, allowing a distal site of anastomosis between the ophthalmic artery and posterior communicating artery. Using an extradural-intradural technique, the ICA just proximal to the ophthalmic artery is then exposed, so that it can be occluded by a clip once the bypass is performed, trapping the pathology proximal to it. Exposure of the

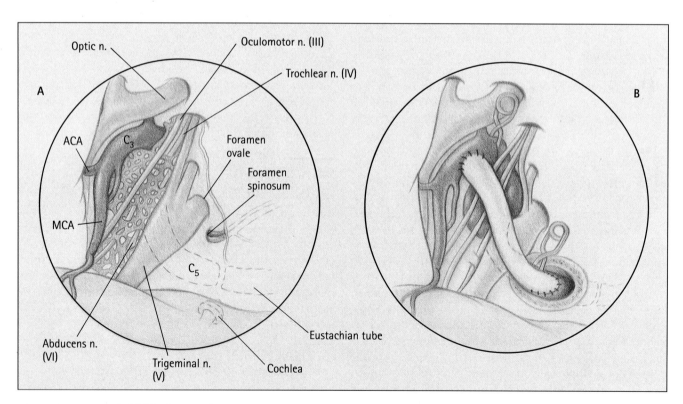

FIGURE 17.8 → **A,** Middle fossa and cavernous sinus surgical anatomic relationships. **B,** Completed petrous carotid–intradural carotid saphenous vein bypass. Note the need for occlusion of the petrous carotid distal to the proximal anastomosis and the internal carotid occlusion proximal to the ophthalmic artery, allowing the bypass to perfuse the eye and brain. (Adapted with permission from Spetzler RF, et al. 1990)

intrapetrous carotid is now carried out with a high-speed drill, just medial to the Eustachean tube and posterior to the foramen spinosum and ovale. After obtaining a complementary-sized segment of saphenous vein from the upper thigh to be used as the graft, the exposed intrapetrous vessel is occluded between a distal permanent aneurysm clip and a more proximal temporary clip. A permanent aneurysm clip is placed on the previously exposed distal ICA, just proximal to the ophthalmic artery origin. Starting just before and during the ICA occlusion, the patient is maintained in EEG burst suppression for cerebral protection, as previously noted. The proximal anastomosis is carried out using 8-0, 9-0, or 10-0 suture. The distal vein graft is then anastomosed with a similar suture to the intradural carotid between temporary aneurysm clips. Once the distal anastomosis is completed, a new vascular channel of similar dimensions has been established, excluding the intracavernous carotid and its associated pathology.

CAROTID-CAVERNOUS SINUS FISTULAS

A small number of symptomatic carotid-cavernous sinus fistulas can present with symptoms of cerebral ischemia. The mechanism for neurologic deterioration in this condition is similar to that in subclavian steal. Retrograde flow of blood in the intradural carotid toward the low resistance fistula effectively "steals" blood from the brain, leading to neurologic deficits. Most of these cases involve high-flow fistulas occuring either spontaneously or following trauma. Currently, direct surgical treatment of these lesions is indicated when percutaneous balloon occlusion therapy cannot occlude the fistula. Occasionally, emergency surgical intervention is necessary to surgically occlude the fistula from the intracranial circulation during an attempted balloon occlusion. The most common scenario involves the inadvertent balloon occlusion of the ICA proximal to the fistula, which further exacerbates the intracranial "steal" because the extracranial ICA no longer feeds the fistula. In these circumstances, the proximal intracranial carotid artery is exposed in a manner similar to that described for petrous carotid-supraclinoid carotid bypass. A permanent aneurysm clip must be placed proximal to the ophthalmic artery, thereby excluding the intracranial arterial and ocular circulation from the fistula. Other surgical options include a direct attack on the fistula within the cavernous sinus, leading to its occlusion, or thrombosis of the cavernous sinus. Exclusion of the intracranial circulation from the fistula usually allows resolution of the patient's symptoms or signs of cerebral ischemia. If the proximal carotid is still supplying the fistula, it can then be ligated or occluded via balloons without worry of distal embolization.

MOYAMOYA DISEASE

Cerebral ischemia is the major manifestation of moyamoya disease in children, while in the adult intracerebral hemorrhage is a more common presentation. This vasculopathy of the circle of Willis and distal carotid circulation results in the angiographic appearance of leptomeningeal and parenchymal shunt vessels associated with occlusion of major intracranial basal arteries. Although no clear etiology has been found for this rare disorder, congenital malformations, acquired vessel occlusions, and combinations of these have been proposed as mechanisms for the development of the disorder. Surgical indications include TIAs, reversible ischemic neurologic deficits, minor strokes, and ischemic convulsions. Surgical treatment is directed at augmenting the delivery of blood to the symptomatic hemisphere by developing new channels for brain perfusion. Surgical methods include the standard STA-MCA bypass, which immediately provides more blood flow to the brain and even increases amounts as the bypass matures. Other methods depend on the spontaneous development of vascular anastomoses between extraarachnoidal vessels and leptomeningeal vessels. These types of shunts require more time to develop but can also eventually supply significant amounts of blood to the brain. Transplantation of vascularized omentum can cover large areas of cerebral cortex. Durapexis, or laying a vascularized pedicle of dura onto the pia/arachnoid has also been effective in developing EC-IC collaterals and relieving patient symptoms. Variations similar to the latter two procedures include encephalomyosynangiosis (EMS), which involves the placement of a vascularized piece of temporalis muscle onto the brain, and encephaloduroarteriosynangiosis (EDAS), in which a segment of galea surrounding either the superficial temporal or occipital artery is placed onto the leptomeninges to allow development of collateral circulation.

INTRACRANIAL VERTEBROBASILAR ARTERY SURGERY

ATHEROSCLEROTIC DISEASE

Vertebrobasilar atherosclerotic disease most often occurs intracranially as opposed to extracranially. The common sites of involvement include the proximal intradural VA and the basilar artery (BA) trunk. Symptomatic stenosis in the former has been treated surgically by endarterectomy, while most other cases are treated medically by anticoagulation. In cases of symptomatic vertebral or basilar stenoses or occlusions that are refractory to systemic anticoagulation, surgical intervention should still be considered. Besides intradural vertebral endarterectomy, procedures developed to increase vertebrobasilar blood flow in these symtomatic patients include: 1) the occipital artery–posterior inferior cerebellar artery (PICA) bypass, 2) the occipital artery–anterior inferior cerebellar artery (AICA) bypass, and 3) the superficial temporal (or saphenous vein graft) to posterior cerebral artery (PCA) or superior cerebellar artery (SCA) bypasses. Patients with vertebrobasilar ischemic episodes should have their entire cerebrovascular circulation evaluated angiographically. If stenosis >70% of one or both extracranial carotids is noted, carotid endarterectomy should be considered as an early option to augment cerebral blood flow. Similarly, a proximal operative procedure should be contemplated if proximal extracranial verterbral disease is present. Many symptomatic patients suffer from symptoms that are directly related to inadequate vertebrobasilar blood flow, becoming symptomatic upon exercising, standing up, or during episodes of mild hypotension. With such clinical findings, these patients need to be optimally managed medically to minimize their operative morbidity and mortality. Despite aggressive medical and surgical interventions, many of these patients succumb to their systemic atherosclerotic disease with a fatal myocardial infarction or stroke.

Specific Surgical Techniques and Considerations

Intradural vertebral endarterectomy is usually performed with the operating microscope after exposing the intracranial and distal extracranial VA via an upper cervical incision and suboccipital craniectomy. Since most of these patients are fully anticoagulated, attention to hemostasis is essential. With the major plaque found just beyond the entrance of the VA into the dura, the dura is opened from the level of C-1 onto the cerebellum, exposing the VA from its entrance into the dura to where it dives under the rostral medulla, uniting with the contralateral vertebral to form the BA. Cutting the rostral two dentate ligaments to the cervical cord assists in visualizing the vessel by allowing the accessory nerve and the C-1 root to be mobilized. The plaque in the vessel often appears as a yellowish-white discoloration of the vessel wall. Angiographic imaging is essential in the preoperative assessment of the plaque's extent. After placing aneurysm clips on the proximal and distal VA, a longitudinal arteriotomy is made across the plaque. The plaque is then carefully dissected from the vessel wall, attempting not to leave an intimal flap. Under high power, the endarterectomy bed is inspected for intimal tags, which if found are removed. The vessel is then closed with 8-0 microvascular suture, paying attention to purging the air from the surgical site prior to opening the distal clip.

Bypass procedures for the vertebrobasilar system together with anterior circulation bypass operations were developed in the late 1970s and early 1980s for treating occlusive cerebrovascular disease not amenable to endarterectomy. With the negative results of the EC-IC bypass study in the mid-1980s, indications for the posterior fossa revascularization procedures became more difficult to defend and the numbers of these procedures being performed has significantly decreased. There remain specific circumstances, however, where these procedures make significant impact on the successful treatment of a patient with unstable vertebrobasilar ischemia.

In the posterior fossa, bypasses were developed to address the specific location of the offending atherosclerotic lesion. For intradural VA disease proximal to the origin of the PICA, patients who remain symptomatic despite systemic anticoagulation should be considered for an occipital artery–PICA bypass (Fig. 17.9). For atherosclerotic disease in the distal VA and BA proximal to the AICA, the surgical procedure of choice becomes the occipital artery–AICA bypass. For both of these procedures, the occipital artery and the recipient vessel need to be visualized on angiography to insure that they are of adequate caliber for anastomosis. The most important other technical point is the need for meticulous dissection of the occipital artery, since it can easily be traumatized and rendered useless during its exposure. The occipital artery is dissected from the retroauricular scalp and, following an ipsilateral suboccipital craniectomy, anastomosed with either the caudal loop of the PICA or the AICA distal to its major pontomedullary perforators. The anastomosis is performed with temporary clips placed on the recipient vessel utilizing the operative microscope and 10-0 suture. Some authors feel that candidates for the occipital artery–AICA bypass are also candidates for STA or venous bypasses to either the PCA or SCA and prefer the latter options to performing the anastomosis in the cerebellopontine angle.

Bypasses involving the STA-PCA or SCA have been developed for reperfusion of the distal BA, as in cases of midbasilar stenoses or occlusions. In these cases, the STA is dissected in a manner similar to that for a STA-MCA bypass but passed subtemporally to be anastomosed with either of the recipient vessels near the tentorial edge (Fig. 17.10). The SCA has been prefered by many since it can be temporarily occluded with less morbidity than the PCA. Again, surgical microscopy and 10-0 suture are required.

Because of the relatively small caliber and blood flow delivered by both the STA and occipital arteries, patients occasionally remain symptomatic following functioning bypasses. The problem appeared to be insufficient flow delivered by these small parent vessels. Therefore, autologous vein bypass grafts, similar to those used in the carotid circulation, have been utilized for their ability to deliver high volumes of blood to the ischemic vertebrobasilar system. With these long vein grafts, harvesting and preparing the

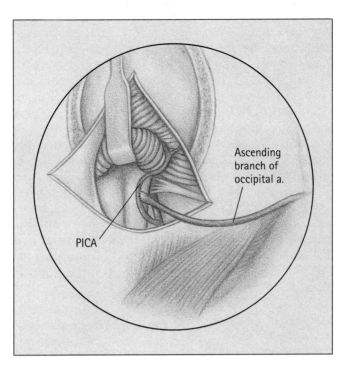

FIGURE 17.9 → The occipital artery–PICA bypass operation takes a branch of the occipital artery from the retroauricular region and anastomoses it with a tonsilar branch of the PICA. (Adapted with permission from Sundt TM Jr, 1987)

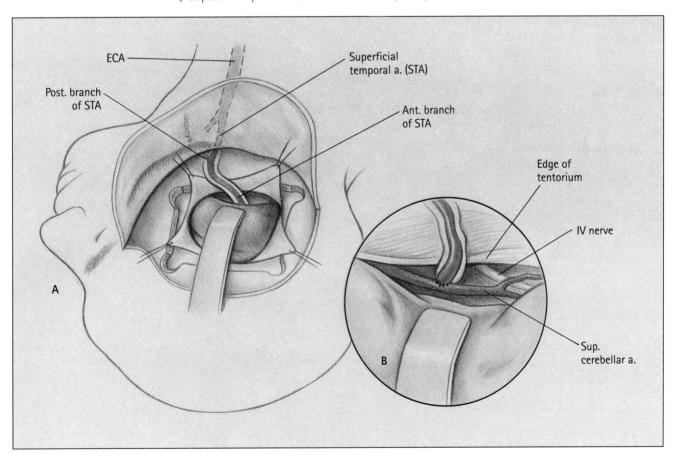

FIGURE 17.10 → **A,** The STA–PCA or STA–SCA bypass operation takes a branch of the superficial temporal artery and anastomoses it via a subtemporal route with either the PCA or SCA.

B, Closeup of completed anastomosis of STA–SCA bypass in tentorial incisura. (Adapted with permission from Sundt TM Jr, 1987)

vein graft are as important as the actual anastomoses. In many cases, the vein is proximally anastomosed to the ECA artery or one of its branches, with the distal anastomosis on either the PCA or SCA (Fig. 17.11). Patients that are neurologically unstable due to inadequate flow may respond dramatically to these high flow grafts. Unfortunately, these grafts and others often promote proximal occlusion of the diseased vessel because of inhibited flow across the stenotic segment, thereby leading to occasional morbidity and mortality.

CONCLUSION

A tremendous number of operative procedures have been designed to treat specific etiologies of cerebral ischemia. Most surgeons feel that medical therapy is a logical step prior to surgery for many conditions of cerebral ischemia not yet evaluated via a randomized clinical trial. Few to date, however, have had the objective evaluation of the EC-IC bypass procedures or carotid endarterectomy. We must not forget that anticoagulation for vertebrobasilar disease has not had a rigorous evaluation either. Surgeons must continue to improve their operative morbidity and mortality data and remain innovative in developing new operative techniques. Future recommendations for the treatment of cerebral ischemia will require even more thorough knowledge of the natural history of the disease, the medical and surgical options, and the associated morbidity and mortality of each option. Physicians in general must welcome and support randomized clinical trials for their medical and surgical therapies in the realization that the patient's well-being is at stake.

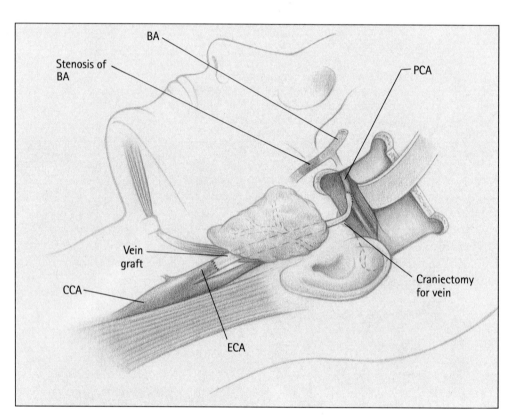

FIGURE 17.11 → A saphenous vein bypass graft utilizes blood flow from the ECA or one of its branches and is anastomosed with a large proximal intracranial vessel, either the PCA (in this case), SCA, or MCA, allowing the immediate development of an anastomosis with a very high flow. (Adapted with permission from Sundt TM Jr, 1987)

REFERENCES

Allen GS, Cohen RJ, Preziosi TJ. Microsurgical endarterectomy of the intracranial vertebral artery for vertebrobasilar transient ischemic attacks. *Neurosurgery.* 1981;8:56–59.

Countee RG, Argila CR. External carotid endarterectomy and surgical management of occluded internal carotoid artery. In: Wood JH (ed). *Carotid Artery Surgery in Stroke,* Philadelphia: Hanley and Belfus. 1989; 201-230.

Eastcott HHG, Pickering GW, Rob C. Reconstruction of internal carotid artery in a patient with intermittent attacks of hemiplegia. *Lancet.* 1954; 2: 994–996.

EC-IC Bypass Study Group. Failure of extracranial-intracranial arterial bypass to reduce the risk of ischemic stroke: results of an international randomized trial. *N Engl J Med.* 1985; 313: 1191–1200.

Eguchi T, Ugajin K. Surgical management of moyamoya disease. In: Schmidek HH, Sweet WH (eds). *Operative Neurosurgical Techniques: Indications, Methods and Results,* 2nd ed. Orlando: Grune and Stratton. 1988: 797–806.

Fisher CM. Occlusion of the carotid arteries. *Arch Neurol Psychiat.* 1954; 72: 187–204.

Fisher CM. Occlusion of the internal carotid artery. *Arch Neurol Psychiat.* 1951; 65: 346–377.

NASCET Collaborators. Beneficial effect of carotid endarterectomy in symptomatic patients with high-grade carotid stenosis. *N Engl J Med.* 1991; 325: 445–453.

Ojemann RG, Crowell RM. *Surgical Management of Cerebrovascular Disease,* Baltimore: Williams and Wilkins; 1983.

Spetzler RF, Fukushima T, Martin N, Zabramski JM. Petrous-to-intradural carotid saphenous vein graft for intracavernous giant aneurysm, tumor, or occlusive cerebrovascular disease. *J Neurosurg.* 1990; 73: 496–591.

Spetzler RF, Martin N, Hadley MN, Thompson RA, Wilkinson E, Raudzens PA. Microsurgical endarterectomy under barbiturate protection: a prospective study. *J Neurosurg.* 1986; 65: 63–73.

Sundt TM Jr. *Occlusive Cerebrovascular Disease: Diagnosis and Surgical Management,* Philadelphia: W.B. Saunders Co. 1987.

Index

A

Excitotoxic-glutamate hypothesis of ischemic injury, 3.5–3.6
External carotid endarterectomy, 17.9, **17.10**
External carotid stump syndrome, 17.9, **17.10**
Extracranial carotid artery
    branches of, 5.3
    surgery for, **17.2–17.5**, 17.2–17.11, **17.7–17.8, 17.10**
Extracranial ICA occlusive disease, 5.1–5.17
    blood supply, target territories, and collateral circulation, **5.3**, 5.3–5.5
    clinical manifestations of, **5.12**, 5.12–5.13
    epidemiology of, 5.3
    hemispheral and retinal infarction, 5.13–5.17, **5.14, 5.16–5.17**
    ICA disorders, **5.4–5.7**, 5.5–5.8
    mechanisms of ischemia, **5.8–5.11**, 5.8–5.12
Extracranial internal carotid embolectomy, 17.7
Extracranial vertebral artery surgery, 17.11–17.13, **17.12**

F

Fabry's disease, 9.18–9.19
Fibrin, 3.10
Fibrinogen, 3.10
Fibrinolysis, 3.11, **3.12**
Fibromuscular dysplasia (FMD), 5.7, 9.9, **9.9, 15.10**
    surgery for, 17.9, 17.13
    in young adults, 10.6–10.7, **10.7**
Free radical inhibitors, 16.10–16.11, **16.10–16.11**
Frontal lobes
    anatomy of, 2.13, **2.13**
Frontopolar branch, of ACA, 2.6

G

Gangliosides, 16.11, **16.12**, 16.13
Glucose supply, to brain, 3.2, **3.2–3.3**

H

HDL-cholesterol, 1.9, 3.17
Hemichorea hemiballismus, 8.11–8.12
Hemimedullary syndrome, 6.15, **6.15**
Hemispheral infarction, 5.13, 5.15
Hemoglobinopathies, 9.14–9.15
Hemorrhage
    intracerebral, 2.18, **2.19**, 10.3, 11.1–11.16
    subarachnoid, 2.17–2.18, **2.18**, 10.3
Hemorrhagic dementia, 13.13

Hemorrhagic transformation, 7.4, **7.7–7.8**, 7.9
Heparin
    in IH therapy, 10.11, 11.15
    for reducing stroke risk, **16.3**, 16.3–16.4
Hereditary AT III deficiency, 9.13, 10.11
Heroin and Talwin use
    as risk factor in stroke, 9.16, 9.18
Homocysteine, 10.13
Homocystinuria, 9.11–9.12
Hydrocephalus, **12.6**, 12.6–12.7
Hypercoagulable states, 9.13–9.14
Hyperdense MCA sign, 7.11, **7.12**
Hypersensitivity vasculitides, 9.8
Hypertension
    prevention and treatment of, 8.17
    as risk factor in stroke, 1.6–1.7, **1.6–1.7**, 4.5, 4.7, 4.9, 8.6–8.7, 11.3–11.4
    as risk factor in vascular dementia, 13.13
Hyperviscosity syndromes, 9.15, **9.16**

I

Idiopathic hypertrophic subaortic stenosis, 9.4
Illicit drug use
    link to IH, 11.8, **11.9**
Imaging techniques. *See* Neuroradiology of stroke
Immune-mediated prothrombotic states, 9.15–9.16, **9.17**
Incidence, of strokes, 1.2
    affect of extracranial ICA occlusive disease on, 5.3
    age and sex variations and, 1.3
    lacunar, 8.2–8.3
    race variations and, 1.3–1.4, **1.4**
    transient ischemic, 4.2–4.5, **4.3–4.6**
    trends in, 1.4–1.6
    in young adults, 10.2, **10.2**
Infarct, 2.19–2.25
    average size of, 7.19–7.20, **7.20**
    border-zone, **13.7**, 13.7–13.8
    cerebellar, **6.14**, 6.15
    clinical categories of, in brain, **8.2**
    diagnosis variables of, **2.21**
    hemimedullary, 6.15, **6.15**
    hemispheral, 5.13, 5.15
    hemorrhagic, 7.4, **7.7–7.8**, 7.9, **15.15**
    lacunar, 2.22–2.23, **2.23**, 11.11, 13.9–13.11, **13.10**
    with large-artery thrombosis, 2.19, 2.21
    lateral medullary, **6.14**, 6.15
    low-perfusion, 5.15
    PCA territory
        bilateral or unilateral, **6.20–6.21**, 6.20–6.23, **6.23**
    retinal, 5.15–5.17

with tandem arterial pathology, 2.22
of unknown origin (cryptogenic), 2.23–2.25, **2.24**
Infection and stroke, 10.7–10.8
Infective endocarditis, 7.17, **7.18**, 7.19, 10.8–10.9
Inflammatory bowel disease (IBD), **9.8**, 9.8–9.9
Initial neurologic deficit, 12.6
Internal carotid artery
    dissections of extracranial, 5.5–5.6, 6.6, **15.9**, 17.9,
        17.11
    supraclinoid segment, 2.4, 5.4
Internal carotid artery occlusive disease, 5.1–5.17
    clinical manifestations of, 5.12–5.13
    conditions affecting, 5.5–5.8
    embolic patterns of strokes in, **5.14**
    epidemiology of, 5.3
    hemispheral infarcts and, 5.13, 5.15
    low perfusion patterns of strokes in, **5.14**
    mechanisms of ischemia, 5.8–5.12
    retinal infarcts and, 5.15–5.17
    target territories of ICA circulation, 5.3–5.5
Intracardiac thrombus formation, **7.2**, 7.3
Intracerebral hemorrhage, 2.18, **2.18**, 10.3, 11.1–11.16
    alcohol abuse and, 11.8
    anticoagulants and, 11.7
    arteriovenous malformations and aneurysms and,
        11.10
    cerebral amyloid angiopathy and, 11.5–11.7
    clinical features of, **11.10**, 11.10–11.11, 11.13
    definition of, 11.1
    hypertension and, 11.3–11.4
    illicit and prescription drugs and, 11.8
    imaging techniques, 15.12, **15.12–15.17**, 15.15,
        15.17
    laboratory testing for, **11.12–11.14**, 11.13–11.14
    medical therapy for, 11.14–11.15
    neoplasms and, 11.7
    nonhypertensive type, 11.5–11.8, 11.10
    prognosis of, 11.16
    surgery for, 11.15–11.16, **11.16**
    thrombolytic agents and, 11.7
Intracranial carotid artery, 2.4, **2.4**. *See also* Internal
        carotid artery occlusive disease
    cavernous segment, 2.4
    petrous segment, 2.4
    surgery for, 17.13–17.15
Intracranial segment, of VA, 2.6
Intracranial vertebrobasilar artery surgery, 17.15–
        17.16, **17.17–17.18**, 17.18
Intradural segment, of VA, 2.6
Intradural vertebral endarterectomy, 17.16
Ionic disturbances, 3.4–3.5, **3.5**
Ischemic-hypoxic dementia, 13.13
Ischemic stroke, 1.12–1.15
    of cardiac origin, 7.3

causes of, in young adults, 10.3–10.15, **10.4–10.9,
        10.13–10.14**
imaging techniques. *See* Neuroradiology of stroke
lacunar. *See* Lacunar stroke
mechanisms of, 5.8–5.12
pathophysiology of. *See* Ischemic stroke patho-
        physiology
prognosis for, 1.14–1.15
recurrence of, 1.13–1.14, **1.14–1.15**
subtypes of, **1.12**, 2.19–2.25, **2.20–2.24**
survival of, 1.12–1.13, **1.13**
territorial susceptibility to, 13.18–13.19, **13.19–
        13.20**, 13.21
therapy for. *See* Ischemic stroke therapy
unusual causes of. *See* Stroke, unusual causes of
worsening after, 1.13
Ischemic stroke pathophysiology, 3.1–3.23
    atherosclerosis and, 3.11–3.23, **3.12–3.23**
    cellular consequences of ischemia, 3.4–3.8, **3.5–
        3.9**
    normal brain physiology, 3.2, **3.2–3.4**, 3.4
    thrombosis and, 3.8, **3.9–3.12**, 3.10–3.11
Ischemic stroke therapy, 16.1–16.14
    acute stroke, **16.4**, 16.4–16.5
    cytoprotective therapy, 16.6–16.13, **16.8–16.12**
    enhanced blood flow, 16.5–16.6, **16.5–16.7**
    for primary intracerebral hemorrhage, 16.13,
        16.13
    for subarachnoid hemorrhage, **16.13**, 16.13–16.14
Isolated angiitis of CNS (IAC), 9.6–9.7

K

Kraepelin, Emil, 13.2, **13.2**

L

Lacunar stroke, 2.22–2.23, **2.23**, 8.1–8.17, 11.11
    clinical features of, 8.6–8.7, **8.6–8.8**
    definition of, 8.2, **8.2**
    diagnosis of
        differential diagnosis of, **8.14**, 8.15–8.16, **8.16**
        laboratory studies, 8.15
    incidence of, 8.2–8.3
    lacunar syndromes, 8.7, 8.9, **8.9**
        ataxic hemiparesis and dysarthria, 8.11, **8.11**
        basilar branch occlusion syndromes, 8.12,
            8.12
        hemichorea hemiballismus, 8.11–8.12
        pure motor hemiparesis, 8.9–8.10, **8.10**
        pure sensory stroke, 8.10–8.11
        sensorimotor stroke, **8.10**, 8.11

vs. lacunar stroke, 8.12, **8.13–8.14**, 8.15
outcome and recurrence of, 8.16–8.17
pathology of, **8.3–8.4**, 8.3–8.6
prevention and treatment of, 8.17
Large-artery thrombosis, 2.19, 2.21
Lateral medullary syndrome, 6.15
signs and symptoms of, **6.14**
sites of infarction, **6.14**
LDL-cholesterol, 1.8, 1.9, 3.16–3.18, **3.18**, 3.20, 3.23
Lesions, 6.13–6.23
of basilar artery, 6.16–6.21, **6.17–6.22**
of cerebral artery, 6.21–6.23, **6.23**
cortical, 13.9, **13.9**
of subclavian artery provimal to VA, 6.6, 6.13
subcortical, 13.9
of vertebral artery, 6.13, **6.14**, 6.15–6.16
white-matter. *See* White-matter lesions
Limb shaking, 5.13
Lime titer, 10.20
Lipids
as risk factor in stroke, 1.8–1.9
Lipid screening, 10.19
Lipohyalinosis, 8.5, **11.3**
Lipoproteins and stroke, 10.4
Low-perfusion state, 5.8, 5.11–5.12
infarcts from, 5.15
patterns of, in carotid territory strokes, **5.14**

M

Magnetic resonance angiography (MRA), 4.11, 14.13–14.14, **14.13–14.15**, 14.16, 15.6
Magnetic resonance imaging (MRI), 7.11, **8.14**, 8.15, 11.13–11.14, **11.13–11.14**, 14.13
for amyloid angiopathy, 15.22
for aneurysms, 15.17–15.18
for arteriovenous malformations, 15.21–15.22, **15.23**
for hemorrhage into tumors, 15.22, 15.24, **15.24**
for intracerebral hemorrhage, 15.12, **15.12–15.17**, 15.15, 15.17
for ischemic stroke, 15.4–15.6, **15.4–15.6**
Malignant atrophic papulosis (Kohlmeier–Degos disease), 9.12
Malignant endotheliomatosis, 9.12
Medial orbitofrontal branch, of ACA, 2.6
Medical therapy
for atherosclerosis, 3.20, **3.21–3.23**, 3.23
for hypertension, 8.17
for intracerebral hemorrhage, 11.14–11.15, **11.15**
for ischemic stroke, 16.1–16.14

for primary intracerebral hemorrhage, 16.13, **16.13**
for subarachnoid hemorrhage, **16.13**, 16.13–16.14
due to saccular aneurysm rupture, **12.11**, 12.11–12.12
for transient ischemic attacks, 4.12, **4.12**, 10.20–10.21
MELAS, 9.12, 10.13
Metastatic lesions, hemorrhagic, 15.22, 15.24, **15.24**
Methylphenidate
link to IH, 11.8
Microatheroma, 8.5
Microembolism, 8.5
Microsurgery, 12.12
Middle cerebral artery, **2.5**, 2.5–2.6, **2.7**, 5.4
cardiac source embolism of, 5.13, 7.11
Migraine-related stroke, 9.19, 10.12, **10.12**
Mitral valve prolapse, 7.15–7.16, **7.16**, 10.8
Mortality rates, 1.2, **1.3, 1.5**
trends in, 1.4–1.6
Moyamoya disease, 9.10–9.11, **9.11**, 15.10, **15.11**
surgery for, 17.15
in young adults, 10.4, 10.6
Multi-infarct dementia, 13.3–13.9, **13.5–13.9**
border-zone infarcts, **13.7**, 13.7–13.8
thalamic dementia, 13.8–13.9, **13.8–13.9**
Multiple cholesterol emboli syndrome, 9.6
Mural plaque, 8.5
Myxomas, 7.19, **7.19**, 10.9

N

Neck bruits and TIAs, **4.8**, 4.9, **4.10**
Neoplasms, 10.13, **10.14**, 11.7
Neurologic deficits, **12.6**, 12.6–12.11, **12.8–12.10**
Neurologic evaluation, 7.11
Neuroradiology of stroke, 15.1–15.24
amyloid angiopathy techniques, 15.22
aneurysm techniques, 15.17–15.19, **15.18–15.22**, 15.21
arteriovenous malformation techniques, 15.21–15.22, **15.23**
hemorrhage into tumors techniques, 15.22, 15.24, **15.24**
intracerebral hemorrhage techniques, 15.12, **15.12–15.17**, 15.15, 15.17
ischemic stroke techniques
computed tomography, 15.2, **15.2–15.3**, 15.4
magnetic resonance angiography, 15.6
magnetic resonance imaging, 15.4–15.6, **15.4–15.6**
vascular imaging, 15.6, **15.6–15.12**, 15.8–15.11

Nicardipine, 16.8
Nimodipine, 12.11, 16.8, 16.14
NMDA channel antagonists, 3.6, **3.7**, 16.8–16.10, **16.9–16.10**
Nonbacterial thrombotic endocarditis, 7.19, 9.2, **9.2**, 10.9
Nonhypertensive intracerebral hemorrhage, 11.5–11.8, 11.10
Nonischemic cardiomyopathy, 7.15
Nonvalvular atrial fibrillation, 7.13–7.14

O

Occipital lobes
  anatomy of, **2.13**, 2.14
Occlusions
  sites of, 7.3–7.4, **7.3–7.6**
  vanishing, 7.4, **7.7**
Ocular plethysmography, 14.9, **14.10**, 14.11
OPC-14117, 16.11, **16.12**
Ophthalmic artery, 5.4
Oral contraceptives
  risk of stroke from, 4.9, 9.11, 10.12
Overlap syndrome, 9.7
Oxygen free radicals, 16.10–16.11, 16.10–16.11
Oxygen supply, to brain, 3.2, **3.2**

P

Paradoxical embolism, 7.3, 7.16, **7.17**, 10.8
Parietal lobes
  anatomy of, **2.13**, 2.13–2.14
Paroxysmal nocturnal hemoglobinopathy, 10.10
Patent foramen ovale, 7.16–7.17, **7.18**, 9.3, 10.8
PC deficiency, 9.13–9.14
Penetrating artery disease, 6.6, **6.9–6.11**, **6.19**, 6.19–6.20
Penumbra, 3.6–3.7, **3.7–3.8**
Pericallosal branch, of ACA, 2.6
Petrous segment, of ICA, 2.4
Phencyclidine (PCP)
  link to IH, 11.8
Phenylpropanolamine
  link to IH, 11.8
Plaque development, 3.12, **3.13–3.17**, 3.14–3.17
Plasminogen disorders, 9.14
Platelet-derived growth factor (PDGF), 3.16–3.17
Platelet-fibrin thrombus, 3.10, **3.10**, 5.10–5.11
Polyarteritis nodosa (PAN), 9.7
Polycythemias, 10.10
Pons
  hemorrhage of, **15.13**

paramedian lesions of, 6.19
Posterior cerebral artery, 2.6, 2.9, **2.11**
  lesions of, 6.21–6.23, **6.23**
Posterior circulation ischemia, 6.1, **6.2–6.5**. *See also* Vertebrobasilar ischemic stroke
Posterior communicating artery, 5.4
Postirridiation arteriopathy, 9.12
Postoperative angiography, 12.12
Pregnancy
  risk of stroke from, 9.14, 10.12
Prescription drugs
  link to IH, 11.8, **11.9**
Prevalence, of strokes, 1.2, 5.12
  age and sex variations in, 1.3
  race variations in, 1.3–1.4
Prevertebral segment, of VA, 2.6
Primary intracerebral hemorrhage
  medical therapy for, 16.13, **16.13**
Prosthetic cardiac valve
  as cause of cardioembolic stroke, 7.15
Protein C/Protein S deficiency, 10.10–10.11
Proximal vertebral endarterectomy, 17.13
PS deficiency, 9.14
Pseudobulbar syndrome, 8.7, **8.8**
Pure motor hemiparesis, 6.19, 8.9–8.10, **8.10**
Pure sensory stroke, 6.19, 8.10–8.11

R

Rebleeding, 16.14
"Response to injury" hypothesis and plaque, 3.15, **3.17**
Retina
  infarcts of, 5.15–5.17
  low-perfusion and ischemia to, 5.11–5.12
Rheumatic heart disease
  as factor in cardioembolic stroke, 7.15
Risk factors, of stroke, **1.6, 1.11**, 1.12, 5.3
  alcohol as, 1.10, **1.10**
  asymptomatic carotid disease as, 1.10–1.11, **4.8**, 4.9, **4.10**
  cardiac disease as, 1.7–1.8, **1.8**
  cigarette smoking as, 1.9–1.10, **1.10**, 4.5, **4.6**
  diabetes mellitus as, 1.8, **1.9**
  hypertension as, 1.6–1.7, **1.6–1.7**, 4.5, 4.7, 4.9, 11.3–11.4
  lipids as, 1.8–1.9
  preventive measures for, 16.1–16.4, **16.2–16.3**
  TIAs as, 1.11
Risk factors, of vascular dementia, 13.13–13.16, **13.14–13.15**

S

Saccular aneurysm, rupture of, 12.1–12.13, **12.2**
    acute subarachnoid hemorrhage, 12.4, **12.4–12.6**, 12.6
    delayed neurological deficits
        cerebral vasospasm, 12.7–12.11, **12.8–12.10**
        hydrocephalus, **12.6**, 12.6–12.7
        rerupture, 12.7
    medical therapy for, **12.11**, 12.11–12.12
    pathophysiology of, 12.3
    prodromal symptoms, 12.3–12.4
    surgery for, 12.12–12.13, **12.13**
Sagittal sinus thrombosis, **15.16–15.17**, 15.17
Sarcoidosis, 9.8
Scleroderma, 9.8, **9.8**
Seizures, 11.11
Senile leukoencephalopathy, **13.14–13.15**, 13.14–13.16
    pathogenesis of, **13.16–13.20**, 13.16–13.21
Sensory motor stroke, 6.19, **8.10**, 8.11
Sickle-cell disease
    risk of stroke and, 9.14, **9.15**, 10.10
Sick sinus syndrome, 7.14–7.15
Small-vessel disease, 3.20, **3.20, 13.9–13.10**, 13.9–13.11
Sneddon's syndrome, 9.12
Spontaneous cervicocephalic arterial dissection (SD), 9.9–9.10, **9.10**
Stagnation thrombus, 5.7
STA-MCA bypass, **17.8**, 17.8–17.9
Stereotactic device, 11.16, **11.16**
Stroke, 1.1. *See also* Stroke, unusual causes of; Stroke in young adults; Stroke subtypes
    cardioembolic. *See* Cardioembolic stroke
    definition of, 2.1
    frequency and distribution of types of, 2.16–2.17
    hemispheral, 5.13, 5.15
    incidence and prevalence of, **1.2**, 1.2–1.4
    ischemic. *See* Ischemic stroke
    lacunar. *See* Lacunar stroke
    localizing, 2.3
    mortality and incidence trends in, **1.4–1.5**, 1.4–1.6
    mortality data on, 1.2, **1.3**
    neuroradiology of. *See* Neuroradiology of stroke
    retinal, 5.15–5.17
    risk factors of. *See* Risk factors, of stroke
    vertebrobasilar ischemic. *See* Vertebrobasilar ischemic stroke
Stroke, unusual causes of, 9.1–9.19
    arteropathic causes of, 9.5–9.12, **9.6**
    in cardioembolic stroke, **9.2**, 9.2–9.5
    hematologic causes of, 9.12–9.18, **9.13, 9.15–9.18**
    miscellaneous causes of, 9.18–9.19

Stroke care unit (SCU), 16.4
Stroke Data Bank, 2.19, 2.21–2.24
Stroke in lupus, 9.8
Stroke in young adults, 10.1–10.21
    causes of
        birth control pills, 10.12
        cardiac and embolic, 10.8–10.9, **10.9**
        drug use, 10.11–10.12
        hematologic, **9.10**, 9.10–9.11
        MELAS, 10.13
        migraine, 10.12, **10.13**
        neoplasms, 10.13, **10.14**
        pregnancy, 10.12
        rheumatologic/autoimmune, 10.11
        vasculopathy, **10.4–10.7**, 10.4–10.8
        venous thrombosis, 10.13, **10.14**, 10.15
    diagnostic evaluation of, 10.15–10.16, **10.15–10.18**, 10.18–10.20
    epidemiology of, 10.2, **10.2**
    prognosis for, 10.15
    treatment of, 10.20–10.21
    types of, **10.2–10.3**, 10.3
Stroke subtypes, 2.16–2.25
    algorithm to classify, **2.20**
    cerebral infarction as, 2.18–2.19
    classification of, 2.16, **2.16**
    distribution of, **2.17**
    frequency discrepancies in, 2.16–2.17
    imaging techniques. *See* Neuroradiology of stroke
    intracerebral hemorrhage as, 2.18, **2.19**
    subarachnoid hemorrhage as, 2.17–2.18, **2.18**
Subarachnoid hemorrhage (SAH), 2.17–2.18, **2.18**, 10.3
    acute major, 12.4, **12.4–12.6**, 12.6
    imaging techniques, 15.17, **15.18**
    medical therapy for, **16.13**, 16.13–16.14
    from saccular aneurysm rupture, 12.1–12.13
Subclavian artery
    lesions of, 6.6, **6.12**, 6.13
Subclavian "steal" phenomenon, 6.13, 15.11, 17.13
Superoxide dismutase (SOD), 16.10–16.11
Supraclinoid segment, of ICA, 2.4
    branches of, 5.4
Surgical therapy, 17.1–17.18
    extracranial carotid artery, 17.2–17.11, **17.3–17.5, 17.7–17.8, 17.10**
    extracranial vertebral artery, 17.11–17.13, **17.12**
    for intracerebral hemorrhage, 11.15–11.16, **11.16**
    for intracranial aneurysms, 12.12–12.13, **12.13**
    intracranial carotid artery, 17.13–17.15
    intracranial vertebrobasilar artery, 17.15–17.16, **17.17–17.18**, 17.18
Systemic lupus erythematosus (SLE), 10.11

W